A Comprehensive Guide to Chinese Medicine

A Comprehensive Guide to Chinese Medicine

editors

Ping-Chung Leung
The Chinese University of Hong Kong, China

Charlie Changli Xue
Royal Melbourne Institute of Technology, Australia

Yung-Chi Cheng
Yale University, USA

World Scientific

NEW JERSEY • LONDON • SINGAPORE • SHANGHAI • HONG KONG • TAIPEI • BANGALORE

Published by

World Scientific Publishing Co. Pte. Ltd.

5 Toh Tuck Link, Singapore 596224

USA office: Suite 202, 1060 Main Street, River Edge, NJ 07661

UK office: 57 Shelton Street, Covent Garden, London WC2H 9HE

Library of Congress Cataloging-in-Publication Data

A comprehensive guide to Chinese medicine / editor, Ping Chung Leung.

p. cm.

Includes bibliographical references and index.

ISBN 981-238-604-1 (alk. paper) -- ISBN 981-238-670-X (pbk. : alk. paper)

1. Medicine, Chinese. I. Leung, Ping-Chung, 1941–

R601.C695 2003

610'.951--dc21

2003063109

British Library Cataloguing-in-Publication Data

A catalogue record for this book is available from the British Library.

Printed in Singapore by Mainland Press

Contents

Contributors

Judy Yuet Wa Chan
Department of Biochemistry
Faculty of Medicine
The Chinese University of Hong Kong
Hong Kong

Yung-Chi Cheng
Department of Pharmacology
Yale School of Medicine
Yale University
USA

Kwok Pui Fung
Department of Biochemistry
Faculty of Medicine
The Chinese University of Hong Kong
Hong Kong

Ting Hor
Anthropologist
11, Clos Désiré I
91120 Palaiseau
France

Pak Kwan Hui
Department of Pathology
Kwong Wah Hospital
Hong Kong

Johnny Chi Man Koon
Department of Biochemistry
Faculty of Medicine
The Chinese University of Hong Kong
Hong Kong

Kit Man Lau
Department of Biochemistry
Faculty of Medicine
The Chinese University of Hong Kong
Hong Kong

Simon Ming Yuen Lee
The Institute of Chinese Medicine
The Chinese University of Hong Kong
Hong Kong

Ping-Chung Leung
The Institute of Chinese Medicine
The Chinese University of Hong Kong
Hong Kong

Chun Guang Li
The RMIT Chinese Medicine Research Group
Faculty of Life Sciences
RMIT University
Australia

Esther Ma
The Institute of Chinese Medicine
The Chinese University of Hong Kong
Hong Kong

Keith Moyle
Drugs, Policy and Services
Department of Human Services
Victorian State Government
Australia

Kylie A. O'Brien
Department of Medicine
Monash University
Australia

Baoyu Xin
The Institute of Chinese Medicine
The Chinese University of Hong Kong
Hong Kong

Charlie Changli Xue
The RMIT Chinese Medicine Research Group
Faculty of Life Sciences
RMIT University
Australia

Qunhao Zhang
Massachusetts General Hospital
Harvard Medical School
USA

Zhen Zheng
The RMIT Chinese Medicine Research Group
RMIT University
Australia

Foreword

This book of essays seeks to assess the place of traditional Chinese medicine (TCM) in the context of the immense advances in scientific medicine. It meets a growing need, as many Chinese observe with keen interest, the advances in TCM methodologies but wonder how scientific they really are. This is particularly true of people who long for a health and wellness approach towards illness in place of one that puts the emphasis on being curative in more invasive ways. Most Chinese have an ambivalence about TCM that can be traced back to the 19th century when Western hospitals were introduced into China and the European colonies. Some Chinese were quick to see their advantages, while others were gradually persuaded that Western methods work better for some kinds of illness. Increasingly, most Chinese realised that doctors who were professionally trained would make more reliable physicians. So much so that TCM practitioners have themselves sought to make their heritage more scientific in order to gain back their credibility. This volume of essays should go a long way towards detailing the valuable relationship between TCM and modern medicine in recent decades.

I recall, when still in high school, I heard that two out of the first three Chinese Queen's scholars from Malaya in the 19th century chose to study medicine in British universities. They were Lim Boon Keng (Lin Wenqing) and Ng Lean Tuck (Wu Liande). I later discovered that this story was similar to the one in Hong Kong where students like Ho Kai (He Qi) not only had a brilliant academic record, but was also one of the founders of the first modern medical college in Hong Kong in 1887. The college produced Sun Yat-sen, one of the first two graduates in Western medicine on Chinese soil, who was to provide a modern world view that changed the course of Chinese history. The college later became the fore-runner of the Faculty of Medicine, University of Hong Kong, now one of the most prestigious medical schools in Asia. Elsewhere too, medical colleges seem to be the first European institutions that Asians everywhere wanted for their children.

Another story reflecting an ongoing ambivalence comes to mind. The famous philanthropist, Tan Kah Kee (1874–1960) wrote in his memoirs how he tried in the 1890s to print copies of the best available TCM prescriptions for distribution among the poor in the villages in China. Decades later, in the 1940s, he remembered with regret how he had failed in his efforts. This was despite his own conversion to the efficacy of Western medicine and his fervent wish for Lim Boon Keng, the graduate of the University of Edinburgh whom he had invited to be the president of Xiamen University, to establish a medical school there during the 1920s. Tan Kah Kee's attitude reflects well a similar deep-seated ambivalence that survives till the present day.

In 1965, while in Kuala Lumpur, I was invited to sit on the Commission of Traditional Medicine. This led me to read more about the subject, and of particular interest was the work of two modern doctors that brought TCM and scientific medicine together in a book entitled *History of Chinese Medicine* (published in 1936). It was written by Wong Chi-min of Hong Kong and Ng Lean Tuck of Malaya, and it clearly represented the classic agnostic approach that still prevails among the Chinese today. But, in the 1960s, there was a hardening of views among the products of Western medical schools in Malaysia. This was so even when those in Europe, North America and Australasia were becoming more open to various kinds of alternative medicines. I recall reading many negative comments about TCM practitioners and challenges to them to have their work scientifically assessed. Nevertheless, our conclusions were not clear-cut. It was felt that popular demand for TCM could not be ignored and that, given the evidence available, we should reach an open verdict on TCM as the most prominent of the alternative systems found in Malaysia at the time.

This volume of essays confirms that the decision reached 35 years ago was an appropriate one. Much has happened since then. Some of the best scientists around the world, not least the large numbers of TCM practitioners and their students in major medical institutions, have begun to test all aspects of Chinese medicine in an increasingly thorough way. The essays show that they are much better placed now to determine what areas are scientifically verifiable, what areas are likely to remain unprovable with current scientific methods, and what are potentially fruitful for future research. The judgments are clear and sharp on some topics and judicious and nuanced for others. They make for a summation of collective wisdom that many readers will find both impressive and reassuring.

Gungwu Wang
East Asian Institute
National University of Singapore

Preface

While food supplements, biological origin preparations and "off-the-counter drugs" are showing genuine rising trends of market sales in Europe and the United States, it is appropriate to point out that those items are not identical to preparations of Chinese medicine. We often hear compatriot Chinese herbal experts and users exclaim that, of the total sales, China owns only a 5% market share. Of course, this is a mistaken view, since botanical origin products outside of China are, most of the time, local leaves and roots traditionally consumed by the native people, not necessarily related to Chinese medicine. *Gingko biloba* from Gingko leaves, for example, is a European product of local consumption, almost unknown to the Chinese, who for centuries used the Gingko nut instead.

Although the bitterness of not owning bigger market shares of herbal medicinal products may not be justified, this fact does however reflect that products of Chinese medicine (which possess much more sophisticated records of clinical effectiveness) can enjoy a good future in the popular world of health promotion.

The 3000-year well-recorded history of the healing art in China has culminated in a comprehensive system of health promotion and maintenance. This system covers a wide range: other than being a special system of health philosophy, it is also a practical guide for healers. On the disease side, there are detailed descriptions on the clinical manifestations and symptomatology, treatment records which extend from case reports to general policies, and a vast documentation on herbal pharmacopaedia. What makes the Chinese system uniquely different from the other traditional healing arts outside China is the use of acupuncture as an important modality of treatment (acupuncture is not utilised in any other ancient healing system), and the great emphasis on the maintenance and promotion of health, i.e. disease prevention.

With this rich background, traditional Chinese medicine will be able to gain international recognition. As there is increasing awareness that efficacy can be proven with modern methodology, we should expect more new herbal products to appear on the world market.

Hong Kong has introduced a system of recognition, from professional registration to educational requirements, for the Chinese medicine practitioners. While other countries are taking stock of the Hong Kong experience and are considering listing Chinese medicine as one of the recommended alternative medicine practices, there is a tendency to exaggerate the scope of efficacy of Chinese medicine at large. There are those, who in their enthusiasm, either as a user or a promoter, claim that Chinese medicine deals with all illnesses and can replace modern medicine. It is true that the comprehensive system of healing in ancient China covers nearly all aspects of human pathology, and accordingly offers treatment. However, in this modern world of advanced science and technology, the diseased should not rely only on the ancient art of healing and isolate himself from scientific investigations and technical treatments. On the other hand, there are those who have enjoyed the fruits of science and technology, and become absolutely convinced that only modern treatments can solve problems. They resist and reject any offer from the traditional factions. Qualified medical practitioners form the majority of the hard core who reject ancient medicine.

Torn between these opposing camps, the sick patient is guided by the more influential group. In the old days, however, we encountered individuals who refused clinical investigations and any formal of modern treatment, relying only on herbal therapy till the very end. Such cases have been rare in the past 30 decades. On the contrary, the reverse of sticking firmly by modern medical treatment in spite of obvious failure is much more common today. The successes of science and technology are probably the reasons why modern medicine is being accepted as the mainstream. Specialisation further promotes the adequate and efficient application of scientific and technological advances to medicine.

Ironically, amidst the sweetness of clinical successes for a large number, bitterness and discontent have grown within a smaller group. This group is increasing in size, and is becoming more unsatisfied with the results of modern treatment, which has so far failed to meet the perfection it claims. They are also unhappy with the deterioration of human care, which is being eroded along with the holistic concept. In the haste to regain more independence in controlling one's own health, this group has started to look for alternative treatments and "off-the-counter" preparations.

One immediate result of this shift of demand for medical care, apart from the addition of cupboards and shelves at the supermarket for "off-the-counter" preparations, is the awareness among the modern practitioners (notably the family physicians) for the need to address alternative/complementary medicine. It is important for every modern practitioner to know something about the alternative form. The blind followers of Hippocrates who advocated that the "proper" healer should not involve in "improper" healing practices should evolve and begin exploring alternative solutions, especially in areas where modern science has failed us.

This book is ideal for the modern practitioners who wish to learn more about Chinese medicine. It can be used as a guide on the basic principles of Chinese medicine, the current situations and the research directions. Its content will enable the reader to be better able to collaborate with the Chinese medicine practitioners.

This book caters also to those trying to decide whether they should utilise Chinese medicine as a form of treatment, as an adjunctive treatment, or as a health promoter and/or for disease prevention. Every patient has a right to know what is good for his/her health and to know the logic behind the justification.

The strength of science and technology remains overwhelming. It does not allow the co-existence of other believes and practices. The popularity of "off-the-counter" preparations and apparent interest on alternative medicine, therefore, can be short-lived. Clinicians and practitioners, in their zeal to help their patients, should put in an extra effort to prove the efficacy of the traditional ways of healing. Their success is the only genuine support to their patients who may be turning towards alternative medicine as a last straw. Their success is expected to bring alternative medicine closer to science and to make science less exclusive.

Ping-Chung Leung
The Institute of Chinese Medicine
The Chinese University of Hong Kong

Chapter 1

Intelligent Use of Traditional Chinese Medicine

Ping-Chung Leung

1.1 Introduction

It is true that all major hospitals in China are providing good services in traditional Chinese medicine on demand (Korn, 2001). It is also noted that 15% of hospital services in the United States are providing different forms of alternative medicine upon request (Eisenberg and Kessler, 1993). In a place like Hong Kong or Singapore where the different cultures meet, there is also an enthusiastic movement for wider recognition of the Oriental art and service (Wong *et al.*, 1993). Nevertheless, it does not mean that the current conventional stream of scientific practitioners should automatically shift towards the apparent trend of using alternative medicine, and either practise more alternative medicine themselves or refer more of their patient clients to alternative treatment. Neither does it mean that patients should give up, or tune down their expectation on modern scientific medicine and obtain a substitute from alternative medicine.

Facing the fact that there is a genuine rising respect and need for alternative medicine, both the service providers and the users, should seriously look at the course of events that has led to the present situation. They should also examine the failures of modern scientific medicine, while at the same time evaluate using modern concepts and with a practical attitude, the traditional concepts and practice of healing. The ultimate aim of this exercise is that eventually, an intelligent use of the traditional practice of cure, can be integrated into modern scientific practice, in a consensual need to bring improved health and well-being to the majority of patients.

1.2 The Successes of Modern Medicine

The major successes of modern medicine occurred all within the last century, of which the most recent 20 years gave the most spectacular advances.

All these advances were based on a thorough successful exploration of the basic medical sciences which supplied detailed understanding of the structures of the human body, its functional mysteries, followed by the exploration of its abnormal structures and functions, viz. the pathological changes (Richardson, 2001). This knowledge has been widening through the years, with advancement from macroscopic to microscopic and from biochemical to molecular. The recent successful correlation between the pathological changes and the gene patterns of the biological entity implies another predictable breakthrough in which treatment of diseases is aimed at the primary cause (instead of treating the outcome pathology). Soon, effective prevention of illnesses at the genetic level will become a reality.

Such successes at the handling of disease problems were previously unheard of. It has led to optimistic speculations that human beings should live to at least 110 years of age, and that the approach to disease management will soon turn towards a preventive or "rooting out" principle.

We, medical or non-medical people, all rejoice over such tremendous advances with admiration (Lieberman *et al.*, 2002).

On a lower level, the day-to-day practice of modern medicine has also made remarkable strides. Just look at the varieties of medication focusing on more and more specific targets in an attempt to accurately correct or supplement, without producing unwanted adverse effects. And the minimally invasive surgeries which brought about less pain and more speedy recoveries. Such advances were also beyond anybody's imagination years ago, not to mention other wonders like organ transplants and technology-related sophisticated investigations.

Whether these successes were a result of day-to-day efforts, achieved step-by-step through years of blood and sweat, or the result of epoch-making innovative inventions, it has been a solid demonstration of the triumph of empirical science working on deductive principles. Identification of the accurate cause of problem naturally led to its solution. Its successful solution led to deduction of parallel approaches and solution of other problems. The history of medical advances has already demonstrated that, when the exact cause of pathology is clearly defined, the solution can be worked out, eventually. Thus, we have appropriate bactericidal agents controlling individual infections and wiping out epidemics. We have substituting agents replacing deficient exocrines and endocrines, and we also have powerful means to remove what is not wanted.

Modern technology has contributed a great deal to the process of problem identification: making the right diagnosis, which is always the first step towards treatment planning. Modern technology has also allowed for various forms of thorough management, which include different methods of treatment and drug manufacturing.

The target-orientated deductive approach has been the key to the success of modern scientific medicine. But at the same time, it has also been the source of numerous problems.

The success of target-orientated deductive medicine depends on a proper narrow focus. Specialisation is the natural outcome. Specialisation is followed by sub-specialisation with an even narrower focus. Treatment of illnesses suffered by the whole human body thus gradually turns into treatment of individual organs and sometimes even tissues. The inseparable relationship between the different organs is often overlooked. Different organs are commonly taken care of by different individual healers or team of healers, who communicate and cooperate with different degrees of enthusiasm and dedication. Holistic care involves caring for the whole human individual as a compact, integrated biological entity. Instead, it has given way to a narrowly focused, specifically targeted, technology-based, well-planned spearhead of treatment. The greatly advocated holistic care is lost, unaware to the healers. Healers are overwhelmed with the successes of the highly targeted treatments, while the less successful examples, not to mention the failures, easily escape their attention (Cheng, 2001).

Science and technology have demonstrated overwhelming successes in all directions of daily living. They have built up an immense atmosphere of satisfaction and pride so that the users feel secure and those lacking appear miserable and helpless. There exists a genuine social pressure via which people are pushed towards modern medicine and its applications. There is also the common assumption that successful outcomes are always related to science and technology.

Those who fail to taste the fruit of success usually stay silent, while those spoiled by the wonders of science dominate the stage, thus depriving others of the opportunity to express dissatisfaction.

However, given the mighty power of science, there are still failures and disappointment. There are those who are only partially cured, many who have been treated but are not fully satisfied, and some who are displeased with the multi-disciplinary care, because care and attention become shallow and segregated. Costs of multi-station consultations, apart from the inhumane aspect of specialist consultation, are likewise a genuine concern. Highly selective focusing has replaced holistic care.

The successes of modern science and technology in the field of medicine has therefore been marred as a result of the declining human care, loss of freedom on more positive choices, and the high health care costs involved.

With the thorough endorsement of human rights, it is true that physicians are giving a lot more information to their patients while treatment is being administered. However, thorough and complete discussions on all available treatment options, be they conventional or supplementary, are not absolutely ensured. After all, the Hippocrates oath recommends that the orthodox attending physician should not liase with the unorthodox. The scientific stream should ignore all other approaches that are outside of their own.

As a result, patients under modern scientific treatment usually stay with their conventional treatment. Alternative medicine will forever remain complementary.

1.3 Traditional Chinese Medicine

Of the four major systems of traditional medicine, viz. Chinese, Indian, Greek (European) and Egyptian, perhaps the most sophisticated one is the Chinese. While solitary plants or simple combinations are used in the Greek and Egyptian systems, both the Chinese and Indian systems (notably the Chinese) are fond of using formulae involving multiple herbs (Kleinman, 1975; WHO, 2000; Goldbeck-Wood *et al.*, 1996).

Although there are insufficient documentations to explain this basic difference between the East and the West, a logical deduction is that all systems start with single herbs. If animal instinct is responsible for domestic animals and household pets to start eating special grass and plants in an attempt to counteract their ailments, the intelligent animal keepers (i.e. human beings) must have also deduced the secret of natural cures, thus applying the same tactic, using the same grass or plant to counteract human ailments. At the very beginning, only one herb was used. Very soon, the Asian healers started using more than one, while their counterparts in Europe kept to their simple single herb application.

A logical explanation to this development of mixed formula was that healers wanted to enhance effects, and at the same time reduce toxicity which, theoretically, could be lowered by adding antidotic herbs. However one of the legendary figures of Chinese medicine, Oriental healer Hua-To, was well known for insisting on using very few herbs, in contrast to his contemporaries who were fond of adopting complex formulae (Hoizey and Hoizey, 1988).

Actually, the wisdom behind the formulae was a lot more sophisticated than the consideration of efficacy enhancement and detoxication. A formula was constructed for efficacy, support, safety and preparation for other directions of achievement (君, 臣, 佐, 使). The formula is created not only for the control of symptoms but also for a transition to health promotion.

While modern, scientific medicine developed according to an understanding of abnormal behaviour in the structure and function of tissues and organs, Chinese medicine developed on the basis of knowledge on the effects of herbs for the control of clinical symptoms.

Apart from the control of symptoms, the Chinese medicine regime aims at the maintenance of function of the organs and tissues that are not directly affected by the pathological mechanisms. The herbalists interpret this aspect of treatment as a measure to consolidate the fundamental vitality, while in modern terminology, this may be interpreted as stimulating the immunological ability of the individual.

1.3.1 *When should the modern clinician consider using Chinese medicine?*

While enjoying and applying the effective means of treatment of modern medicine, should the modern clinician also consider using Chinese medicine? He does not need to, if he can fulfill his objectives. However, if he has tried very hard to solve a problem and yet fails to do so, it is his duty to look for other alternatives, otherwise he has not fulfilled his ethical obligation to his patient.

Are there areas where modern medicine has failed to offer adequate solutions?

Indeed there are plenty. Deductive science works very well when the course of events, i.e. the structures involved, the functional derangements, the pathological changes, etc. are clearly known. For instance, straightforward infections can be easily cured, deficiencies can be skillfully supplemented and simple tumours effectively removed. However, when the course of events is not easily understood or when the exact pathological changes are unknown or are too complicated, an effective cure is beyond reach and even controlling symptoms can become haphazard.

Thus, allergic conditions often involve unknown agents via uncertain pathways, causing a multitude of involvements — handling and treatment become most difficult. There are anti-allergic agents and other means of controlling allergic reactions. However, it is not uncommon to find that treatment stays at a level of symptomatic control, remains transient or partial. Examples include skin diseases like atopic eczema, some other dermatitis and respiratory problems like allergic rhinitis and asthma (Kaptchuk and Eisenberg, 1998).

Viral infections involve ultra-microorganisms which do not easily expose themselves. Therefore, even identifying their pathological existence requires time. In addition, their pathological manoevres may involve unusual pathways, so that symptomatology becomes bizarre and complex, making identification and explanation very difficult. How viruses invade cells and how they multiply are complicated issues. While fully understanding these basic phenomena takes time, creating a means of controlling the mechanisms is even more difficult. As a result, most viral infections still do not have reliable treatment methods (He *et al.*, 2002). Some examples are common cold, influenza, hepatitis and acquired immune deficiency syndrome (AIDS).

The next group of diseases that scientists have yet to conquer involves diseases of the auto-immune system. While odd patients develop rejection against their own proteins, their presentations are lack of uniformity and the pathological changes also demonstrate great varieties of behaviour. In spite of the extensive research input, the reward is very much outweighed by the resources put in. The helplessness and perplexity involved in the management of autoimmune conditions therefore, remain as frequent frustrations among physicians. Hence, the rheumatological conditions remain a broad group of diseases lacking in efficient control (Wiener, 1975).

Chronic problems represent either accumulation of unsolved acute problems or complicated ailments without solutions. While acute problems exhibit clear target orientations i.e. the tissues or organs involved are clearly defined, making solution possible and straightforward, the unsolved components and the multiple involvement of tissues and organs in chronic situations present the most difficult challenges to the healers. Where should they begin the treatment? Where is the priority? What are the correlations between the different pathological presentations?

Chronic painful conditions therefore persist as difficult challenges for clinicians. Diseases related to the mind have so many possible linkages and correlations — exocrinal, endocrinal, psychological, social and immunological — that not only make solution nearly impossible, but constantly lead to the appearance of fresh, new problems (Ezzo, 2000; Tulder and Cherk, 1999).

Last but not least, there are the cancers. Cancer treatment has always been designed as the elimination of cancer cells. As the methods used are not exclusive, and the target chosen is not absolutely specific, one expects the following:

- Unnecessary destruction of normal cells and tissues during the stage of cancer cell elimination, causing additional symptoms and suffering.
- Normal cells and tissues may be more extensively affected than cancer cells and tissues.
- Prolonged period of recovery and rehabilitation.

- Recurrence resulting from residual tumour cells.
- Recurrence resulting from the breakdown of defense mechanism.

Technology and pharmacological inventions have improved the results of cancer control in the past decade. However, there are still no specific means available for counteracting the adverse effects of destructive methologies in cancer treatment.

In conclusion, conditions where modern scientific medicine have failed to provide effective solutions include the following:

Allergies — Atopic ecezema, hay fever, asthma
Viral infections — Influenza, hepatitis, AIDS
Autoimmune diseases — Rheumatogical conditions
Chronic problems — Pain, mental disorders
Cancers — Adverse drug effects, late stages and recurrences

Physicians and surgeons may thoroughly explain to their patients about their limitations in their attempts to offer the best treatment under those circumstances. They have the ethical duty to explore for alternative or additional means of treatment, in order to be more responsible, unless patients themselves do not care for more comprehensive treatment.

1.3.2 *When should the patient consider alternative medicine?*

Every modern city enjoys a good provision of modern hospitals and clinics offering effective, scientific treatment for patients. The average individual today, therefore, should be fully aware of the promises of modern medicine. They should be appreciative and thus satisfied.

But, where are the promises?

They occur in the following areas:

(1) Emergency medicine

When life is being threatened, emergency medicine has a lot to offer. Airway obstructions need to be cleared immediately. Cardiac arrests can be counteracted by simple means of resuscitation. Bleeding from different sources requires direct, focused haemostatic manoevres. Every modern hospital is proud of its ability to deal with these life-threatening conditions and the past decades of emergency practices have accumulated excellent experience on effective procedures known to all working personnel belonging to the relevant services today. One perfect example is blood replacement which has saved millions of lives.

(2) Emergency surgery

Life-saving practices are often related with surgical procedures which bring about immediate solutions. Examples are found in haemostasis, airway maintenance, cardiac resuscitation, urine and bowel diversion, etc.

(3) Where investigations are required, either to identify the pathology or to guide the treatment

Investigations can be simple and straightforward like urine and blood tests. On the other hand, they can be technology-orientated like radiographs, scannings or using other gadgets. When investigations indicate simple pathology, it is clear that simple means, either effective pharmaceuticals or surgery, can offer the solution.

(4) Straightforward pathology

Good examples are bacterial infections and benign tumours. What can be more effective than the antibiotics that get rid of the germs responsible for a nasty bout of pneumonia or cellulites? What other methods can be more effective than the simple surgical removal of a cyst, or lipoma or a tumour-like pathology?

The average individual of today is fully aware of these basic modern medical facilities and will not hesitate to use them when the need arises. Should he or she therefore ever resort to alternatives?

While accepting modern medicine as the standard service for emergency and straightforward modalities of disease treatment, the individual should also be aware of other alternatives under the following circumstances:

(1) Modern medicine fails to offer a cure. Such circumstance occurs when the modern physician finds difficulties satisfying the client. Thorough discussions have just been given under the previous section.

(2) The individual becomes disappointed with modern scientific, specific treatment. The target of modern treatment so frequently aims at a narrow specific target which excludes a divergence into other possibly related areas. The attending modern practitioner does not apply the holistic approach. When the individual seeks treatment in areas outside of the specific area, he is usually referred to another specialist. The holistic care expected by the individual is thus not given. Under such circumstances, only some unscientific alternatives can be considered as a substitution.

(3) Related or unrelated to the absence of holistic care, the individual wants more control over his/her problems. Individual freedom and personal choice are considered issues of utmost importance to the apparently helpless patient. One way of reverting to self-determination is to adopt alternative forms of treatment. Whatever the choice, it must be provided with clear instructions, explanations and persuasions for utilisation, thus earning respect and a good chance of adoption. Friends, relatives and colourful advertisements will then become influential guides in the choices. The final decision is made at the dispensary where off-the-counter shelves display promising varieties of choices.

(4) Lastly, every individual is able to feel for his/her own state of health. The inner feeling can be weak or strong, and is expressed objectively as increase or decrease in weight, exercise tolerance, quality of sleep, duration of working hours, etc. The feeling is also expressed subjectively as loss of energy, loss of enthusiasm, emotional imbalance, failure to achieve certain personal standards or low self-esteem. Such feelings are often affected by personal observations and knowledge of disease entities. The fact that relatives or friends fall sick or similar knowledge of mortalities and morbidities naturally cause concern for one's own health. Unfortunately, apart from what is widely practiced in public health for disease prevention, modern medicine and specialists offering specific care are not putting sufficient emphasis on preventive care. It is true that lifestyle, personal habits and the need for exercise are currently widely emphasised. But the source of emphasis comes from the media, general health workers and groups, and ironically, from off-the-counter drug producers, not medical professionals.

It becomes natural, therefore, that when individuals want to do something to promote personal health, or to prevent mishappenings, they look towards alternative herbal treatment. They would try various means, including dietary or food supplements and off-the-counter offers. With a rapidly increasing ageing population, the need for health promotion and disease prevention becomes more and more important.

1.3.3 *What does Chinese medicine offer?*

When Chinese medicine is mentioned, herbs, herbal decoctions and acupuncture come to one's mind. In fact Chinese medicine offers a special philosophy of health and disease treatment, which is just as important as the herbs and acupuncture.

Herbal healers not only believe in curing, they also put importance in disease prevention. They use a special term "treating the undiseased" (治未病) which carries a special connotation in classical or modern medical treatment concept. "Treating the undiseased" is more than a general means of disease prevention. It is a concept of supporting and boostering the unaffected organs and functional systems during a disease period, so that the diseased organs and systems are given more chances to heal. It is also a comprehensive programme catered for the individual to avoid specific diseases and to maintain good general health. Hence, the programme can be highly specialised with a specific target, or it can simply be for general health promotion. What then are the advocations? They range from personal lifestyle, eating habits, to special food or herbal supplements. The supplements are closely related to considerations of qualities of life unique to the philosophy of Chinese medicine.

In the modern health concept, quality of life refers to the individual's sense of wellness, for example, activities of daily living, sleep conditions, social activities, etc. Chinese medicine healers, in addition to the approach adopted based on conventional common sense, have their own special way of interpreting the quality of life. The human body maintains its state of internal harmony by balancing the counteracting forces of Yin and Yang. These counteracting forces are felt by the individual as being cold or hot, superficial or deep, and soft or solid.

	Cold ↔ Hot	
Yin	Superficial ↔ Deep	**Yang**
	Soft ↔ Solid	

It is not possible to give objective data to explain these opposing vital forces. Although modern scientists have tried to quantify them using physiological research models, they have not been successful (Hor, 2003). The Chinese people, however, with some basic explanation, thoughtful adaptation and effort, are able to understand and "feel" the opposing forces. Possibly, there exists a cultural heritage which allows for this understanding. However, with an open mind, even those foreign to the culture should be able to appreciate, albeit to different extents. It is common knowledge that when body temperature is high, the normal feeling of hotness, can, at some instance, be substituted with that of cold. Likewise, the feeling can be felt as superficial or deep, and soft or hard.

The differentiation between Yin and Yang guides the Chinese medicine healer on a detailed choice of treatment. The feeling of the opposing forces guides, to different extents, the individuals to make their own choices on disease prevention and adoption of specific programmes for avoidance of certain ailments.

From this unique philosophy of healing, the simple person in the commonplace household obtains the instructions for self-care. From a similar philosophy, the experienced healer works out his sophisticated scheme of treatment (Campion, 1993).

There are scholars inside and outside of China who deny the importance of the healing philosophy and adopt the view that the main value of Chinese medicine lies in the provision of herbal treatment and the large varieties of herbal formulae documented for specific uses.

But how do the herbs work?

Herbs were used for the control of symptoms in the early days during which no one cared to learn about the mode of action. As long as the effects were seen, there was little concern about how and why they came about. When basic laboratory research on herbal medicine began, pharmacological concepts were utilised and herbal effects were compared with known pharmacological effects of synthetic drugs. A broad understanding of herbal action for symptom relief can probably be simplified into two main categories, viz. direct and indirect action.

Direct actions

Although never as specific and systematic, herbal choices are known for the control of fever, pain, inflammation and specific symptoms like vomiting, diarrhea, constipation; and even less common symptoms like bleeding, rash, pallor and shortness of breath.

In Chinese communities, proprietor drugs of Chinese medicine origin are well known and commonly used in the average household for headache, stomachache, diarrhea, vomiting and constipation. Most of the time, these give good satisfaction and have been adopted as traditional practices passed down from generation to generation. Few will question the value, and even less will worry about possible adverse side effects.

On a higher level of demand for healing, the Chinese medicine practitioner must differentiate between the different degrees of fever, inflammation or pain. Herbs which have both symptom control effects as well as anti-viral or anti-bacterial properties are available. They are used like antibiotics. Likewise, potent pain-killers like the opiates are selectively used. Anti-fungal and anti-helmetic agents are known and used to produce direct control of infestations. Sophisticated means are available to bring about bowel motion relevant to the need (WHO, 2000).

The use of herbs for direct purposes follows what appears to be pharmacological principles, and such items can be developed into pharmaceuticals. Thus, Ma-huang (麻黃), a well-known herb used in the treatment of asthma was extracted to produce ephedrine, which was widely used for bronchial asthma treatment until more sophisticated drugs with less adverse effects were invented. On a more modern front, Qing-hao was produced from a plant. It was used specifically against one type of malarial parasites (Bensky and Gamble, 1993).

Indeed pharmacocognostics is a whole section within the boundaries of pharmacy which deals with plants and other natural products that can be used as prototypes for specific drugs. There are some examples of modern day pharmaceuticals used with extreme specificity that are actually chemical products produced as a result of extensive laboratory studies on their original parent plants. That is why today's scientists continue to focus their resources on plants believed to be providing therapeutic remedies to natives in villages throughout the world, with the aim of identifying effective pharmaceutical components. In this area, French chemists have been particularly successful as have been exemplified in their manufacture of Vincristine, a powerful cytotoxic drug from a flower called periwinkle, and another equally promising drug of the same family, Taxol, from the bark of the Yew tree (National Centre for Scientific Research France, 1999).

The Chinese herbalist, apart from using herbal preparations on specific, direct needs of symptom control, also makes use of their indirect abilities. The lack of scientific knowledge about the human structure and function motivated the ancient healers to adopt a direction emphasising on a maintenance of the undiseased organs while the diseased organs struggle to heal under the influence of body defense. Body defense, with modern understanding is equivalent to immunological well-being and resistance to diseases.

A great deal of research interests on herbal medicine in the past decades have been focused on the possible immunostimulant effects of different herbs (Fairfield *et al.*, 1998).

In Europe and America, there are flower extracts and pollen preparations widely used as immunostimulants because consumers feel rejuvenated and less susceptible to ailments and diseases. In Chinese communities, mushroom extracts, Lingzhi and Yunzhi are more widely consumed after serious major diseases, during and after cancer treatment, and among the general population for promotion of good health and enhancement of ability to resist pathological invasions.

Animal studies and isolated human trials have given indications that the herbs or herbal extracts under study do provide positive effects on immunological support, and thus presumably, promote health (Leung, 2001).

There is no intention here of guiding the reader on a choice of health promotion products, therefore there is no provision of details on the completed studies. People should realise that Chinese medicine and its uses, in spite of attempts to modernise it, has not reached the strict evidence-based stage.

1.4 Conclusion

The use of Chinese medicine is undergoing significant changes. There are good reasons to believe that we are drawing closer towards the evidence-based scientific demand such that one day in the near future, definite recommendations can be made.

At this present time, we are aware of five major applications. Some are obviously historical (habitual or cultural), some are moving towards science (insistently or conceptually), while others are practical. We need not adopt strong opinions for or against such practices because we are as yet totally uncertain of the direction. However, it is time for the user to know what he or she wants and to understand the limitations and problems.

Five different types of Chinese medicine users:

(1) Household users

They use proprietor preparations or "grandmother's" herbal formulae for commonplace ailments and symptoms as the first line of defense.

(2) Seekers for herbalist care

They believe that the herbalist can do a better job for special symptoms. The previous assumption that this group must consist of elderlies and the uneducated is proven wrong in a recent survey on herbalist users. Professionals and middle-rank executives are found to be the main users. These individuals firmly believe in the freedom of choice (Studlert *et al.*, 1998).

(3) Modern users

Professionals who enjoy the fruits of science and insist on scientific pursuits. Yet they follow the advice and recommendations expressed by health scientists, odd modern practitioners and clever advertisements that upgrade proprietor drugs into quasi-scientific preparations (assumably pharmaceuticals).

(4) Preventive users

The concern and fear of health deterioration and pathological changes in otherwise normal and healthy individuals have driven thousands of upper-middle class people on health pursuits, using different modalities of preparations and programmes available on the market.

(5) Research users

Clinical scientists will feel more comfortable if they can obtain positive data from evidence-based trials on the various herbal preparations claiming efficacy. Since the World Health Organization and National Institutes of Health in the United States endorsed the approach of proving efficacy using scientific standard methodology (NIH, 2001), clinicians have been devoting more time in the search for some apparently unscientific means to solve their difficult problems. One is looking forward to the results of many ongoing clinical trials. Positive results are expected to open up many new fields of problem-solving research. The future trustworthy guidelines should come mainly from this group.

1.5 Limitations of Chinese Medicine Research

The research users are having a difficult time — while they want to follow strict scientific methodologies so as to maintain the highest credibility, they have found it to be practically impossible. They rely on herbs where there is yet no way to ensure uniform quality. They very often use a combination of herbs. Not even individual herbal contents and functions are clear, and they know very little about their interactions. They observe clinical and laboratory data, and confirm the changes without knowing why and how. They make assumptions about the efficacies, but do not have any idea about the pharmacokinetics and pharmacodynamics. These are the obvious limitations.

If one insists on the clearance of these limitations before embarking on the research planning and commitment, one has to wait for decades. The only compromise therefore is to assume that the best quality of herbs are already available, that herbal interactions are uniform, and that the reasons behind the clinical and laboratory changes will be revealed sooner or later. Likewise, assumptions should be made that the pharmacokinetics and pharmacodynamics would not affect the final choices.

The intelligent use of Chinese medicine should therefore be individualised. It is used when modern medicine fails to offer what is desired. We should not assume that Chinese medicine can substitute modern medicine. We can however recognise Chinese medicine as a separate specialty of medicine that supplements other specialties.

Reference

Ayurveda Medicine (2000) *World Health Organization: Strategic Plan on the Promotion of Folk Medicine*. WHO Publication.

Bensky, D. and Gamble, A. (1993) *Chinese Herbal Medicine Materia Medica.* Eastland Press, Seattle.

Campion, E.W. (1993) Why unconventional medicine? Editorial. *New Engl. J. Med.* **328**, 282–283.

Cheng, Y.C. (2001) A personal perspective on bringing Chinese medicine into mainstream medicine of the 21st century. In: *2001 Traditional Chinese Medicine and National Products, China.* Era Resources Publisher, Hong Kong, pp. 27-35.

Eisenberg, D.M. and Kessler, R.C. (1993) Unconventional medicine in the United States. *New Engl. J. Med.* **328**(4), 246–252.

Ezzo, J., Berman, B.M. and Hadhazy, V.A. (2000) Is acupuncture effective for the treatment of chronic pain? A systemic review. *Pain* **38**(4), 346–354.

Fairfield, K.M., Davis, R.B. and Eisenberg, D. (1998) Patterns of use: expenditures and perceived efficacy of complementary and alternative therapy in HIV-infected patients. *Arch. Intern. Med.* **158**, 2257–2264.

Goldbeck-Wood, S., Dorozynski, A. and Gunnar, L. (1996) Complementary medicine is booming worldwide. *BMJ* **313**(7050), 131–133.

He, Y., Yuan, F. Y. and Wang, J. B. (2002) Clinical study on treatment of liver fibrosis of chronic hepatitis B patients with ginkgo leaf. *Chin. J. Integr. Trad. West. Med.* **8**(2), 90–94.

Hoizey, D. and Hoizey, M.J. (1988) *History of Chinese Medicine*. Edinburgh University Press.

Hor, T. (2003) Anthropology of Chinese medicine. In: *A Comprehensive Guide to Chinese Medicine.* World Scientific Publishing Co., Singapore, London.

Kaptchuk, T.J. and Eisenberg, D.M. (1998) The persuasive appeal of alternative medicine. *Ann. Intern. Med.* **129**, 1061–1065.

Kleinman, A. (1975) *Medicine in Chinese Cultures: Comparative Studies of Health Care in China and Other Societies*. U.S. Department of Health, Education and Welfare, Washington D.C.

Korn, D (2001) *Report After a Special Visit to China to Understand the Situation of Chinese Medicine in China*. Internal Publication, University Grant Council, Hong Kong.

Leung, P.C. (2001) Editorial: seminar on Chinese medicine. *J. Hong Kong Med. Assoc.* **7**, 352–353.

Lieberman, J.R., Daluiski, A. and Einhorn, T. (2002) The role of growth factors. *Biol. Clin. Appl.* **84**, 1032–1044.

National Centre for Scientific Research France (1999) *Report on the Successes of Development of Drugs from Botanical Plants*. Special Report CNRS, France.

National Institutes of Health USA (2001) *National Centre for Complementary and Alternative Medicine: Five-year Strategic Plan. 2001–2005*. NIH USA.

Rees, L. and Weil, A. (2001) Integrated medicine: imbues aothodox medicine with the value of complementary medicine. *BMJ* **322**(7229), 119–120.

Richardson, W. (2001) *Crossing the Quality Chasm: A New Hhealth System for the 21st Century*. The National Academic News.

Studlert, D.M., Eisenberg, D.M. and Miller, F.H. (1998) Medical malpractice implications of alternative medicine. *JAMA* **280**(19), 1610–1615.

Tulder van, M.W. and Cherk, D.C. (1999) The effectiveness of acupuncture in the management of acute and chronic low back pain: a systemic review within the framework of the Cochrane collaboration. *Spine* **24**(11), 1113–1123.

Wiener, C.L. (1975) The burden of rheumatoid arthritis: tolerating the uncertainty. *Soc. Sci. Med.* **9**, 97–104.

Wong, T.W., Wong, S.L. and Donnan, S.J. (1993) Traditional Chinese medicine and Western medicine in Hong Kong. *J. Hong Kong Med. Assoc.* **45**, 278–284.

Chapter 2

Modalities of Chinese Medicine

Charlie Changli Xue & Kylie A. O'Brien

2.1 Introduction

Chinese medicine uses a number of modalities or therapies for both prevention and treatment of disease. The most commonly used modalities are acupuncture and Chinese herbal medicine. Others include *moxibustion* (a technique of applying heat to the body that is often used in conjunction with acupuncture), *tuina* (Chinese remedial massage), cupping (a technique in which glass cups are applied to the body), exercise therapy (including qigong and taichi) and diet therapy (the appropriate application of food as a supplementary method for clinical treatment to enhance health and therapeutic outcomes). These all may be used as forms of treatment and as ways of preventing ill health and achieving better health.

Regardless of the type of therapy used, they are all guided by the fundamental theories of Chinese medicine. All forms of treatment are used to help the body return to its natural state of harmony of Yin and Yang. This chapter will provide a brief description of various forms of therapies used in Chinese medicine. Further reading is recommended for readers who would like to know more about individual therapies.

2.2 Chinese Herbal Medicine

Chinese herbal medicine uses herbs that are combined in a prescription according to Chinese medicine theory. The term "herb" includes not only plants but also various minerals and animal products. Different parts of plants may be used as herbal medicine, including leaves, roots, stems, flowers and seeds. Interestingly, different parts of the same plant may have very different therapeutic actions, such as the root and twigs of *Ma huang* (Herba Ephedrae). In addition, the part of the plant used in herbal medicine can differ between Chinese herbalism and Western herbalism, i.e. in Western herbalism, the leaves may be used whereas in Chinese medicine, it may be the root that is considered to have therapeutic actions and values. Mineral substances can include shells such as abalone shell, oyster shell and turtle shell, and minerals such as amber, haematite and iron filings. Animal products include such substances as cicada moulting, flying squirrel faeces, deer horn, and in the past, more exotic substances such as tiger bone and rhinoceros horn. Fortunately, most countries now do not condone the use of endangered species of wildlife and plant life, so the use of many animal products and plants that are endangered is decreasing.

There are approximately 500 different Chinese herbs in the *Chinese Materia Medica*, the Chinese medicine pharmacological reference book, and a typical outpatient clinic uses around 350–400 of these. Herbs may be processed using a variety of methods (discussed in more detail later). Obviously, the most complex aspect of the clinical use of herbs is the combination of them. This will be discussed briefly in the following sections.

2.2.1 *How is Chinese herbal medicine understood?*

Herbs are categorised primarily in terms of their action on the body. Their action depends on the properties of the herbs that include the flavour (or taste) and temperature characteristics. Herbs are designated as hot, warm, neutral, cool or cold, and there may be varying degrees of temperature, e.g. slightly cold or slightly warm (Bensky and Gamble, 1993). In terms of taste or flavour, herbs are classified as acrid, bitter, sweet, sour, salty, bland and astringent (Bensky and Gamble, 1993; Lin *et al.*, 1985). The temperature characteristics and tastes can be classified into Yin and Yang also. Acrid, sweet and bland herbs are considered Yang and sour, salty and bitter herbs are considered Yin (Lin *et al.*, 1985). Yin herbs are those that are cool or cold and Yang herbs are those that are warm or hot.

In terms of how the properties of the herbs help determine the action, cool or cold herbs (that correlate with Yin) are generally used to treat conditions in the body in which there is heat associated. Heat may manifest when there is a deficiency of Yin leaving a relative excess of Yang (heat), called a *deficient-heat* condition or syndrome (since the root cause is deficiency of Yin), or when there is an absolute excess of Yang (heat), called an *excess-heat* condition or syndrome. Yin herbs may also be used in a formula to down-regulate or moderate the characteristics of warm or hot herbs used in a formula to strengthen Yang: in this way, the formula is not excessive in one therapeutic direction. In contrast, warm or hot herbs are classified as Yang and are used to treat conditions characterised by cold. These conditions may be deficiency-type conditions where there is a deficiency of Yang leading to a relative excess of Yin (cold), termed a *deficiency-cold* condition or syndrome (since the root cause is deficiency), or when there is an absolute excess of Yin (cold), termed an *excess-cold* condition. Similarly, Yang herbs may also be added to formulae that contain predominantly Yin herbs in order to moderate the action of the Yin herbs, i.e. balance the formula.

The flavours also help determine the specific effects of the herbs on the body. For example, bitter herbs are said to drain and dry (Bensky and Gamble, 1993) and so may be useful in draining heat from the body (heat can manifest in many ways including sore throat, sores, swellings, fever) or draining dampness in the body (that can manifest as fluid accumulation, including oedema) or drying dampness in the body (dampness can manifest as excessive discharges from the body such as leucorrhoea or other disorders such as diarrhoea, for example). Sweet herbs like licorice root (the Chinese herb *gan cao*) or ginseng nourish and tonify, and may be useful in treating conditions in which there is deficiency of qi, for example. Bland herbs such as poria (Chinese herb *fu ling*) can leach out dampness and promote urination: many are diuretics that help eliminate water from the body (Lin *et al.*, 1985; Bensky and Gamble, 1993). Sour herbs have an astringent action and help prevent the loss of fluids and essence and qi from the body (Lin *et al.*, 1985). Salty herbs have an affinity with the Kidney and have the action of purging and softening hardness (hardness may manifest, for example, as masses in the body such as tumour). Many of the mineral herbs, particularly shells, are salty in flavour. Examples include oyster shell, abalone shell, pearl, mother of pearl and magnetite. Most herbs are characterised by one to two flavours.

Chinese medicine theory also holds that herbs enter specific meridians. It is understood that each individual herb has an affinity with one or more specific organs and it is this tendency to travel to specific organs via the meridians that helps explain the therapeutic effect of an herb on conditions associated with those organs. This is probably the earliest form of understanding of receptors and target organs. For example, the herb *jie geng* enters the *Lung* meridian and is often used to treat conditions such as coughing with excessive phlegm, the Lung organ being the involved *zang-fu* organ.

The affinity of certain herbs for particular internal *zang-fu* organs is also related to the flavours of the herbs. The sour flavour is believed to have an affinity for the Liver, the sweet flavour for the Spleen, saltiness for the Kidney, bitterness for the Heart and acridity for the Lung (PCC, 1997).

Herbs are also said to have a directional tendency: they tend to rise or float, sink or fall (Bensky and Gamble, 1993). Flowers tend to ascend and are often used to treat conditions of the head including headache and sore throat. An example is the herb *ju hua* or chrysanthemum flower that is often used to treat headache. This herb is acrid, sweet, bitter and slightly cold and also enters the Lung and Liver meridians. The eye is the sense organ associated with the Liver. *Ju hua* is commonly used in prescriptions that treat eye disorders because of its ability to target the eyes. Descending substances can move qi downward (Bensky and Gamble, 1993); many of the mineral herbs have a descending action.

Putting the flavour and temperature characteristics of an herb together, along with information on meridians entered, we begin to understand the action of the herb. For example, the herb *lian xin* (lotus plumule) is bitter and cold and enters the Heart and Pericardium meridians (PPC, 1997). It may be used to drain Heart-fire that can manifest as insomnia and restlessness.[1]

In general, each herb has a number of actions, one of which is usually its primary action. For example, the primary action of the herb *yu xing cao* is to clear heat and toxicity and to reduce swellings and abscesses

[1]According to Chinese medicine.

for conditions such as cough with thick yellow sputum or Lung abscess (Bensky and Gamble, 1993). However, it also has the action of draining damp-heat and promoting urination and can be used to treat conditions including diarrhoea and urinary tract infection (Lin *et al.*, 1985; Bensky and Gamble, 1993).

The actions of Chinese herbs may be explained in terms of modern biomedical concepts. For example, herbs belonging to categories such as "*herbs that drain fire*", "*herbs that cool the blood*" and "*herbs that clear heat and relieve toxicity*" generally have antipyretic (i.e. reduce fever), anti-inflammatory and anti-microbial or anti-infection actions (Lin *et al.*, 1985; Bensky and Gamble, 1993). Many of the herbs in the category of "*herbs that drain dampness*" have a diuretic action (Lin *et al.*, 1985). They are used to treat conditions in which there is an accumulation of fluids (for example, oedema) or internal dampness in the body that may be combined with heat that may manifest as conditions such as urinary tract infections, excessive vaginal discharge, and weeping skin ulcers (Bensky and Gamble, 1993). The modern pharmacological actions of many of the herbs are in fact well known.

Examples of other categories of herbs include: "*herbs that stop bleeding*", "*herbs that relieve cough and wheezing*" (used in the treatment of cough and/or asthma), "*herbs that invigorate blood*" (these are herbs that promote blood circulation and are used in conditions where there is blood stasis) and "*herbs that transform phlegm-cold*" (used in the treatment of cough with phlegm, bronchial disorders and Lung abscess). "*External application herbs*" are used to treat skin disorders and "*herbs that extinguish wind and stop tremors*" may be used in the treatment of hypertension, stroke, migraine, arthritis (including joint pain), dizziness and spasms that are caused by "*internal wind*" according to Chinese medicine theory (Lin *et al.*, 1985).

2.2.2 *How are the herbs used?*

Chinese herbs are rarely used individually. They are usually combined into a prescription of typically two to 12 herbs. This prescription is called a "medicinal formula". The choice of herbs follows Chinese medicine theory and the prescription is individualised according to the patient's condition, constitution, age, gender and for females, time of the menstrual cycle. The dosage of each herb is very important: all herbs have a recommended dosage range within which the herb will have a therapeutic action but is considered safe. As a general rule, the dosage range for herbs should not be exceeded, particularly for those herbs that are considered to have toxicity associated. On the other hand, using too little of an herb may result in it having no therapeutic effect. Dosage of individual herbs is always tailored to the individual. For herbs that are considered strong in action, the dosage used will be less for an individual who is elderly or very young, or of weak constitution. Certain herbs that are toxic are contraindicated (i.e. should be avoided) in certain patients including those who are pregnant.

Herbs are often processed using a variety of methods including dry frying, baking and frying with other substances such as wine or salt or vinegar. The reasons that herbs are processed include increasing the potency of the herb, decreasing toxicity and minimising side effects, and changing the herb's properties and thereby its therapeutic action (Lin *et al.*, 1985). For example, frying an herb with salty water is believed to increase that herb's actions on the Kidney organ and frying wine will enhance an herb's ability to promote blood circulation.

2.2.3 *How are Chinese herbal medicinal formulae developed?*

The art of prescribing herbs is built on a solid knowledge of the guiding theories of Chinese medicine, the actions and properties of the herbs and on years of clinical experience. Following diagnosis of disease and syndrome (symptom/sign pattern complex) that is achieved through the analysis of the signs and symptoms and presenting complaint in terms of Chinese medicine theory, the treatment principle(s) is formed. From this, the key representative medicinal formula is chosen or the formula developed.

There are hundreds of known medicinal formulae that treat many diseases and their various syndromes. Practitioners may simply choose the key representative formula for a given condition and syndrome or use a formula as the basis of their own formulae and modify it according to the patient's presenting condition. Alternatively, practitioners may also develop their own medicinal formulae based on their understanding of the disease aetiology (cause) and mechanism (pathogenesis), knowledge of the actions and properties of the herbs and clinical experience. Regardless of which option is chosen, Chinese medicine theory guides the choice and formulation of the medicinal formula.

The structure of a medicinal formula is precise and was originally described in terms of positions within the imperial court hierarchy (Zhang and Rose, 1995). There are four classes of herbs that generally make up the structure of an herbal formula. The first is the *chief* herb(s) or *king*: usually one or two herbs that produce the main therapeutic action of the formula. The *deputies* or *ministers* are those herbs that support the main actions of the chief herb(s). The *assistants* or *adjuvants* are the herbs that treat other secondary signs and symptoms, moderate or lessen any toxicity or harsh properties associated with the main herbs and assist the chief herb(s) and deputies in achieving their therapeutic aims (Bensky and Gamble, 1993). The assistants may also be used to balance the formula (Bensky and Gamble, 1993). For example, in a formula where the main aim is to tonify Yang, the herbs will be predominantly warm and may also be drying, so one or two Yin-nourishing herbs (predominantly cool or cold and moistening) may be used to moderate the warming and drying action of the Yang herbs, so that overall, the formula is not too warm or drying. The fourth category of herbs is the *guide herb* or *envoy* or *courier* (Bensky and Gamble, 1993). It has the action of guiding the other herbs in the formulae into a particular meridian or area of the body and/or harmonising the herbs in the formula so as to eliminate any side effects that could occur in combining the herbs. In the development of a formula, this structure is not always strictly adhered to, however, it provides general principles for the formation of an herbal medicinal formula. And historically, the use of the metaphor of positions of the court (to describe the structure of an herbal formula) was a reflection of the influence of Confucian philosophy and social order at the time on the development of Chinese medicine (Zhang and Rose, 1995).

In general, the formula is chosen or developed to address the primary presenting complaint. The practitioner must decide whether he/she will treat the root cause (ben), the (secondary) manifestations (biao) or both. The relevant formula is chosen and necessary modifications made: herbs may be added or subtracted from the base formula and the dosage of the herbs will be tailored to the individual. The balance of herbs used in treating the root cause (ben) and its manifestations (biao) will depend on the individual condition. Sometimes if the manifestations are the more urgent issue, the formula will use a majority of herbs to address these and in subsequent formulae, the underlying root cause is addressed. For example, in the case of bleeding haemorrhoids, there may be an underlying deficiency condition that is the root cause of the bleeding. However, the most pressing issue is to stop the bleeding first and *herbs that stop bleeding* will form the bulk of the prescription. Once the acute episode is over, subsequent formulae may be used to address the underlying root cause that is a deficiency condition to prevent future episodes. Signs and symptoms in addition to the presenting complaint are often taken into account and herbs may be added to the main formula to address these problems.

Certain herbs are contraindicated in combination since the combination can lead to toxicity and cause adverse reactions or because the addition of one reduces or negates the positive effect of the other. Conversely, there are combinations of herbs that are advantageous, the combination accentuating the action of one or more of the herbs or reducing undesirable toxicity or side effects of one of the herbs.

In practice, certain categories of herbs are often used together. For example, *herbs that regulate qi* are often used in combination with *herbs that tonify* to moderate the rich and sometimes cloying nature of these tonifying herbs so that the qi of the body does not become stagnant. Herbs in the *stop bleeding* category are often used in combination with *herbs that cool blood* since the root cause of bleeding in its acute stage is often "heat in the blood".

2.2.4 *What are the forms of herbal medicine?*

There are many different forms of herbal medicine. These include decoction, tablets, pills, powder, granules, medicinal wines, tinctures and herbal plasters. In ancient times, herbal decoction was the primary method of preparation of the herbs and is considered the fastest acting of the forms of internal medicine. In a decoction, the raw herbs are boiled in water for about 30 to 45 minutes until the volume of liquid is reduced, then the thickened liquid drunk warm. Decoction is still used today, but is time-consuming and not always convenient. It has the advantage that the formula can be tailored or individualised according to the patient's condition in terms of selection of the kinds of herbs and dosage.

Granules are a more modern form of Chinese herbal medicine and are dissolved in hot water and drunk. Powders may be placed on the tongue and chased down with water. Single herbs in granulated or powder form may be combined in a formula that is individualised for the patient. Chinese medicine in the form of pills and tablets are forms of proprietary medicines and are convenient to use though their action is considered slower than that of decocted raw herbs. The disadvantage with propriety forms of herbal medicine is that the combination and dosage of the herbs is fixed and cannot be altered. Medicinal wines are made by steeping herbs in, typically, rice wine for a number of months. Wine is thought to promote blood circulation. Tinctures and herbal plasters are used for external application, for example in the treatment of sprains and to help broken bones mend.

2.2.5 *What types of conditions are herbs used for?*

Chinese herbal medicine has been used for over 2500 years to treat a wide range of disorders from skin diseases to internal diseases of the body. Herbal medicine is used to treat mild disorders such as the common cold or flu and more serious diseases including heart disease, hepatitis (liver disease) and cancer. Some examples of conditions that may be treated with herbal medicine include period pain, arthritis, angina, urinary tract infection, infertility, prostate hyperplasia, stomach ulcer, irritable bowel syndrome, cough, sore throat, asthma, haemorrhoids, chronic fatigue syndrome and stomach pain.

The effectiveness of Chinese herbal medicine in treating different diseases varies and is beginning to be investigated and established scientifically. Obviously some diseases are better treated with Western medicine, particularly certain acute diseases and those that require surgical intervention. Chinese herbal medicine shows particular promise in the treatment of many chronic diseases that are not effectively treated with Western medicine.

2.2.6 *What are the benefits of Chinese herbal medicine?*

Chinese medicine is relatively safe with few side effects in comparison with Western medicine. With its long history of clinical use, Chinese herbal medicine has established its unique role in health care, particularly in China and most of the Asian countries. The increasing popularity of Chinese herbal medicine, more recently in Western countries, is due to the public belief that Chinese herbal medicine is milder and safer.

In considering the benefits of Chinese medicine, the practice has been criticised for lack of scientific evidence of efficacy (i.e. that it works). Currently, Chinese medicine is not well understood by the Western medicine fraternity. However, *no evidence of effect* is different from *evidence of no effect*. Research that assesses Chinese herbal medicine according to scientific research methodology is still in its infancy due to various constraints including lack of funding, the small numbers of researchers trained in Chinese medicine and a lack of receptivity within orthodox medical circles. Despite this, extensive laboratory research has been conducted into herbs and a number of recent clinical trials have demonstrated the value of Chinese herbal medicine for a variety of clinical conditions, for example, irritable bowel syndrome, hayfever and hepatitis C.

Experiential evidence of safety and efficacy over thousands of years of practice is a strong form of evidence. It is therefore somewhat naïve to say that there is inadequate evidence to support clinical efficacy and safety of herbal medicine. In fact, the majority of current Western medical interventions also lack "scientific evidence" with regard to efficacy and safety but are routinely used in everyday practice. The concept of evidence-based medicine that demands that a treatment or substance be investigated according to scientific principles has only been popularised in the last ten to 20 years. In contrast, Chinese medicine has been in practice for over 25 centuries. With more research being conducted, the overall role of

Chinese herbal medicine in the management of common clinical conditions will be better understood.

2.2.7 *Cautions and contraindications*

Although herbs are generally safe, a number of herbs are toxic, and the toxicity ranges from mild to strong. Certain herbs are toxic in the raw state but rendered relatively safe when correctly processed. It is thus important that the practitioner is properly trained in the use of herbal medicine. Herbs that are strongly toxic are not commonly used and in some countries such as Australia, use of certain toxic herbs is prohibited by law.

As discussed previously, certain herbs should not be used in combination with each other as certain herbs can either negate the action of the other herb or the combination can cause adverse effects. Interactions of Chinese herbs with Western medications can occur and whilst some of these have been documented, in general, there is not enough known about such interactions.

Care must be taken with pregnant women. Certain categories of herbs, for example, those that are purgatives or have a strong draining action, those that promote blood circulation and all of the toxic herbs are contraindicated in pregnancy. Care should also be taken in the case of elderly patients, children, those of delicate constitution or those who have been suffering prolonged illness and are weak. Herbs with strong actions and toxic herbs are usually avoided in such cases.

2.2.8 *What issues need to be addressed in the future?*

Research is needed to establish the safety, quality and effectiveness of herbal medicines in the treatment of different conditions. Thousands of years of traditional use or experiential evidence is a form of evidence of safety and effectiveness that should not be minimised. However there is now a shift in Western medicine towards evidence-based practice that demands that a treatment or medicine be tested using scientific methodology. Chinese medicine is not the same as a Western pharmaceutical and the practice of Chinese medicine is vastly different to Western medicine. Therefore, laboratory studies and clinical trials that test Chinese herbal medicine in ways that stay true to the underlying principles and practice of the medicine will be necessary.

The issue of safety and quality of herbal medicines needs to be addressed and there is not a simple solution. Proprietary medicines (i.e. tablets and pills) are more readily controlled than raw herbs in terms of quality via the requirements of Good Manufacturing Practice (GMP) set down by governments in different countries. However, the quality control of raw herbs remains an issue. Problems with quality control include misidentification of herbs and incorrect labelling, substitution of herbs, contamination (for example, with heavy metals) and adulteration with Western medications. There can be variations in the quality of herbs in terms of the amount or concentration of active constituents within the herb. This can vary from season to season or between regions that the herbs are grown in. This is a particularly important issue with respect to toxic herbs. In addition, certain herbs have a shorter shelf-life than other herbs (for example, those herbs containing volatile oils like *bo he* or field mint) and may lose their therapeutic effect if not used in a timely manner. Quality control systems will need to be put in place in the future.

Research into interactions between Chinese herbal medicine and Western medications is necessary. There are a number of known interactions such as that between Warfarin (an anti-coagulant) and the herb *Dan shen* (Salvia root). Furthermore, adverse event reporting is a critical issue that needs to be addressed to ensure public safety.

2.3 Acupuncture

Acupuncture is a technique that uses very fine needles to puncture the surface of the skin at specific points along energy channels or pathways known as *meridians and collaterals*. These sites are called *acupoints*, and are chosen according to Chinese medicine theory in order to elicit specific therapeutic effects. Following diagnosis of the disease and syndrome (symptom/sign complex), the treatment principle and acupuncture prescription is formulated. Needles are inserted and manipulated using a variety of techniques, each having a specific therapeutic effect.

2.3.1 *What theory guides acupuncture practice?*

The practice of acupuncture is guided by the major theories of Chinese medicine including Yin-Yang Theory, Zang-Fu Theory, Five-Element Theory and in particular, the Theory of Meridians and Collaterals. These will be discussed in Chapter 3. According to theory, acupoints are points through which the meridian qi and qi of the zang-fu organs are transported to the body's surface (Qiu *et al.*, 1993; Cheng, 1987). The number of acupoints on each meridian varies from nine on the Heart and Pericardium meridians to 67 on the Bladder meridian.

Acupoints can have a local effect and/or a distal effect, i.e. an effect on another part of the body remote from the acupoint (Cai *et al.*, 1997). Acupoints on the same meridian share common functions, however in addition, each acupoint has its own specific function(s). For example, the acupoint *Quchi* (Large Intestine 11)[2] near the elbow shares common functions with several other points on the Large Intestine meridian including the treatment of pain, numbness and motor impairment (such as immobility and spasm) of the lateral arm and shoulder (Cheng, 1987; Deadman *et al.*, 1998). However, its special function is relieving fever and is usually the acupoint of choice for conditions with high fever. Each regular meridian[3] has specific points with functions that are common to all meridians. For example, each meridian has a *Yuan* or *Primary point* that is used to treat deficiency-type conditions, and a *Xi-Cleft point* that is used to treat acute-type disorders.

In treatment, a variety of points may be chosen. Acupoints are usually chosen from the affected side of the body, however, in some cases, acupoints from the opposite side may be chosen (this is called cross-needling) (Deadman *et al.*, 1998). Local points are those that overlie or are very close to the diseased area of the body (Deadman *et al.*, 1998). Adjacent points are those nearby. Distal points of the regular meridians

---

[2]Acupoints are named after features in nature, animals, utensils and architectural structures (Cheng, 1987). Quchi means "crooked pool" (Cheng, 1987). They are also named in chronological order according to the meridian they belong to. Quchi is the 11th point on the Large Intestine meridian.

[3]The term *regular meridian* refers to the 12 meridians of the body but is often used to include the two meridians along the midline of the body — the Du and Ren meridians.

have actions on parts of the body remote from their location (Qiu *et al.*, 1993). Distal points are located below the elbow and knees and are primarily chosen from the meridian involved in the disorder, being commonly used to treat conditions of the head, chest, abdomen and back (Deadman *et al.*, 1998). For example, the acupoint He Gu (Large Intestine 4) on the hand is commonly chosen to treat conditions of the head, face and eyes such as headache, sinusitis, conjunctivitis, toothache and facial paralysis (Maciocia, 1989). In practice, a combination of local, adjacent and distal points are commonly chosen to treat pain and disorders of the zang-fu organs (Deadman *et al.*, 1998).

According to Zang-Fu Theory, each zang organ (considered deeper in the body) is connected or paired with a more superficial fu organ, and the connection is provided by the respective meridians (this is described as an interior-exterior relationship). In the treatment of a disorder of a particular zang-fu organ, points from its paired meridian may also be chosen. For example, in the treatment of a Lung disease, a point from the Lung meridian's paired meridian, the Large Intestine meridian, may be chosen. Empirical points are those that have a historically established and specific effect that does not necessarily bear a relationship with its course. For example, *Lieque* (Lung 7) is traditionally used to treat headache even though the Lung channel does not pass to the head (Deadman *et al.*, 1998). There are also combinations of points that historically have been found to be effective.

Acupoints may be chosen according to many principles that include:

- From the front of the body to treat the back and vice versa.
- From the lower body to treat the upper body and vice versa.
- From one meridian to treat its interior-exteriorly related meridian.
- Selection of empirical points or empirical combinations.
- From the opposite side of the body (cross-needling).
- Treatment of the root cause (ben) and the secondary manifestations (biao) (Deadman *et al.*, 1998).

2.3.2 *How is acupuncture performed?*

Following the formulation of an acupuncture prescription, the patient is generally asked to lie on the treatment couch. The skin is cleaned and swabbed with an alcohol swab and an appropriate sterile needle chosen. Acupuncture commonly uses very fine filiform needles that have a handle at one end and the needle at the other. A modern variation on traditional needles is the addition of plastic guide tubes that may be supplied with the needles that limit the initial depth of insertion of the needle into the skin: once inserted, the guide tube is removed and the needle inserted deeper and/or manipulated. The needles vary in length and thickness. For insertion into an area of abundant muscle such as the buttocks, a needle of greater length and usually greater thickness is chosen, whereas for insertion into, for example, areas on the face where only superficial insertion is needed, a shorter and finer needle is generally chosen.

The angle, direction and depth of needle insertion are all important factors in acupuncture technique. The needle may be inserted at right angles (90°) to the body surface, or inserted obliquely (approximately 45° to the body surface) or transversely (at an angle of 15°) (Cai *et al.*, 1997). A transverse insertion is usually used where the muscle coverage is thin, such as acupoints on the head and face (Qiu *et al.*, 1993). An oblique insertion is usually used when the needle is to be inserted into acupoints near important organs or close to bones (Cai *et al.*, 1997). A perpendicular insertion is used in areas where soft tissue is thick and on the limbs (Cai *et al.*, 1997).

Direction of insertion depends on where on the body the needle is to be inserted and is related to angle of insertion (Cai *et al.*, 1997). Depth of insertion depends on where on the body the needle is to be placed and the overlying musculature and fat. Extreme care with depth of insertion must be taken when needling acupoints close to or overlying vital internal organs. Depth of insertion is less for a thin person with little body fat and muscle, for example, than someone who has a lot of muscle. Shallow insertion is suitable for those with a poorer constitution or who are weaker, for example, elderly people, whereas deeper insertion is suitable for those with a strong constitution, and generally young and middle-aged people (Cai *et al.*, 1997).

The therapeutic effect of needling depends on achievement of the "arrival of qi" or "de qi". This is a subjective sensation felt by the practitioner and the patient. The patient may feel as sensation of heaviness around where the needle is inserted. In some cases, the sensation may be like a tiny electric shock that travels along the course of the meridian (that the acupoint belongs to). The practitioner feels a sensation akin to the needle having been *grasped* by the tissue.

Once the needle is inserted, the needle is generally left in the body for 15–30 minutes, although for certain conditions, the needle retention time is only a matter of seconds (usually in acute conditions such as pain syndrome and in conditions such as hay fever). During the period of needle retention, the practitioner may manipulate the needle. Again, there are a variety of manipulation techniques that have different therapeutic effects. For example, the needle may be lifted up and thrust down again, or twirled and rotated continuously. Another technique is to shake the needle or cause it to vibrate. Force and speed of needle manipulation, depth of insertion, and amplitude of rotation of the needle have therapeutic significance. For example, in order to *reinforce* in the case of a deficiency-type condition,[4] the needle is rotated gently and slowly using a small amplitude: this is called a *reinforcing technique*. In comparison, in order to *reduce* an excess-type *condition*,[5] the needle is rotated rapidly using a large amplitude: this is called a *reducing technique*.

At the end of the treatment, the needle is removed from the patient. Again, technique of removal has therapeutic significance. For example, in a reinforcing technique, the removal of the needle is gentle whereas it is more forceful in a reducing technique. The acupoint is generally pressed with a sterile cotton swab or ball after removal of the needle in order to prevent swelling around the site that may be caused by bleeding beneath the skin or to stem spot bleeding from the acupoint if it occurs.

There are other kinds of acupuncture needles and techniques. For example, the dermal hammer is a hammer-shaped instrument with many fine needles in the head. It is tapped against the skin to cause superficial bleeding. It is used to treat mainly musculoskeletal conditions in which there is blood stasis.

---

[4]A deficiency condition denotes a deficiency of antipathogenic qi. More specifically, there can be a deficiency of qi, blood, body fluids, yin, yang and jing (essence).

[5]An excess condition is one in which the pathogenic factors are strong and the body is fighting back strongly.

2.3.3 *What kinds of conditions is acupuncture used for?*

Acupuncture is used for a wide range of conditions including digestion problems, women's health problems, pain relief, treatment of musculoskeletal problems (such as lower back pain, sprains and strains, frozen shoulder, tennis and golfer's elbow), asthma, chronic fatigue syndrome, urinary dysfunction, infertility, common cold, fever, sore throat, constipation and diarrhoea — to name only a few.

2.3.4 *What are the benefits of using acupuncture?*

The purpose of acupuncture is to bring the body back into internal balance, harmonising the yin and yang and qi and blood of the body. In Chinese medicine, acupuncture is believed to have immediate action on the vital energy via the meridians and collaterals. In the past, acupuncture was believed to be one of the most effective methods in treatment of medical emergencies. This role obviously has been diminished due to the advancement of Western medicine, however, it is still frequently used for acute pain management. Recent research has also demonstrated the value of acupuncture for the management for disorders including various pain syndromes (acute and chronic), urinary tract infection, nausea, vomiting, morning sickness and hay fever.

2.3.5 *What are the risks of using acupuncture?*

Risks of acupuncture are minimised by correct technique and adherence to infection control guidelines. Problems can include broken or bent needles, stuck needles and haematoma (swelling around the acupuncture site due to bleeding beneath the skin) (Cheng, 1987). Fainting can also occur, particularly in patients who are very nervous, over-fatigued, or have a weak constitution. For this reason, the practitioner should monitor the patient's response carefully, and in general, first-time patients should be needled lying down, not sitting up. More serious problems can include puncture of major body organs such as the lung (e.g. pneumothorax), and infection of the local acupuncture site or even introduction of pathogens deeper into the body. There are risks to the practitioner too.

These can include needle-stick injury where the practitioner accidentally pricks himself/herself with a needle that has been used on the patient. Aseptic technique is vital in order to avoid infection of the body. The use of disposable single use needles (instead of re-usable needles) is recommended in order to decrease the risks of contamination and spread of infection. Blood-borne diseases including HIV-AIDS and Hepatitis B and C can be spread with contaminated needles.

2.3.6 *Precautions/contraindications*

Care must be taken with first-time patients and those who are particularly nervous or of weak constitution to avoid fainting. Acupuncture should be avoided in patients who are over-fatigued, over-hungry or intoxicated (Qiu *et al.*, 1993; Cheng, 1987). Strong needling techniques should not be used in patients who are very weak and deficient in qi or blood. Certain acupoints are contraindicated in pregnant females, particularly those on the abdomen or lumbo-sacral areas (lower back region) and those that stimulate blood circulation (Qiu *et al.*, 1993). There are points that can stimulate uterine contraction and obviously these must be avoided in pregnancy. Acupuncture should also be avoided during menstruation unless it is for the purpose of regulating menstruation (Qiu *et al.*, 1993). Acupuncture should not be performed on patients who are prone to spontaneous bleeding and is also contraindicated in local areas where there are skin infections, ulcers or other lesions, broken skin, some rashes, scars or tumours (Qiu *et al.*, 1993).

2.4 Electro-Acupuncture

Electro-acupuncture is a relatively modern variation on acupuncture in which electrodes are attached to the handles of the filiform needles once inserted into the body, and a small electrical current applied. In terms of the Western biomedical model, application of the electrical current has the effect of altering ion concentration and distribution in the body tissues and can be used to regulate the functioning of the body, promote analgesia and regulate muscle tone (Qiu *et al.*, 1993). In terms of Chinese medicine theory, it is able to promote the circulation of qi and blood (Qiu *et al.*, 1993). Different wave forms of electrical activity may be applied and each has its own therapeutic action.

Electro-acupuncture has a similar wide range of indications as regular needling (Qiu *et al.*, 1993). However, it is contraindicated in patients with pacemakers and caution must be taken to avoid the current loop passing the heart for persons with heart disease (Qiu *et al.*, 1993). It is generally not recommended for use in pregnant females.

2.5 Magnetic Therapy

In modern times, the use of magnets as a form of acupuncture therapy has become popular. Magnets in the form of beads or sheets are applied to an acupuncture point, setting up a magnetic field (Cai *et al.*, 1997). Magnetic sheets may also be placed opposite each other, for example, on either side of a limb (Cai *et al.*, 1997). Such placement allows the magnetic force to penetrate deep into the tissue (Cai *et al.*, 1997). Magnetic therapy is used for a range of disorders including hypertension, sprains and muscular strains, heart disease, asthma, joint pain, period pain and dizziness (Cai *et al.*, 1997).

2.6 Ear Acupuncture

Based on the principle that since all the meridians directly or indirectly communicate with the ear and each meridian is related to a zang-fu organ, theory holds the ear is closely related with the zang-fu (Qiu *et al.*, 1993). The body structures are mapped onto the surface of the ear in the shape of an inverted foetus (Qiu *et al.*, 1993). Not only are there areas on the ear surface that correspond to body parts, but there are also specific points that have particular therapeutic functions. For example, the ear acupuncture point *Shenmen* is commonly used for insomnia because of its therapeutic function of calming the Heart and mind (Chen and Cui, 1991). According to Chinese medicine theory, sleep (quality and quantity) depends on the state of the *shen* (spirit) or mind (Maciocia, 1994) and the Heart is the zang-fu organ that controls the mind.

Acupuncture needles are inserted into points in the ear. Alternatively, small seeds backed with sticking plaster are taped onto specific ear acupuncture points. They are generally left on the ear for two to three days and pressed daily two to three times per day in order to stimulate the point and elicit the therapeutic effect. Like in regular acupuncture, an acupuncture prescription is formulated following diagnosis of disorder and differentiation of syndrome according to Chinese medicine theories (Chen and Cui, 1991). Acupoints may be chosen according to:

- Chinese medicine theory (e.g. for disorders involving the Spleen, the *Spleen point* is chosen).
- Disease location (e.g. for bronchitis or cough, the *Lung point* is chosen).
- Modern medical knowledge (e.g. the *Sympathetic point* is chosen for disorders involving the sympathetic nervous system).
- Clinical experience (e.g. *Shenmen* is chosen for insomnia or manic depression) (Qiu *et al.*, 1993).

Ear acupuncture is not only used as a treatment option. Knowledge of the ear acupoints can aid in diagnosis. For example, when there is disease, corresponding areas on the ear may become tender or show a change in colour or form (Qiu *et al.*, 1993). Ear acupuncture is indicated for a wide range of disorders, including palpitations, insomnia, hypertension, hypotension, tonsillitis, dysmenorrhoea, epilepsy, constipation, various skin disorders, headache and sciatica (Chen and Cui, 1991).

2.7 Scalp Acupuncture

Scalp acupuncture differs from regular acupuncture or ear acupuncture in that areas on the scalp rather than specific points are stimulated. In general, the areas overlie specific regions of the brain that they have a therapeutic effect on (and after which they are named). For example, there is a sensory area overlying the *Sensory Area* of the brain (indicated for sensory disorders such as numbness, migraines and vertigo), a *Motor Area* (indicated for disorders such as paralysis of the lower limbs), a *Speech III Area* overlying the parietal area of the skull used for treatment of sensory aphasia (disturbance in understanding speech), and a *Visual Area* overlying the occipital lobe of the brain used to treat cortical (brain-related) visual problems (Qiu *et al.*, 1993).

Electro-acupuncture is commonly used to treat cerebral or encephalic disorders such as stroke, epilepsy, chorea, paralysis, aphasia and vertigo (Qiu *et al.*, 1993). It may also be used to treat different kinds of neuralgia, lower back and leg pain, nocturnal eneuresis and other disorders (Qiu *et al.*, 1993).

Electro-acupuncture may be applied to stimulate the specific regions of the scalp. Alternatively, manual manipulation of the needle may be performed: following rapid needle insertion, the needle is rotated very rapidly at a frequency of approximately 200 times per minute for approximately 30–60 seconds (Qiu *et al.*, 1993). This manipulation is usually followed by a break of several minutes then the manipulation/break sequence is repeated twice (Qiu *et al.*, 1993).

2.8 Moxibustion

Moxibustion is a form of therapy in which heat is applied to the body in the form of a cone or stick of the herb *Artemisia vulgaris* (Chinese herb *Ai ye*), an acrid, bitter and warm herb. This cone or stick of herb is known as moxa or moxa "wool": its consistency is a little like that of unspun wool. In some forms of moxa, other herbs are added to *Ai ye*. The moxa stick or cone is ignited and allowed to smoulder. As a consequence of the properties of the herb *Ai ye*, moxa may be used to warm the meridians and dispel cold and dampness, promote the flow of qi and blood in the meridians, relieve swelling and pain, penetrate into muscles and strengthen the yang qi of the body and prevent illness (Cheng, 1987; Cai *et al.*, 1997).

If a moxa stick is used, it is usually held above the area or acupuncture point to be treated until the area becomes warm. The stick is usually moved around above the body so that it does not over-warm the area of skin. Moxa may be used in conjunction with acupuncture: a piece of moxa wool is placed over the handle of the acupuncture needle and ignited. This transfers the heat to the acupuncture point. Care must be taken that the ash from the moxa does not drop onto the patient's skin.

An ancient method of using a moxa cone was to apply it directly to the skin, ignite it and allow it to burn out, leaving blisters: this was called *scarring moxibustion* (Cheng, 1987). Alternatively, before the cone burned down completely, it was removed and another placed on the body: this was called *non-scarring moxibustion* (Cheng, 1987). Direct moxibustion, particularly the scarring form, is not used much in modern Chinese medicine. Indirect moxibustion involves placing an insulating material such as a slice of ginger or garlic between the body and the moxa cone, then igniting the cone (Cheng, 1987).

Moxibustion must not be used (i.e. is contraindicated) when there is excessive heat in the body, for example, when there is fever, or when there is an excess-type syndrome (Cheng, 1987). Moxibustion on the abdomen and lumbar and sacral areas of the (lower) back of pregnant women is also contraindicated (Cheng, 1987). Scarring moxibustion must not be used on the face, head or over areas near large blood vessels or certain vital organs (Cheng, 1987).

Moxibustion is used in the clinic to treat many different kinds of disorders, providing the syndrome differentiated is one in which moxibustion is suitable. Such disorders can include arthralgia (joint pain), vertigo, amenorrhoea (absence of periods in a woman who has not reached menopause), mastitis, prolapse of the uterus or anus, protracted diarrhoea, vomiting, diarrhoea and abdominal pain (Cai *et al.*, 1997).

2.9 Cupping

Cupping is a form of therapy in which a cup, usually made of glass or bamboo, is placed on the skin, usually in an area of abundant muscle, after a negative pressure is created inside the cup by passing a flame into it. The negative pressure created draws the skin and underlying tissue up into the cup. The purpose of cupping is to relieve areas of blood and qi stagnation: cupping warms and dispels cold and stimulates or facilitates the flow of qi and blood in the meridians (Cheng, 1987). It is commonly used to treat musculoskeletal problems and may be used in combination with acupuncture where the needle is inserted into the skin first then the cup placed over the needle, or it may be used prior to or following acupuncture. The after-effect of cupping is usually a localised area of blood stasis manifesting as a red-purple circular area of bruising that subsides after several days. In general, the greater the amount of blood stasis, the darker the "bruised" area.

Cupping may also be used in combination with a technique called "blood-letting" in which the skin is pierced with a lancet or three-edged needle or dermal hammer and the cup placed over the area. This has the effect of drawing out the blood in areas where there is blood stagnation and is used to treat acute sprains where there is blood stasis (Cheng, 1987).

Cupping may be used as a form of massage: oil is applied to the body and a cup applied, creating a vacuum. The cup is then moved or dragged over the surface of the skin; again the purpose is to encourage the flow of qi and blood in the meridians in areas where it may be stagnant, and to warm the area and dispel cold.

In cases where cupping is used in conjunction with needling or blood-letting, glass cups must be re-sterilised or disposed of after use. Bamboo cups are generally considered unsuitable for use from the point of view of infection control since they cannot be adequately cleaned and sterilised.

Cupping is contraindicated in patients prone to spontaneous bleeding, on areas where skin is broken or ulcerated, in patients with oedema or high fever, and over the sacral area and abdomen of pregnant women (Cheng, 1987). Strong cupping should be avoided in patients who are very weak.

2.10 Tuina (Chinese Massage)

Tuina is used as a treatment modality and a form of preventive medicine and is guided by Chinese medicine theory.

One of the major differences between tuina and Western forms of massage is that it is traditionally done through the patient's clothes, a reflection of the reserve that characterises Chinese culture. Herbal liniments may be used when necessary, but massage oils are not commonly used and *essential oils* (extracted from various flowers and plants) that are favoured in Western massage are absent.

Chinese massage developed throughout the many dynasties of Chinese history and numerous schools of massage were formed, each characterised by its own special manipulations or "chief manipulations" plus several auxiliary techniques (Zhang, 1990). The numerous schools and academic branches of massage in China include: one-finger meditation massage, rolling massage, digital acupoint pressure massage, paediatric massage, organ and channel massage, sports massage, bone-setting massage and chiropractic therapy, to name but a few (Zhang, 1990).

The major schools and forms of massage include the following:

- *One finger meditation massage:* Focuses on massage of acupoints along the meridians and in addition to its primary technique of using the radial side, tip and whorled surface of the thumb, uses 11 other hand techniques (Zhang, 1990).
- *Rolling massage:* Uses a rolling action as the chief hand-technique and uses a large manipulation area and strong force (Zhang, 1990).
- *Internal exercise massage:* One of the more interesting forms, requiring the practitioner to be schooled in *Shaolin*[6] *internal* exercise. The practitioner directs qi inside whilst performing the massage and at the same time, the patient should also practise *Shaolin internal exercise* during the massage to strengthen their resistance (Zhang, 1990). Thus, both the outer and inner are treated. A large number of hand-techniques are utilised.
- *Digital point therapy* developed from the actions of traditional Chinese martial arts; the basic hand techniques include energetic and swift digital pressing, hitting, thumping and patting (Zhang, 1990).
- *Finger-pressing massage* uses the finger tip to press acupoints and tender points (termed Ashi points) (Zhang, 1990).

The effectiveness of massage depends on the quality of the manipulation, i.e. the practitioner's technique, and the therapeutic effect related to the stimulation of the meridians, acupoints and other locations chosen

[6]Shaolin monks in the Shaolin Temple in China are renowned for their amazing feats of physical strength that have, as a foundation, a fierce strength of mind and spirit.

(Zhang, 1990). Massage has a local effect on promoting blood circulation in soft tissue and muscles and helps the soft tissue, tendons, joints and bones recover from injury (Zhang, 1990). Massage also works by regulating yin and yang, regulating the function of the meridians and collaterals, and influencing the state of the body's vital substances (such as qi, blood and body fluids), internal organs and the emotions via its action on the meridians and collaterals and specific acupoints (Zhang, 1990).

2.11 Diet Therapy

In ancient China, medicine and diet were believed to be the same (Zhao, 1996). Diet therapy, the use of foods to sustain or improve health or treat illness, was used by ordinary people and in the imperial court of China as far back as 2000 years ago (Zhao, 1996).

Certain herbs used in medicinal formula are also used as foods in soups or other dishes and families passed down recipes to younger generations to help alleviate various illnesses. For example, the herb *dang gui* (Chinese angelica root, a herbs that nourishes blood) can be added to chicken soup: this is particularly nourishing for women following childbirth and for those patients who are weak following long-term illness. The herb *gou qi zi* (Chinese wolfberry fruit, a herb that nourishes the Liver blood and Kidney yin) can be cooked with pork (which also strengthens the Kidney) in order to help strengthen the Kidney organ system. The herb *shan yao* (Chinese yam) can be cooked with rice: the combination helps strengthen the Spleen organ system and may help those who have hyper- or hypo-acidity of the stomach.

Like medicinal herbs, everyday foods are understood and categorised according to Chinese medicine theory. The properties of the foods — the temperature characteristics and flavours — help determine the action of the foods on the body. Foods have different actions on the body as understood in terms of Chinese medicine theory. Some foods tonify qi, others tonify yin and yang and nourish blood, others still may clear heat or are diuretics. Foods can have specific effects on certain zang-fu organs. For example, apricots are sweet, sour and neutral in flavour and "moisten the Lung" and "nourish the Stomach yin": they may be used in the diet to help alleviate a dry cough and in conditions associated with Stomach yin deficiency such as gastritis (inflammation of the stomach). Grapes are sweet, slightly sour and neutral in flavour and act particularly on the Stomach, Kidney and Liver zang-fu organs. They also help strengthen deficient qi and nourish blood for conditions of qi and blood deficiency and can help generate body fluids. Pork helps strengthen the Kidney, chicken helps strengthen the Lung, beef helps strengthen the Liver and lamb helps strengthen the Heart.

Foods should be eaten in the season in which they naturally grow. During winter, warm foods should be eaten and cold and raw foods that can damage the Spleen and Stomach zang-fu organs (responsible for digestion in Chinese medicine) should be avoided.

Not all foods have a positive effect on the body, and how the body reacts depends on the individual. Mangoes and bananas, for example, are believed to contribute to internal dampness; in Chinese medicine, dampness can manifest as abnormal discharges. Certain foods can aggravate or exacerbate conditions. A good example is alcohol. Alcohol can contribute to the formation of internal heat in the body. Internal heat or fire that flares upwards can lead to headache and red eyes and contribute to hypertension. Alcohol can also lead to "internal dampness" that can manifest in some women, for example, as stomach bloating and thrush, an itchy vaginal discharge.

The knowledge of the properties and action of foods on the body can thus be utilised in two ways:

- To ascertain whether there are foods in the diet that are aggravating or causing the patient's condition.
- To suggest dietary modifications including the addition of certain foods that may be beneficial to the patient.

A Chinese medicine practitioner will question a patient about diet and following diagnosis of disease and syndrome involved, will provide advice on foods that should be avoided and those that may be beneficial to add to the diet. Chinese medicine theory guides this dietary analysis and advice. There are many diet therapy books containing recipes that are indicated for certain internal diseases or ailments. Recipes also exist for external treatment of various skin diseases including psoriasis, eczema and tinea (Zhao, 1996).

2.12 Exercise Therapy

Taichi and qigong are two of the major forms of exercise therapy of Chinese medicine. In both qigong and taichi, the breath and body movements are coordinated and the mind focussed internally in order to promote the unobstructed flow of qi and blood around the body, calm the spirit, regulate the emotions, and strengthen the body's qi and internal zang-fu organs.

Taichi has also been described as "an approach to following the earlier form of Taoist philosophy in movement" (Crompton, 1990: p. vii). Taichi consists of a series of slow, controlled, gentle movements and postures in a specific sequence. There are several different schools of taichi and several forms of taichi also. For example, in the Yang style (school) of taichi, the "long form" consists of 108 separate postures/movements linked together in a flowing sequence. However gentle these movements appear, the individual movements are actually martial arts moves. Taichi is essentially a fighting form practised, as a rule, alone i.e. no partner is necessary for most of the forms of taichi, although there are some forms such as *pushing hands* in which a partner is necessary. There are also several forms of taichi involving weaponry such as swords (taichi jian). Taichi can be practised as simply a form of physical exercise or as a deeper meditative practice: it is often called "meditation in movement" (Crompton, 1990: p. vii).

Qigong (or chikung) means "cultivation of internal energy" (or qi) (Crompton, 1990: p. 82). Taichi is believed to have developed out of qigong (Crompton, 1990). Qigong has both static forms in which different stationary postures are adopted, and dynamic forms in which postures are sequenced. Different postures and movements are thought to be beneficial to specific zang-fu organs. *Qigong self-massage* is another kind of therapy in which the hands are placed on certain parts of the body, particularly over a point below the navel believed to be a focal point of qi (Crompton, 1990). Different exercises may be prescribed by a practitioner in order to specifically improve the functioning of certain organs.

2.13 Conclusion

Chinese medicine has a rich variety of modalities with which to promote wellness, prevent illness and treat ill health. Different modalities may be utilised depending on the patient's condition and preference for treatment. In practice, a combination of several of the modalities allows for a holistic treatment.

References

Bensky, D. and Gamble, A. (1993) *Chinese Herbal Medicine Materia Medica.* Eastland Press, Seattle, Washington.

Cai, J., Chao, G., Chen, D., *et al.* (eds.) (1997) *State Administration of Traditional Chinese Medicine: Advanced Textbook on Traditional Chinese Medicine and Pharmacology, Vol. 4.* New World Press, Beijing, China.

Chen, K. and Cui, Y. (1991) *Handbook to Chinese Auricular Therapy.* Foreign Languages Press, Beijing.

Cheng, X. (ed.) (1987) *Chinese Acupuncture and Moxibustion.* Foreign Languages Press, Beijing, China.

Crompton, P. (1990) *The Elements of Tai Chi.* Element Books Ltd., Shaftesbury, Dorsett.

Deadman, P., Al-Khafaji, M. and Baker, K. (1998) *A Manual of Acupuncture.* Journal of Chinese Medicine Publications, East Sussex, England.

Lin Y.K., *et al.* (1985) *Chinese Materia Medica.* Shanghai Science and Technology Press, Shanghai, China.

Maciocia, G. (1989) *The Foundations of Chinese Medicine. A Comprehensive Text for Acupuncturists and Herbalists.* Churchill Livingstone, New York.

Maciocia, G. (1994) *The Practice of Chinese Medicine. The Treatment of Diseases with Acupuncture and Chinese Herbs.* Churchill Livingstone, New York.

The Pharmacopoeia Commission of China (PCC) (1997) *Pharmacopoeia of PR China* (Vol. 1 in English). Chemical Industry Press, Beijing.

Qiu, M.L., Zang, S.C., Yu, Z.Q., *et al.* (1993) *Chinese Acupuncture and Moxibustion.* Churchill Livingstone, Edinburgh.

Zhang, E. (ed.) (1990) *Chinese Massage.* Publishing House of Shanghai University of Traditional Cinese Medicine, Shanghai.

Zhang, Y.H. and Rose, K. (1995) *Who Can Ride the Dragon? An Exploration of the Cultural Roots of Traditional Chinese Medicine.* Paradigm Publications, Brookline, Massachusetts.

Zhao, M. (1996) *Chinese Diet Therapy.* China Esperanto Press, Beijing.

Chapter 3

The Theoretical Framework of Chinese Medicine

Kylie A. O'Brien & Charlie Changli Xue

3.1 Introduction

Chinese medicine is a unique medical system. An in-depth understanding of the theoretical framework of the Chinese medical system including its philosophical underpinnings is essential in order for Chinese medicine to be practised effectively. In order to arrive at a diagnosis, the practitioner must be able to systematically collect and analyse the symptoms and signs according to Chinese medicine theories. The theories provide a framework in which to understand the cause of disease (aetiology) and what happens in the body during the course of the disease, and are used to guide treatment. The treatment principles follow directly from the diagnosis and an acupuncture and/or Chinese herbal medicine prescription is subsequently formulated and/or advice given to the patient. Figure 3.1 depicts the foundations of the practice of Chinese medicine.

This chapter will describe the features of the Chinese medicine system, philosophical underpinnings and theories of Chinese medicine that guide practice, how Chinese medicine understands both the workings of the human body and causal factors of disease, and what goes into the clinical decision-making process. Chinese medicine places a strong emphasis on prevention of illness, thus a brief introduction to this topic is also included.

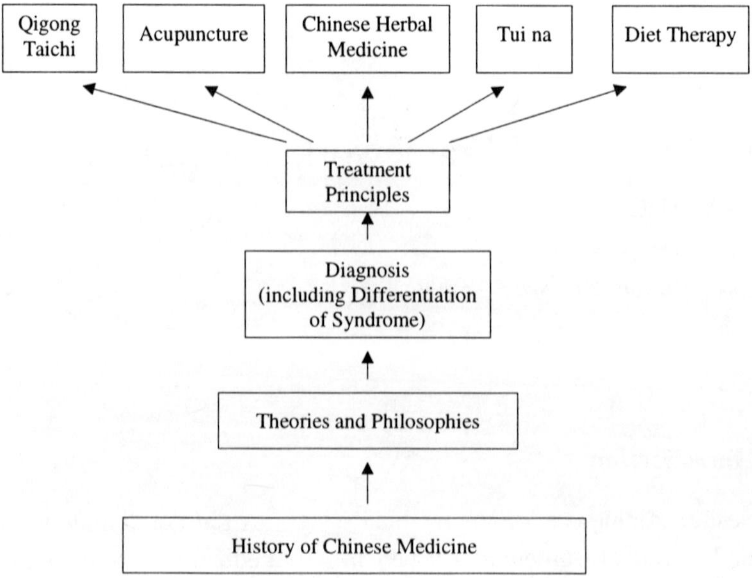

Figure 3.1. Basis of the practice of Chinese medicine.

3.2 Features of Chinese Medicine

It could be argued that the influence of Eastern systems of thought within the area of health in Western countries stems predominantly from China and India. Many newer forms of complementary medicine are using concepts and ideas that have their roots in the ancient medical systems of traditional Chinese medicine and Indian traditional medicine (Ayurveda). There are several features of the Chinese medicine system that together make it a unique medical system.

3.2.1 *Holistic ideology*

Underpinning the theoretical system of Chinese medicine is the ideology of holism (Cai *et al.*, 1995).[1] This holistic philosophy has its roots in

---

[1]Holism is the view that certain things or phenomena "are more than merely the sum of their parts — that they can be understood only be examining them as a whole" (Martin, 2002: p. 146).

ancient China, when humans were seen as a smaller universe (microcosm) of the greater surrounding universe (macrocosm) (Beinfield and Korngold, 1991).

Chinese medicine theory holds that the human body is an organic entity composed of different organs and tissues, each having their own distinct functions but existing in a mutually inter-dependent relationship with each other (Cai *et al.*, 1995). The body's organs, tissues and other parts are connected into this organic whole by the *meridian system*, a system of channels of the body in which the body's *vital substances*, including *qi* (commonly described as a form of vital energy in the West) and blood, circulate (Cheng, 1987; Deadman, 1998). The body's internal (physiological) balance is maintained by the harmonious functioning of the organs and vital substances (Cai *et al.*, 1995) and when the body is in balance internally, similar to haemostasis, there is good health. However, because of the inter-dependent relationship between organs, if disease should occur, the organs may be mutually affected (Cai *et al.*, 1995). It follows that in treatment of disease, consideration needs to take into account not only the tissue or organ directly involved, but other organs and/or tissues that may also be or become affected.

The philosophy of holism extends to the intimate relationship between humans and nature. Humans do not live in a vacuum, instead, they live within the natural and increasingly unnatural environment, and environmental change can have a significant impact on the body either directly or indirectly. The body can either adapt or a pathological response can occur (maladaption) (Cai *et al.*, 1995). Different seasons tend to be associated with different types of factors that cause disease (Cai *et al.*, 1995). These will be discussed in more detail later. Treatment takes into account many environmental factors including geography, climate and season and artificial environments (for example, air-conditioned offices) in addition to other individual factors such as gender, age and constitution (Cai *et al.*, 1995).

3.2.2 *The mind-body continuum*

Many complementary medicine practices are underpinned by an understanding of the connection between the mind and body and the flow of energy through the mind-body system (O'Brien, 2002). The roots of this understanding can be found in traditional medical systems including Chinese medicine (O'Brien, 2002). In Chinese medicine, the mind, emotions and body are not seen as separate but as a continuum. A person's emotional and mental states are seen as having a significant impact on the body and *vice versa*. Furthermore, the physiological basis for the mental processes and emotions are the same substances that make up the body: *qi*, a form of vital energy, essence and blood (explained in detail later) (Maciocia, 1989).

The mind-body concept is being substantiated within the Western medical system where the field of psychoneuroimmunology is making in-roads into identifying neurotransmitters associated with emotions and effects on the immune system. In many ways, the concepts involved in this field are not so far removed from those of Chinese medicine, but the language is different. *New* mind-body or "vibrational medicine" paradigms describe human beings in terms of energetic systems, and Chinese medicine concepts are being utilised and incorporated into newer theories in order to understand the human state of existence (Gerber, 1988).

3.2.3 *Concept of health and illness*

Also flowing from the holistic philosophy, good health is seen as a reflection of internal harmony of the body: harmony between the organs, tissues, vital substances, structures, mind and emotions, and harmony of man/woman within their environment. Illness occurs when there is a disturbance of the internal harmony within the body.

3.2.4 *Other key features of the Chinese medicine system*

There are several other key features of Chinese medicine. These include:

(a) *Differentiation of syndromes:* Diseases or conditions are subcategorised into "syndromes" or patterns of disease by analysis of the signs and symptoms according to Chinese medicine theory.

Each disease or condition typically has three to five "syndromes" or subcategories that represent the manifestations of disease and pathology at a certain stage in the course of a disease.

(b) *Terminology:* Much of the language of Chinese medicine developed from analogies drawn through observation of nature and differs greatly from that of Western medicine. However, many of the terms can be readily understood in terms of Western medicine.

(c) *Individualisation of treatment:* The treatment and prescription (e.g. acupuncture points or herbs) is tailor-made for the individual, and takes into account the individual's constitution, age, gender, syndrome, primary complaint and accompanying signs and symptoms, season of occurrence of the disease and geographic location.

(d) *Emphasis on prevention of disease:* It is said that "the superior doctor provides measures of prevention and the average doctor provides treatment" (Wang, 1995). Chinese medicine places a heavy emphasis on prevention of disease and promotion of health.

3.3 What Thinking Underpins Chinese Medicine?

Chinese medicine developed under the influence of two important and ancient theories: the Yin-Yang Theory and the Five Element Theory. The world and life were seen as being the result of a dynamic balance between the two vital forces, namely, Yin and Yang. In addition, the formation and development of the material world were seen as being based on the inter-relationship between the five types of basic materials occurring in nature: wood, fire, earth, metal and water. From these simple observations of nature, philosophers began to draw analogies about other areas of life. These ways of interpreting reality were developed into systems of thought that were applied in many different social areas of life. These same systems of thought began to be applied to explain the way the body behaves.

3.3.1 *Yin-Yang Theory*

The Yin-Yang Theory is the single-most important and fundamental theory underlying the practice of Chinese Medicine. It is a dialectic[2] and materialistic ideology based on the belief that the world is material and results from the mutual action of two complementary but opposite material forces, termed *Yin* and *Yang* (Kaptchuk, 1983; Cai *et al.*, 1995).

The Yin-Yang theory was formed during the Yin (16th century–11th century B.C.) and Zhou (11th century–221 B.C.) Dynasties and was developed to its highest degree by the "Yin Yang School" during the Warring States Period (476–221 B.C.), a time when many schools of thought arose (Cheng, 1987; Maciocia, 1989).

It is thought that the Yin-Yang Theory originated from peasants' observations of the cycle of day and night and the changes of light and shade on the side of a mountain as the sun moved across the sky (Maciocia, 1989; Beinfeld and Korngold, 1991). The sunny side of the mountain was classified as Yang in comparison with the shady side that was Yin; day was Yang and night was Yin (Beinfeld and Korngold, 1991; Cai *et al.*, 1995). As the day turns into night, Yang becomes Yin, and as night becomes day, Yin becomes Yang.

From these original observations, the theory of Yin and Yang developed. According to the theory, the world results from a unity of opposites forces, Yin and Yang, and that changes in the universe come about through the motion of these opposites (Yin *et al.*, 1992). Everything in the natural world was seen as having the opposing aspects of Yin and Yang (Yin *et al.*, 1992). Yin and Yang were originally classified on the basis of paired opposites; for example, darkness (Yin) and brightness (Yang) (Cheng, 1987). See Table 3.1 for a list of characteristics that correspond to Yin and Yang.

This thinking was eventually subsumed into Chinese medicine, appearing in the most important Chinese medicine text, the *Huang Di Nei Jing* ("Inner Canon of the Yellow Emperor"), and was used to describe

---

[2]Dialectic is used in the sense of meaning the conflict of opposites that requires resolution (Honderich, 1995). It also questions which is first in the development of reality: matter or consciousness (Honderich, 1995).

Table 3.1. Characteristics corresponding to Yin and Yang.

Yin	Yang
Cold	Heat
Interior	Exterior
Inward	Outward
Downward	Upward
Heavy	Light
Stillness	Activity
Day	Night
Darkness	Brightness
Earth	Heaven

the human body and how it works (its physiology) and pathological processes that occur in disease (Cheng, 1987; Cai *et al.*, 1995).

There are four aspects of the Yin-Yang relationship:

(i) Opposition of Yin and Yang: Yin and Yang represent the characteristics of two opposite but complementary aspects of a phenomenon, or the characteristics of two mutually related objects or phenomenon, or opposite stages of an alternating cycle.

(ii) Inter-dependence of Yin and Yang: Yin and Yang depend on each other for existence and form a unity. Without Yang, there is no Yin and *vice versa*.

(iii) Mutual transformation of Yin and Yang: Yin and Yang can transform into each other under certain conditions.

(iv) Dynamic equilibrium of Yin and Yang: Yin and Yang are constantly changing, waxing and waning, mutually consuming and supporting each other, and under normal conditions, exist in a state of relative equilibrium (Maciocia, 1989; Cai *et al.*, 1995; Cheng, 1987).

If the equilibrium between Yin and Yang is disturbed, it can lead to four possible states of imbalance:

(i) An absolute excess of Yin: When this happens, it will consume Yang leading to a decrease in Yang.

(ii) An absolute excess of Yang: When this occurs, it will consume Yin leading to a decrease in Yin.
(iii) A relative excess of Yin: Yang is deficient so Yin is in relative excess.
(iv) A relative excess of Yang: Yin is deficient so Yang is in relative excess (Maciocia, 1989; Cheng, 1987).

The Yin-Yang Theory only makes sense when considering two objects that are mutually related or two opposite aspects of the one phenomenon. If these conditions do not exist, the theory cannot be used to explain their relationship (Cai *et al.*, 1995).

Role of Yin-Yang Theory in Chinese Medicine

The Yin-Yang Theory permeates all facets of Chinese medicine. All other theories relate back in some way to the Yin-Yang Theory and the theory itself guides clinical practice. The following are examples of how the Yin-Yang Theory is used.

Classifying body structures

Body structures may be classified according to Yin and Yang (see Table 3.2). The internal organ structures and material substances of the body (such as blood, body fluids and mucous) are classified Yin and the functional activities of the organs and movement of qi are classified as Yang (Beinfield and Korngold, 1991; Cheng, 1987).

Table 3.2. Classification of body structures according to Yin and Yang.

Yin	Yang
Interior of body	Body surface
Zang organs	Fu organs
Yin meridians	Yang meridians
Lower body	Upper body
Medial aspect of body	Lateral aspect of body

Explaining how the body works and pathological changes in disease

The theory is used to explain the body's normal physiological functioning and pathological changes in disease. Nutrient substances in the body are classified as Yin and functional activities as Yang (Cheng, 1987). The activities (Yang) of the internal organs produce nutrient substances (Yin) that in turn nourish them and allow their functioning (Yang) (Cheng, 1987). Thus, Yin relies on Yang and *vice versa*.

Good health relies on the dynamic balance of Yin and Yang within the body. Fundamentally, disease occurs because of a loss of balance of Yin and Yang in the body due to either an excess or deficiency of one or the other (Cheng, 1987).

Yin and Yang may be used to classify the external and internal causative agents of disease, termed *pathogenic factors* (described later), according to their nature (Yin *et al.*, 1992). External causative agents of disease or *exogenous pathogenic factors* are abnormal manifestations of climatic factors occurring in nature: wind, cold, dampness, fire, dryness and summer-heat. Fire and dryness are examples of Yang pathogens and dampness and cold are Yin pathogens.

The application of the theory to explain pathological processes is complex. For example, a Yang *pathogenic factor* can lead to an excess of Yang (i.e. above its normal level) and heat that leads to a consumption of Yin and fluids (Maciocia, 1989; Yin *et al.*, 1992). A deficiency of Yin within the body can lead to a relative excess of Yang and internal heat. Under certain conditions, a Yang syndrome may transform into a Yin syndrome and *vice versa* (Yin *et al.*, 1992). An example of this latter situation is sometimes seen in the common cold, where the body is attacked by an external cold (Yin) pathogen that invades the body and turns into a heat (Yang) pathogen leading to sore throat and raised temperature.

Explaining clinical manifestations

Clinical manifestations may be analysed in terms of Yin and Yang in order to guide diagnosis. Table 3.3 sets out examples of clinical manifestations classified in terms of Yin and Yang. Yin and Yang are the foundation for the differentiation of disease syndromes according to the *Eight Guiding*

Table 3.3. Classification of clinical manifestations according to Yin and Yang.

Yin sign or symptom	Yang sign or symptom
Low energy level	Hyperactive
Sleepiness	Insomnia
Soft, feeble voice	Strong voice
Slow pulse	Rapid pulse

Principles, a set of eight principles applied in the analysis of signs and symptoms in order to categorise patterns of disease (Yin/Yang, Cold/Heat, Interior/Exterior and Deficiency/Excess). This is described later.

Guiding treatment

The Yin-Yang Theory is used to guide treatment. A deficiency of either Yin or Yang can lead to a *relative* excess of the other. In such a case, the deficient Yin or Yang is nourished or strengthened using herbs and/or acupuncture. If there is an *absolute* excess of Yang or Yin and the corresponding Yin or Yang is not damaged, then the excess is eliminated. For example, in the case where there is an internal *excess heat syndrome*, herbs of a cold (Yin) nature may be given to clear the heat and drain the internal fire. In addition, the theory is also used to categorise the nature or temperature characteristic, flavour/taste and action of medicinal herbs (Cai *et al.*, 1995). Herbs that are warm or hot in terms of temperature characteristic, for example, *rou gui* (cinnamon bark), are Yang. In contrast, herbs that are cool or cold such as *jin yin hua* (honeysuckle flower) are Yin.

3.3.2 *The Five Element Theory*

Wu Xing or *Five-Element Theory* (also called *Five Phase Theory*) developed in ancient China around the time of the Yin (16th century–11th century B.C.) and Zhou (11th century–221 B.C.) Dynasties from observations of five elements essential to life: Wood, Fire, Earth, Metal and Water (Cheng, 1987). The elements were seen as symbolising patterns of motion, characteristics or states of phenomena or kinds of processes, and it was believed that all things came into being because of the motion and change of these five elements (Yin *et al.*, 1992; Kaptchuk, 1983; Maciocia, 1989). The five elements were seen as existing in a dynamic and balanced relationship with each other. By way of analogy, phenomena and matter were classified in terms of the five elements (Cheng, 1987). The symbolism of the elements is as follows:

- Fire: Warm or hot; flaring; ascending
- Earth: Nourishing; growth-promoting
- Wood: Germination; growth; flourishing
- Metal: Descending; clearing; astringing
- Water: Cooling; flowing downward (Yin *et al.*, 1992; Cai *et al.*, 1995; Cheng, 1987).

The five elements or phases can also be seen as stages of the cycle of seasons and of human life (Beinfeld and Korngold, 1991; Maciocia ,1989). The Wood phase (associated with Spring) is akin to birth and the phase of rapid growth during childhood (Beinfeld and Korngold, 1991). The Fire phase (associated with Summer) is the prime of life when adulthood is reached (Beinfeld and Korngold, 1991). The ripening phase of Earth (associated with late Summer) is experienced as a maturing process, and the metal phase (the Autumn years) the stage of ageing and degeneration (Beinfeld and Korngold, 1991). The Water stage (associated with Winter) is reached when, on dying, there is a return to a state of dissolution (Beinfeld and Korngold, 1991).

The theory developed as a conceptual means for understanding phenomena and was applied in Chinese medicine (Cheng, 1987).

Role of Five Element Theory in Chinese Medicine

The Five Element Theory is not usually used in isolation but in conjunction with the other theories that guide Chinese medicine. It is used to explain how the body works (physiology) and the pathological changes in disease. It also guides treatment.

Explaining how the body works

The Five Element Theory is used as a model to explain the functions of the body's internal (zang-fu) organs and tissues in terms of the characteristics of the five elements, and analyse the dynamic relationship between the organs (Yin *et al.*, 1992). This forms the basis of understanding of how the body works (its physiological functioning) and also what happens in disease (pathological processes).

Correlations between functions of the five internal *zang* organs and attributes of a particular element were made (Yin *et al.*, 1992). For example, the Kidney corresponds to the element of Water since it regulates water metabolism (Cai *et al.*, 1995). Each element is associated with an internal organ, tissue, sense organ, season, colour, direction, smell and taste, embodying the unity of man and nature (Yin *et al.*, 1992). See Table 3.4.

According to theory, there exist defined relationships between the elements and by association, the zang-fu organs, that explain the physiological functioning of the body. The five processes or patterns of motion within the body represented by the five elements interact, promote and control each other to maintain a balanced system. Pathology in the body may arise when the relationships between the five processes and organs becomes unbalanced or distorted. Since the body is an organic whole,

Table 3.4. Classification according to the five elements.

	Wood	Fire	Earth	Metal	Water
Season	Spring	Summer	Late summer	Autumn	Winter
Climate	Wind	Heat	Dampness	Dryness	Cold
Flavours	Sour	Bitter	Sweet	Pungent	Salty
Colours	Green	Red	Yellow	White	Black
Zang organ	Liver	Heart	Spleen	Lung	Kidney
Fu organ	Gallbladder	Small Intestine	Stomach	Large Intestine	Bladder
Sense organ	Eye	Tongue	Mouth	Nose	Ears
Tissues	Tendons	Blood vessels	Muscles	Skin	Bones
Emotions	Anger	Joy	Overthinking	Melancholy	Fear
Sounds	Shouting	Laughing	Singing	Crying	Mourning

Source: Cai *et al.* (1995).

when one organ is affected in a disease process, other organs and tissues may become affected via the interconnections described by the theory (Cheng, 1987). There are several disharmonious relationships between the elements that can be used to explain these pathological changes.

Major harmonious relationships between the elements

Two major relationships between the elements and, by association, between the zang-fu organs exist under normal physiological conditions in the body:

(i) The Generation Cycle (mother-son sequence): The promoting relationship that describes the generation, nourishment and support given by the "mother" in the sequence (always the preceding element or organ) to its son (the next element or organ in the sequence). For example, Fire (Heart) is the son of Wood (Liver) and mother of Earth (Spleen), and so on (Fig. 3.2).

(ii) The Restraining Cycle: The relationship that describes the dynamics of restraint or control between elements or organs (Beinfield and Korngold, 1991), represented by the arrows between elements/organs in Fig. 3.3. This provides the means by which the zang-fu organs keep each other in check (Cheng, 1987). For example, Earth (Spleen) controls Water (Kidney) and is itself controlled by Wood (Liver) (Fig. 3.3).

Disharmonious relationships between the elements

Several disharmonious relationships can occur when there is imbalance between the elements/zang-fu organs, usually as a result of an excess or deficiency of one or more of the elements (Cheng, 1987). Such imbalances can lead to disease. Disharmonious relationships in the Restraining Cycle are:

- *Over-acting:* The zang organ (element) that normally controls another in the *Restraining Sequence* excessively controls that zang organ (i.e. over-controls it), disturbing the organ's functioning (Cheng, 1987). This can more readily occur if the organ that is normally controlled becomes weakened or deficient (Fig. 3.4).

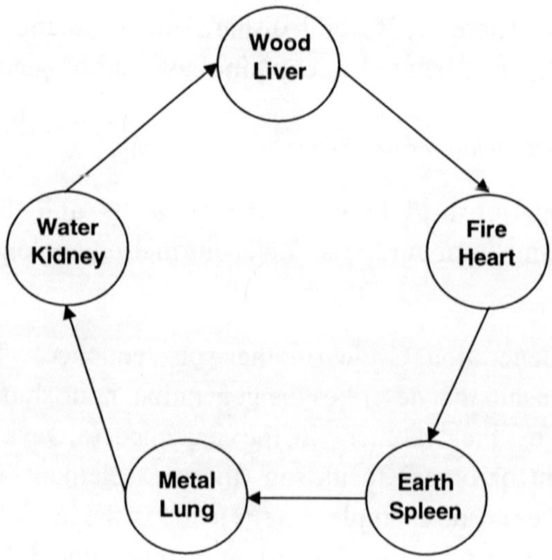

Figure 3.2. Five element generation cycle.

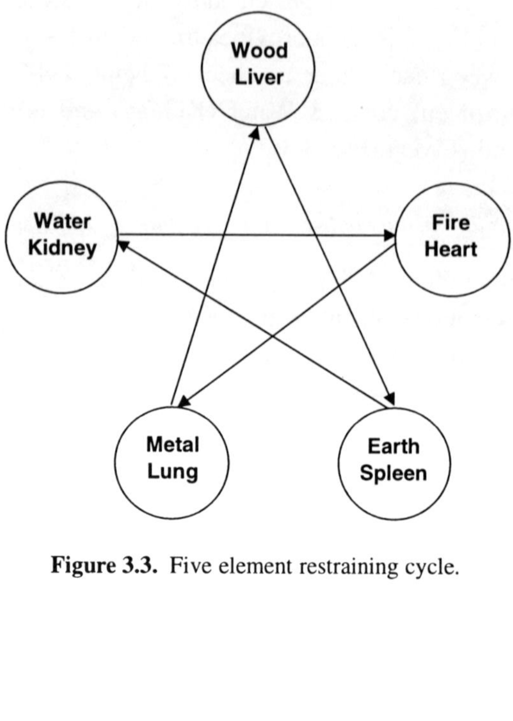

Figure 3.3. Five element restraining cycle.

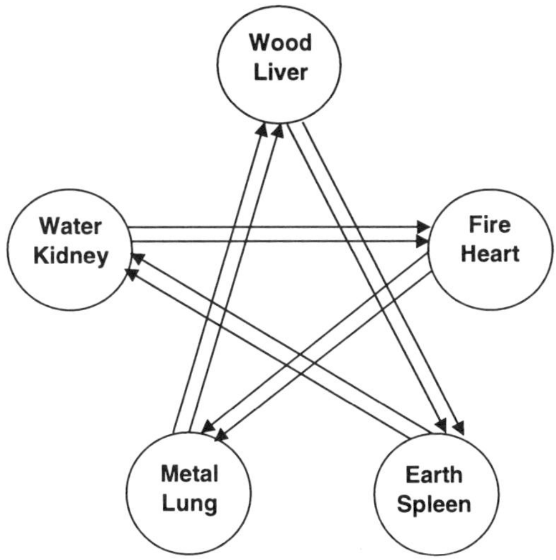

Figure 3.4. Five element overacting cycle.

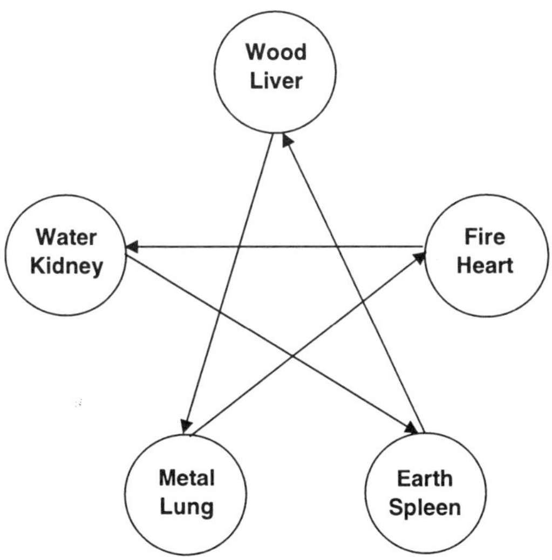

Figure 3.5. Five element counteracting cycle.

- *Counter-acting:* The zang organ (element) that is normally controlled in the *Restraining Sequence* becomes the controller and attacks the organ (element) that would normally control it (Fig. 3.5).

The abnormal relationships in the Generation Cycle (mother-son sequence) may manifest as:

- Disorders of "the mother affecting the son", and
- Disorders of "the son affecting the mother" (Cheng, 1987).

Guiding clinical diagnosis and treatment

The theory may be applied in analysis of signs and symptoms in order to reach a diagnosis. Use is made of the correspondences between organs, elements, sense organs, emotions, colours, tastes and other attributes. For example, a person with red, swollen eyes and bitter taste in the mouth is likely to have a problem in the Liver, since a bitter taste is associated with the element Wood and the eye is the sense organ related to the Liver.

The theory may be applied in clinical treatment. For example, if the Liver is *overacting* on the Spleen, herbs may be given to calm the Liver and strengthen the weakened Spleen. Acupuncture points may also be chosen according to Five Element Theory. For example, specific acupuncture points are selected according to the theory to "reinforce the mother" in the case where the "son" element is weak.

3.4 How Does Chinese Medicine Understand Human Physiology?

Chinese medicine believes that good health is due to a kinetic balance between both Yin aspects (*vital substances*) and Yang aspects (functional activities) of the human body. Generation of the body's *vital substances*, including essence, qi, blood and body fluids, is reliant on the normal physiological functioning of various internal organs, collectively termed *zang-fu organs*. The *vital substances* are distributed to the various parts of the body, from the body surface to the internal organs, so that they can function normally and generate more vital substances. The whole system connecting the organs and transporting the vital substances is the *meridian system*.

This section will describe the vital substances within the body and the major theories to describe the physiological functioning of the body, the Zang-Fu Theory and the Meridian Theory.

3.4.1 *The vital substances: essence, qi, blood and body fluids*

According to Chinese medicine theory, essence (jing), qi, blood and body fluids, collectively referred to as *vital substances*, are the four substances within the body that are fundamental to life and provide the material and functional basis of the body (Cai *et al.*, 1995; Cheng, 1987). A deficiency in any of these can lead to dysfunction of various organs or systems in the body.

Essence

Essence or *jing* is the essential material that provides the foundation for the physiological functioning of the body (Cai *et al.*, 1995). It is fluid-like and determines our basic constitution (Maciocia, 1989). Inception of human life depends on good quality *essence* from a healthy male and female. Adequate essence is required for normal growth, development and reproduction, and a deficiency can manifest in problems such as developmental delays. Essence may be congenital or acquired (derived from food) and is stored in the Kidneys (Maciocia, 1989).

Qi

In ancient China, philosophers believed that *qi* was the fundamental substance that made up everything in the world and that all things came into being through the movement and flux of qi (Yin *et al.*, 1992; Cai *et al.*, 1995).

The concept of qi is both simple and profound. Qi is a philosophical concept that permeated the arts and literature as well as medicine (Zhang and Rose, 2001). Qi was referred to in Daoist writings, in which developed the idea that "the world begins with qi" (Zhang and Rose, 2001: p. 26). The philosophical understanding of qi was subsumed into Chinese medicine, where it was used to explain the vital forces that give life to humans and control the physiological functioning of the body (Zhang and Rose, 2001). More than 270 classifications of qi were recorded in the Huang Di Nei Jing (Yellow Emperor's Classic of Internal Medicine), one of the most important medical texts in Chinese medicine history (Zhang and Rose, 2001). Zhang and Rose believe that "the clearest and simplest explanation of qi is that it is the interchange of yin and yang" (Zhang and Rose, 2001: p. 26).

At a basic level, qi is both a material and functional concept. In the material sense, it refers to a type of rarefied, subtle, vital energy that is the material basis of the body and is used to perform normal physiological functions (Cheng, 1987). Qi, along with body fluids, also forms the material basis of blood (Yin *et al.*, 1992). In a functional sense, qi refers to the activities of the zang-fu organs (Cheng, 1987; Maciocia, 1989).

Qi is thought to circulate within special pathways of the body called *meridians* and in blood. Western literature often equates qi with "energy", though the scientific notion of energy is not entirely adequate. Qi can assume a range of states, from a denser, tangible state (matter in its solid state) to a rarified, non-material state (Maciocia, 1989). The sources of qi are both congenital and acquired (from food) and are inter-dependent.

There are several different types of qi. Qi has several different functions including protecting the body against attack of external pathogens; promoting growth and development, functioning of the internal organs and tissues, and qi and blood circulation; generating and distributing blood and body fluids; warming the body and regulating body temperature; and regulating water metabolism, sweating, digestion and seminal emission (Yin *et al.*, 1992; Cai *et al.*, 1995).

Signs and symptoms of qi deficiency can include dizziness, blurred vision, lack of energy, shortness of breath, sweating with little exertion, weak voice, pale complexion and tongue, weak pulse, and susceptibility to colds and flu (Yin *et al.*, 1992).

Blood and body fluids

According to theory, blood is formed primarily from nutrient qi[3] and body fluids and blood circulation is promoted by qi (Yin *et al.*, 1992).

[3]There are several types of qi. Nutrient qi is that derived from food.

Blood and qi provide the material foundation for the body's vital activities and in particular, blood nourishes and moistens the body's organs, muscles, tendons and tissues (Cheng, 1987; Cai *et al.*, 1995). Blood also provides the main material foundation for the mental processes (Cheng, 1987).

A deficiency of blood may be caused by acute conditions such as haemorrhage or by more chronic conditions, often due to insufficient blood production and prolonged illness. Signs of chronic blood deficiency may include pale complexion and lips, dry and brittle hair and nails, dry skin, fatigue, poor concentration and memory, dizziness, numbness and in severe cases, motor impairment of the limbs (Yin *et al.*, 1992; Cai *et al.*, 1995). Anaemia may or may not be present. Blood deficiency does not always imply anaemia, however, if there is anaemia, there is blood deficiency.

Body fluids are the normal fluids of the body including saliva, gastric juices, sweat and synovial fluid in joints (Cai *et al.*, 1995; Cheng, 1987). Body fluids have the function of warming and nourishing parts of the body such as muscles and moistening joints and skin (Cheng, 1987). Pathological problems associated with body fluids may include retention of body fluids (for example, oedema) and deficiency of body fluids. Signs and symptoms of deficient body fluids include thirst, dry lips, throat and skin, dry tongue coating, dry cough, scanty and concentrated (dark yellow) urine (Deng, 1999).

Inter-dependence of essence, qi, blood and body fluids

The inter-dependent relationship between essence, qi, blood and body fluids is complex and provides the basis for understanding the physiology of the body and pathological changes occurring in disease.

For example, qi and blood provide the material basis of vital activities, blood carries qi and qi provides the motive force to drive blood circulation. Qi deficiency can lead to blood deficiency and poor circulation since qi is a component of blood and deficient qi is unable to adequately drive blood circulation. Since qi also "holds" the blood within blood vessels, haemorrhages may also result from deficient qi.

3.4.2 *The vital organs: Zang-Fu Theory*

The Zang-Fu Theory is the principal theory that explains the physiological functions, inter-dependent relationships and pathology of the internal organs by observing how they manifest externally in the body (Cai *et al.*, 1995).

The concept of "organ" in Chinese medicine is not equivalent to that in Western medicine. Although the internal organs, collectively known as *zang-fu organs*, do share some of the functions as the same-named organs as understood in Western medicine, there are major departures in terms of function and inter-relationships. Zang-fu organs are better thought of as complex functional systems.

Zang-fu organs

The internal body organs are divided into three sub-categories, namely:

- Zang organs
- Fu organs
- Extraordinary organs

According to theory, the zang organs are solid organs that perform major functions including production, transformation, regulation and storage of the *vital substances*: qi, blood, body fluids and essence (Kaptchuk, 1983). There are five zang organs: Heart, Lung, Kidney, Liver and Spleen[4] (Cheng, 1987). Fu organs are hollow organs that are functionally related and play a role in the processes of digestion, absorption and excretion (Cheng, 1987). There are six fu organs: Small Intestine, Large Intestine, Bladder, Gallbladder, Stomach and the Triple Jiao.[5] The

[4]Plus the Pericardium that is considered as an attachment to the Heart rather than an independent zang organ (Cheng, 1987).

[5]The Triple Jiao or Triple Burner controls the qi in the body including qi circulation and activity. It also serves as the pathway for qi and water throughout the body (Cai *et al.*, 1995). The Triple Jiao encompasses all organs and consists of the upper jiao located above the diaphragm, middle jiao located between the umbilicus and diaphragm, and lower jiao located below the stomach (Cai *et al.*, 1995).

fu organs are generally considered to be more external to the zang organs (Kaptchuk, 1983; Cheng, 1987).

The internal organs have their own distinct functions, but exist within a mutually inter-dependent relationship with all other organs, connected by the *meridian system* (Cheng, 1987).

Pairing of Zang and Fu organs

Each of the zang organs is structurally and functionally connected to and paired with a fu organ by the meridian system, forming an organic whole (Cheng, 1987; Cai *et al.*, 1995). The functional properties of the zang-fu organs are symbolised by one of the *five elements* (Table 3.4).

Extraordinary Fu organs

The six *extraordinary fu organs* include the uterus, brain, marrow, bones, blood vessels and gallbladder (the gallbladder is also a fu organ and thus occurs in two categories). They are called *extraordinary fu organs* because they are hollow like fu organs but function like a zang organ in storing the body's vital substances (Maciocia, 1989).

Related sense organs and body tissues

Each zang organ pair is connected with a sense organ and body tissue via the meridian system. The physiological functioning and pathological changes in the zang-fu organs may be reflected exteriorly in the condition and/or functioning of the related tissue or sense organ (Cheng, 1987; Maciocia, 1989) (Table 3.4).

For example, the Liver is related to the eyes and the tendons and its condition is reflected in the nails (Cai *et al.*, 1995). Observation of the appearance and condition of the nails and eyes and functioning of the eyes and tendons can give clues as to the state of the Liver organ system. Pathology of the Liver organ system may manifest in signs and symptoms including dry and/or red eyes, blurred vision, weak and thin or dry, chipped nails, numbness or tremors of limbs, tendon weakness, muscle cramps and joint dysfunction (Cheng, 1987; Maciocia, 1989).

Relationship between organs and emotions

Although Western medicine ascribes emotions and mental processes to the functions of the brain, according to the Zang-Fu Theory the emotions are also intimately related to the functioning of the zang organs (Maciocia, 1989; Yin *et al.*, 1992). Each zang organ is associated with a particular emotion (Table 3.4) and qi, blood and essence are seen as the basis for emotional and mental processes (Maciocia, 1989; Cai *et al.*, 1995; Cheng, 1987). Excessive emotions can adversely affect the physiological functioning of the zang organs by disturbing the balance of qi and blood (Cai *et al.*, 1995). According to Chinese medicine theory, the Heart has the overall role in controlling mental activity and emotions (Yin *et al.*, 1992).

Functions of the zang organs

In brief, the functions of the zang organs are as follows:

- **Heart:** Controls blood circulation and emotions and mental processes including consciousness, memory, perception and thinking (Cai *et al.*, 1995; Maciocia, 1989).
- **Liver:** Regulates the blood volume (storage of blood) and menstruation, and ensures the smooth flow of qi in the body (which in turn affects the functioning of the other organs) (Maciocia, 1989).
- **Lungs:** Controls respiration and regulates the circulation of qi throughout the body (Maciocia, 1989; Cai *et al.*, 1995).
- **Spleen:** Plays a major role in the digestion and absorption of food and production of nutrient qi that is distributed to the whole body (Yin *et al.*, 1992).
- **Kidney:** Stores essence and is the foundation of Yin and Yang of the whole body; responsible for growth and development and reproduction (Yin *et al.*, 1992). It plays an important role in water metabolism and in coordinating respiration in conjunction with the Lung (Yin *et al.*, 1992).

Inter-relationships of the zang-fu organs

The body is an organic whole maintained by the functioning of the zang-fu and the vital substances (essence, qi, blood and body fluids)

(Cai *et al.*, 1995). The physiological functions of the organs are intimately inter-related and complex. For example, the Heart is said to govern blood circulation and the Liver said to store blood and regulate blood volume (Cai *et al.*, 1995). If the Liver is deficient in blood, this can lead to a deficiency in Heart blood and problems such as palpitations, insomnia and dizziness. In addition, the Heart regulates the emotions but this also relies on the Liver's ability to free flow qi. The Spleen/Stomach as a functional system is responsible for digestion of food and also relies on the Liver's ability to ensure the free flow of qi for this to occur effectively. The Spleen in turn produces nutrient qi that nourishes the Liver and allows it to function.

Application of Zang-Fu Theory

The relationships between the individual zang organs, between individual fu organs and between zang and fu organs and their related sense organs and tissues form the basis for understanding how the body works and the causes of and pathological changes in disease.

Knowledge of this theory is essential in understanding aetiology and pathogenesis of disorders and in order to arrive at a diagnosis and treatment strategy. Because of the close physiological relationships and connections provided by the meridian system, pathology of a zang organ may affect its paired fu organ or other zang organs or related sense organs and tissues. Similarly, pathology of a fu organ can affect other fu organs or zang organs (Cheng, 1987).

Syndromes of disease may be differentiated according to Zang-Fu Theory. Each zang and fu organ has several disease syndromes associated with pathology of that organ, each of which is characterised by certain signs and symptoms. Observation of the body's exterior including sense organs and tissues and their functioning informs clinical diagnosis.

Treatment principles follow diagnosis of the disease and syndrome and take into account not only the principle organs that are involved but also the other organs that may be involved or vulnerable via the close inter-relationships. Both acupuncture and herbal medicine treatments are guided by the theory. The action of herbs is understood and explained predominantly in terms of their specific effects on specific zang-fu organs (Bensky and Gamble, 1993).

3.4.3 *The connecting system: Meridian Theory*

Meridian Theory describes the distribution and physiological functions of the *meridian system* and its inter-relationship with the zang-fu organs, providing the basis for understanding physiology and pathology of the human body and the basis for the treatment modalities of acupuncture and Chinese herbal medicine.

The *meridian system* (*Jing Luo Xi Tong*) is the system of interconnecting pathways throughout the body in which qi and blood circulate, connecting all parts of the body into an organic whole (Cai *et al.*, 1995; Cheng, 1987; Qiu *et al.*, 1993). It is comprised of meridians (channels or *jing*) and collaterals (*luo*), collectively known as *Jingluo*. The meridians run longitudinally and more deeply within the body whilst the finer collaterals, the branches of the meridians, run transversely and more superficially connecting the meridians with the connective tissue and skin (Deadman *et al.*, 1998; Cheng, 1987). The jingluo connect the interior zang-fu organs, related sense organs, tissues, orifices, interior and exterior and upper and lower parts of the body (Qiu *et al.*, 1993; Deadman *et al.*, 1998).

There are 12 regular meridians replicated on each side of the body that traverse the trunk, upper and lower limbs and head, plus two meridians running along the body midline (Du and Ren meridians) (Qiu *et al.*, 1993). There are also several other types of meridians including divergent meridians that branch out from the regular meridians (Cheng, 1987).

Each regular meridian connects internally with a specific zang or fu organ, after which the meridian is named, and its related sense organ. For example, the *Kidney meridian* connects the Kidney organ with its related sense organ, the ear. There are also 12 musculo-tendinous regions and 12 cutaneous regions where qi and blood nourish the muscles/tendons and skin respectively (Cheng, 1987). The 12 regular meridians also connect with the ear either directly or indirectly, forming the basis for ear acupuncture (Qiu *et al.*, 1993).

The 12 regular meridians are connected to each other in a cyclical sequence beginning with the Lung meridian and ending with the Liver meridian (see Fig. 3.6 below). The order of the sequence depicted horizontally on the diagram below also reflects the interior-exterior pairing of the zang-fu organs. For example, the Lung and Large Intestine form a zang-fu pair, and the Spleen and Stomach form another pair, and so on. Each meridian is associated with a two-hour period in which the qi is most active.

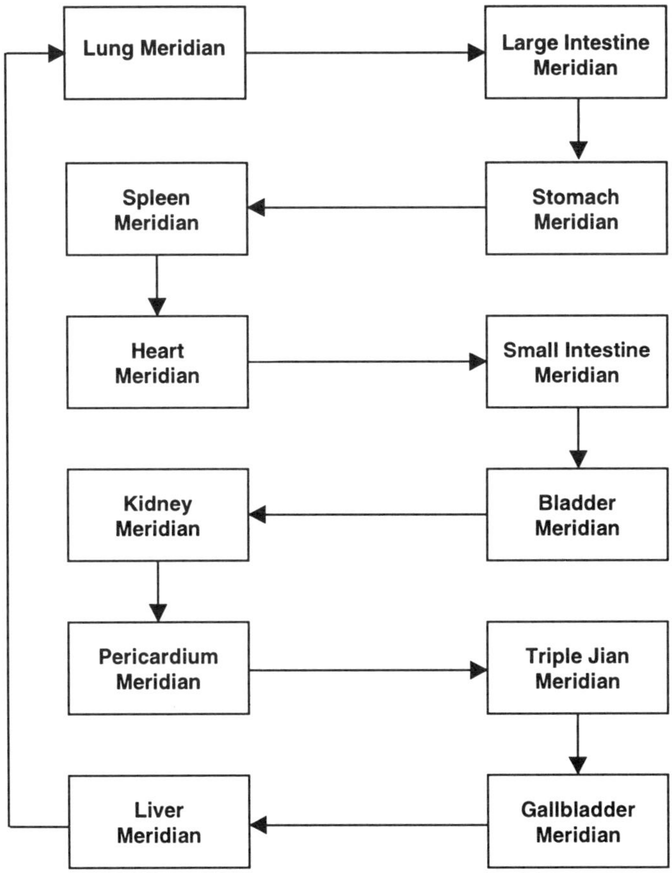

Figure 3.6. Meridian cyclical flow of Qi.

Acupoints

Each meridian has specific points called acupoints. The Chinese characters for acupoint translate to "transportation hole" (Cheng, 1987). Acupoints are defined points on the body surface where the qi of the zang-fu organs and meridians is transported to the body's surface (Li *et al.*, 2000; Cai *et al.*, 1997; Qiu *et al.*, 1993). Each acupoint has specific therapeutic actions and in addition, acupoints on the same meridian share a generalised action on that meridian. There are many categories of acupoints. For example, each regular meridian has a *Primary* (*Yuan*) *point* that is used primarily to treat chronic *deficiency-type* disorders.

The therapeutic effect of acupuncture is thought to be dependent on achievement of the *needling sensation* or "de qi": a subjective sensation felt by both practitioner and patient. The practitioner may feel a tightening sensation around the needle, as if it has been grabbed. The patient may feel it as a localised sensation of heaviness or in some cases, like a small electric shock along the course of the meridian.

Application of Meridian Theory

The meridians:

- Link the body parts into an organic whole
- Carry qi and blood
- Protect against exogenous pathogens
- Transmit the needling response associated with therapeutic effect (Cai *et al.*, 1995)

By understanding the functions and the anatomy of the meridian system, the Meridian Theory can be used to:

- Explain aetiology, location and pathogenesis of disease
- Guide diagnosis
- Guide treatment

Explaining cause, location and mechanism of disease

Each meridian connects with a zang or fu organ and its related tissue and sense organ, and the meridians inter-connect all organs and parts of the body. The inter-connections provided by the meridians provide a means by which exogenous pathogens may transmit from the exterior to the body's interior in disease, and the means by which diseases of the zang-fu transmit to each other and to their sense organs and tissues (Qiu *et al.*, 1993).

Diseases associated with meridians and/or zang-fu organs produce characteristic sign/symptom complexes. Recognition of these key signs and symptoms and knowledge of the course of the meridians and inter-relationships between meridians and organs aids in locating the disease, understanding its aetiology and mechanism (pathogenesis) and, ultimately reaching a diagnosis. For instance, where there is a disorder of a meridian or a zang-fu organ, acupoints on the related meridian *may* be tender or the overlying skin may show changes (Qiu *et al.*, 1993; Deadman *et al.*, 1998). Knowing the time of onset or exacerbation of symptoms and/or signs and peak time of meridian activity can often aid in diagnosis.

The following case illustrates the above points. A patient primarily complains of headache at the vertex of the head. Questioning elicits the fact that he also has pain in the hypochondriac region, red eyes, and bitter taste in the mouth. The symptoms and signs tend to manifest once or twice a week following outbursts of anger and have been occurring for three months. He is frustrated with his life and angry that his wife left him several months ago. His symptoms point to pathology in the Liver system. Bitter taste and the emotion of anger are associated with the element Wood (Liver). Eyes are the sense organs connected to the Liver via the Liver meridian; redness of eyes would suggest Liver-fire (heat). The Liver meridian traverses the hypochondriac region of the body and an internal branch travels to the vertex of the head. In summary:

- Location of the disease: Liver
- Aetiology: Internal damage to the Liver organ as a result of unresolved anger
- Pathogenesis/Mechanism: Liver-fire flaring upwards to the head and eyes
- Diagnosis: Headache due to flaring Liver-fire

Guiding treatment

In an acupuncture treatment, needles are inserted into acupoints that are chosen according to Meridian Theory in order to regulate the functions of the meridians and qi and blood, and restore the balance of yin and yang (Qiu *et al.*, 1993; Cheng, 1987; Cai *et al.*, 1997).

If there is disease of a meridian, zang-fu organ or related sense organ, points on that meridian are usually chosen. Local points or distal points (usually distal to the elbow and knees) or combinations may be chosen depending on diagnosis of the disease and syndrome. If other meridians or organs are involved, points may be chosen to treat those also. Meridian Theory is used in conjunction with other theories including Five Element Theory, Zang-Fu Theory and Yin-Yang Theory to understand the disease and guide selection of acupoints.

Many different principles guide the choice of acupoints following the correct differentiation of the syndrome. For example:

- Acupoints on one meridian may be chosen to treat disorders of that meridian or that meridian's related zang-fu organ or sense organ or its paired meridian's organ (Cai *et al.*, 1997).
- Certain empirical acupoints or combinations of acupoints that have historically been found to be effective may be chosen (Deadman *et al.*, 1998).
- Distal points are important in the treatment of disorders of the chest, abdomen, back and head (Deadman *et al.*, 1998).

The Meridian Theory also has relevance to Chinese herbal medicine: Chinese herbs have affinities for particular meridians and zang-fu organs. The therapeutic actions of the herbs are attributed to the meridian and organ specificity (Bensky and Gamble, 1993; Cai *et al.*, 1995). Thus following diagnosis of syndrome, herbs that *enter* the relevant meridian(s) may be chosen. This idea is further developed in the concept of a "guide herb". In an herbal medicine formula, a guide herb that has a particular affinity with a part of the body, meridian or zang-fu organ, may be used to guide the action of the other herbs in the prescription to that area (Bensky and Gamble, 1993; Bensky and Barolet, 1990).

3.5 How Does Chinese Medicine Understand the Occurrence of Diseases?

Aetiology, the cause of disease, and pathogenesis, the processes involved in development of disease, can be understood in terms of many different and complex theories. However, there are some fundamental underlying beliefs. These will be discussed briefly.

3.5.1 *Cause of disease (aetiology)*

Chinese medicine holds the view that diseases occur when the balance between Yin and Yang is lost, thus anything that causes an imbalance is identified as a causal factor. This concept is distinctively different from Western medicine, as aetiological or causal factors that help establish the diagnosis are normally tangible, such as viruses or bacteria. In contrast, the causal factors in Chinese medicine are normally not tangible and are recognised by their clinical manifestations. For example, disorders occurring abruptly and being of a short duration are often related to wind, analogous to its nature. Thus, totally unrelated conditions such as hay fever and acute cerebral haemorrhage share the same nature as wind-related conditions.

At a basic level, in order for disease to manifest, two situations usually need to occur:

(i) The person's *antipathogenic qi* is deficient.
(ii) A *pathogenic factor* presents.

The term *antipathogenic qi*, also called *zheng qi*, refers to the body's functional activities and ability to resist disease (Cai *et al.*, 1995). Antipathogenic qi does not equate directly with the immune system in Western medical terms. It is a much broader concept, however it does include this. When the antipathogenic qi is strong, the body can resist most pathogens but when the antipathogenic qi is deficient, the body may become susceptible to disease. An exception to this may be resistance to those extremely infectious and virulent pathogens associated with epidemic infectious disease, termed *epidemic pathogenic factors* (Maciocia, 1989). In the presence of such pathogens, even someone with strong zheng qi may succumb. Many factors affect the condition of a person's antipathogenic qi including constitution, mental/emotional state, lifestyle, environment and diet (Cai *et al.*, 1995).

The concept of *pathogenic qi* is broad and may include external pathogens outside the body and internal pathogenic factors. Both are discussed in the sections following. It includes the Western concepts of bacteria and viruses.

The cause of disease can be broken into three main groups:

- External causes
- Internal causes
- Other causes

External causes: climatic factors

External causes are those that arise from outside the body. In nature, there are *six climatic factors*: wind, cold, damp, summer-heat, dryness and fire that typically correspond with the seasons. If these climatic factors are excessive, occur out of season or change too rapidly, and the body is susceptible or relatively weak in relation to one or more of the factors, they can become harmful (pathogenic) and are termed *six exogenous pathogenic factors* (Maciocia, 1989; Yin *et al.*, 1992; Cai *et al.*, 1995).

The normal correspondence between the climatic factors and seasons is:

- Wind: spring
- Fire: summer
- Summer-Heat: summer
- Dampness: late summer
- Dryness: autumn
- Cold: winter

Perhaps more important clinically, the six exogenous pathogenic factors denote patterns of disease characterised by symptoms and signs in the body analogous to that climate in nature. For example, pathogenic dampness may cause signs such as abnormal sticky discharges and a subjective feeling of heaviness in the body. Cold as a causal factor may produce symptoms such as a cold sensation and pain in the joints. Since cold causes contraction and obstruction of the flow of qi and blood within the meridians of the body, pain results.

Internal causes

Internal pathogenic factors are those that arise within the body and include *endogenous* pathogenic fire, heat, damp, dryness, wind and cold. They can manifest with similar signs and symptoms as those caused by external pathogens, but they are caused by dysfunction of the internal body organs (termed *zang-fu organs*) and disturbances in the body's *vital substances* (Cai *et al.*, 1995).

Mind, emotions and body are inseparable, part of an integrated whole (Maciocia, 1989). Experiencing emotions is part of being human and in general, a healthy individual is able to experience a range of emotions without ill effects. However, emotions can become internal causes of disease if become deficient or excessive, occur suddenly, are prolonged, suppressed or unacknowledged, or when one or more become predominant (Maciocia, 1989; Ross, 1985). Certain emotions have a tendency to preferentially affect particular internal zang-fu organs. For example, anger affects the Liver, fright or fear affects the Kidney (see Table 3.4 for correspondences). Conversely, particular emotional states may be caused by dysfunction of particular zang-fu organs (Maciocia, 1989). According to theory, the Heart is the "king of organs" and "houses the spirit". This means that the Heart is the most important organ with respect to a person's spirit, mind and emotions. Consequently, it tends to be affected first by emotional upsets. In general, a positive state of mind and emotional balance will contribute to strong antipathogenic qi whereas a negative state of mind or emotional disharmony will contribute to weakening of the antipathogenic qi.

Other causes

Many other factors causing disease are due to lifestyle choices and include poor or irregular diet, excessive mental activity, excessive physical work, insufficient, incorrect or excessive physical exercise, and excessive or irregular sexual activity. Poor constitution contributes to susceptibility to disease. Other aetiological factors include trauma, incorrect treatment, Western medication (iatrogenic disease), pestilence and poisons (Maciocia, 1989; Ross, 1985).

3.5.2 *Mechanism(s) of disease (pathogenesis)*

The understanding of the mechanism of development of disease (pathogenesis) is complex and relies on a comprehension of all of the basic theories of Chinese medicine. Since the body is an organic whole made up of inter-dependent organs and tissues, an imbalance in one organ may affect others.

Fundamentally, the pathogenesis of a disease is understood in terms of a conflict between the person's antipathogenic qi and the pathogenic factor(s). When the pathogenic factor is strong and the body's defence system is fighting back strongly, this is termed an "excess" type of disorder or *excess syndrome* (Cai *et al.*, 1995). Excess syndromes typically occur in early stages of disease and in acute disorders (Cai *et al.*, 1995). However, when the antipathogenic qi is weak and deficient, the body's struggle is weak. This is termed a "deficiency" type of disorder or *deficiency syndrome* and is typically seen in chronic, prolonged or advanced stages of disease (Cai *et al.*, 1995).

3.6 Clinical Decision Making: Diagnosis

In the clinical setting, diagnosis and treatment are guided by the aforementioned theories. Diagnosis includes data collection and analysis that leads to a determination of the disease and identification of the pattern of disease (syndrome). The treatment principle follows diagnosis and a treatment plan is subsequently formulated. At this point, a variety of treatment options will be considered such as acupuncture, Chinese herbal medicine, dietary therapy or exercise therapy. Preventive advice may also be given as to how to promote health and recovery and prevent the condition from deteriorating.

The following section will discuss methods applied in clinical diagnosis and will introduce how treatment principles are formed.

3.6.1 *Data collection*

Data collection begins the moment the patient walks through the clinic door. There are four basic components of data collection:

- Case history taking
- Inspection
- Auscultation and olfaction
- Palpation

The case history involves systematically questioning the patient about their health complaints, history of illness, signs and symptoms, any current medications and treatment, previous conditions, family history of disease and any other relevant factors.

Inspection involves observation of the physical body including general appearance and demeanour, posture and movement, complexion, skin, hair, vitality, sense organs, and importantly, the tongue. Tongue diagnosis is one of the more peculiar features of Chinese medicine diagnosis. The normal tongue body is neither too thick nor too thin, and is pink-red in colour with a thin and white coating. An abnormality of the appearance of the tongue body and coating is reflective of pathology in the body. For example, when there is excess heat in the body, the tongue body may be red and the coating yellow. Changes in the disease course may be charted by observing the tongue.

Auscultation involves listening to the sound of the voice, breathing, and other sounds such as coughing (Deng, 1999). For example, in a deficiency syndrome, the voice will typically be soft and weak. Abnormal body smells can also reflect the nature of disorders.

Palpation involves not only palpation of parts of the body as necessary, but pulse diagnosis. According to theory, the formation of the pulse is strongly related to qi, blood and the zang-fu organs, and changes in the pulse may reflect disease or disharmony in the body (Cai *et al.*, 1995). In contrast with pulse taking in Western medicine, the radial pulse of both wrists is felt in three adjacent positions, each position corresponding to a different organ. The pulse depth, speed, character, width and force are all noted and help the practitioner ascertain the disease location, nature and prognosis. For example, a rapid pulse may indicate heat and a superficial pulse indicates the disease is in the exterior level of the body.

Once the data is collected, it is analysed according to the many theories and the disease and syndrome differentiated.

3.6.2 *Data analysis: differentiation of syndromes*

Diseases are sub-categorised or differentiated into *syndromes* or patterns of disease according to many theories, including those described in the preceding sections. The *Eight Guiding Principles* are vital to syndrome differentiation.

Eight Guiding Principles

The *Eight Guiding Principles* are a set of principles used to systematically analyse signs and symptoms in order to categorise syndromes on the basis of nature and location of the disease and the relative strength of the antipathogenic qi and pathogenic factors.

They are:

- Yin/Yang: The chief principles that summarise the other six principles
- Cold/Heat: Establishes the nature of the disease
- Interior/Exterior: Establishes the depth of the disease
- Excess/Deficiency: Determines the relative strength of the antipathogenic qi and pathogenic factors (Cai *et al.*, 1995)

The last six principles can be classified as either Yin or Yang:

Yin: Cold, interior, deficiency
Yang: Heat, exterior, excess

Interior diseases are usually caused by internal disharmonies of the zang-fu and vital substances (Cai *et al.*, 1995; Kaptchuk, 1983). Interior diseases usually have a more gradual onset and a longer time-course and are often chronic and more serious (Ross, 1985). Exterior diseases are those caused by invasion of the six exogenous pathogenic factors where the disease is in the exterior level of the body (Ross, 1985). Exterior diseases usually occur suddenly and are of short duration i.e. they tend to be acute (Cai *et al.*, 1995; Ross, 1985).

Deficiency diseases are those in which there is a deficiency of antipathogenic qi. There may be a deficiency of qi, blood, body fluids, or yin or yang of the organs and body due to a hypofunction of the zang-fu organs (Kaptchuk, 1983). Deficiency diseases are often chronic. Excess syndromes are often acute and are those in which the pathogenic factors are predominant and the body is waging a strong fight (Cai *et al.*, 1995).

In cold syndromes, there is a predominance of Yin whereas in heat syndromes, there is a predominance of Yang.

There can be combinations of the above six pairs of characteristics. For example, there can be excess cold syndromes that are interior or exterior, excess or deficiency heat syndromes, and so on. To further complicate matters, there can be a mixture of deficiency and excess or heat and cold in complex disease patterns. All diseases can be eventually reduced to either Yin or Yang in terms of their essential nature.

Once a diagnosis is reached, the Eight Guiding Principles may also be used to guide formulation of the treatment principles.

3.6.3 *Diagnosis and treatment principles*

At the end of the differentiation process, the pattern of disease or syndrome(s) will be determined. At this point, the practitioner is able to describe the location, causal factors and mechanism (pathogenesis) of the current disorder or condition.

With this in mind, a specific treatment plan tailored for the patient is then formulated based on nature of the disorder and the individuals' constitution, age, gender, season and geographical conditions.

Treatment principles follow the diagnosis of the syndrome and are couched in terms of the theories used in diagnosis. Treatment ultimately aims at restoring the balance of Yin and Yang, restoring the functions of the zang-fu organs, regulating qi and blood and takes into account individual factors described above.

Fundamentally, Chinese medicine treatment relies on understanding the aetiology and pathogenesis of the disease. The root cause (*ben*) and secondary manifestations (*biao*) must be diagnosed. Treatment ultimately addresses both and which is addressed first depends on the relative strength of the body's antipathogenic qi and the pathogenic factor(s). For example, in cases where the body's antipathogenic qi is strong, the treatment principle may simply be to eliminate the pathogenic factor(s). However, if the antipathogenic qi is weak, strong treatment to eliminate pathogens could further weaken the body, so the treatment principle may be to strengthen the antipathogenic qi first and then eliminate the pathogenic factor(s) later.

In formulating treatment principles according to the Eight Guiding Principles, for example, in the case of an interior cold syndrome, the treatment principle would be to "warm the interior" (Cai *et al.*, 1995). How this is done using various modalities of Chinese medicine such as herbal medicine and/or acupuncture is the subject of another chapter.

3.7 Prevention

One of the most valuable pieces of guidance a practitioner can give a patient is how to prevent illness and promote positive health. Good health relies on a balance of Yin and Yang in the body that is achieved by the harmonious functioning of the zang-fu organs. In good health, the mind is centred and the mind-body has sufficient adaptability to cope with life. In ancient China, Chinese medicine was a preventive practice: imbalances in the body were detected before they could create serious problems and measures were taken to address the imbalances.

If a disease has manifested, prevention of deterioration of the condition is essential (Cai *et al.*, 1995). This includes consideration of the internal organs that may not be affected now, but are at risk due to the interrelationships between zang-fu organs. This may involve the prophylactic use of herbal medicine, acupuncture or other treatment modalities.

At a basic level, emotions, diet and lifestyle choices are factors that are important in achieving balance of the mind-body and ensuring good health. A lifestyle that includes sufficient sleep, exercise and regular eating patterns is necessary for good health to be maintained. A healthy, varied diet, choosing foods according to the seasons and avoiding certain foods known to cause problems, will help ensure that the body has sufficient nutrients to achieve optimal functioning of the body.

Physical exercise is important in achieving health. Over-exercising may cause injuries to muscles and tendons and overstrain the internal organs and deplete qi (Cai *et al.*, 1995). Exercise helps stimulate the flow of qi and blood around the body that in turn aids the functioning of the internal organs and helps harmonise the emotions and calm the mind. Unremitting over-working needs to be avoided. Excessive mental activity can consume blood and lead to mental fatigue. Sexual activity should be enjoyed in moderation. Excessive sex can deplete the Kidney qi and jing — not a good thing when the Kidney is the source of the Yin and Yang of the whole body.

Mind and body are not separate. Time needs to be taken on a daily basis to relax the mind, particularly for those who expend a lot of mental energy. Physical exercises such as taichi and qigong can help both body and mind to relax, strengthen health and prevent illness. Regular time needs to be given back to the self to explore its inherent spiritual nature. Happiness builds strong antipathogenic qi, helps prevent disease occurring and can speed up recovery from illness. We do not live in isolation from each other and positive mental energy and happiness shared can also help strengthen another's body and soul.

3.8 Conclusion

In conclusion, Chinese medicine is a unique medical system which views the world and the human body very differently from Western medicine, and is guided by a unique philosophical conceptual framework. These concepts have a significant impact on the understanding of human physiology and pathology and underpin the clinical decision-making process. In particular, it holds the view that prevention should come first and that good health is the result of a comprehensive approach to maintaining the harmony within the body and between the human and environment.

Treatment is aimed at correcting the imbalance within the human body. However, the body has its limits and once these are reached, the illness can become incurable or chronic with poor prognosis.

Individuals have a significant degree of responsibility to themselves to achieve and maintain their own health. Chinese medicine is a system that offers many keys to wellness.

References

Beinfield, H. and Korngold, E. (1991) *Between Heaven and Earth. A Guide to Chinese Medicine.* Ballantine Books, New York.

Bensky, D. and Barolet, R. (199) *Chinese Herbal Medicine Formulas and Strategies.* Eastland Press, Seattle, Washington.

Bensky, D. and Gamble, A. (1993) *Chinese Herbal Medicine Materia Medica.* Eastland Press, Seattle, Washington.

Cai, G., Chao, G., Chen, D., *et al.* (eds.) (1995) *State Administration of Traditional Chinese Medicine, Advanced Textbook on Traditional Chinese Medicine and Pharmacology Vol. I.* New World Press, Beijing.

Cai, J., Chao, G., Chen, D., *et al.* (eds.) (1997) *State Administration of Traditional Chinese Medicine, Advanced Textbook on Traditional Chinese Medicine and Pharmacology Vol. IV.* New World Press, Beijing, China.

Cheng, X. (ed.) (1987) *Chinese Acupuncture and Moxibustion.* Foreign Languages Press, Beijing, China.

Deadman, P., Al-Khafaji, M. and Baker, K. (1998) *A Manual of Acupuncture.* Journal of Chinese Medicine Publications, East Sussex, England.

Deng, T. (1999) *Practical Diagnosis in Traditional Chinese Medicine.* Churchill Livingstone, Edinburgh.

Gerber, R. (1988) *Vibrational Medicine.* Bear and Co., Sante Fe.

Honderich, T. (ed.) (1995) *The Oxford Companion to Philosophy.* Oxford University Press, Oxford, New York.

Kaptchuk, T. (1983) *Chinese Medicine: The Web That Has No Weaver.* Rider, London.

Li, W.X., Xue, C.L. and Li, J.H. (2000) *Easy Locating of Acupuncture Points, 4th Ed.* Shanghai Book Company Ltd, Hong Kong.

Maciocia, G. (1989) *The Foundations of Chinese Medicine. A Comprehensive Text for Acupuncturists and Herbalists.* Churchill Livingstone, New York.

Martin, R.M. (2002) *The Philosopher's Dictionary*, 3rd Ed. Broadview Press, Ontario, Canada.

O'Brien, K. (2002) Problems and potentials of complementary and alternative medicine. *J. Intern. Med.* **32**, 163–164.

Qiu, M.L., Zang, S.C., Yu, Z.Q., *et al.* (1993) *Chinese Acupuncture and Moxibustion.* Churchill Livingstone, Edinburgh.

Ross, J. (1985) *Zang Fu. The Organ Systems of Traditional Chinese Medicine*, 2nd Ed. Churchill Livingstone, Edinburgh.

Wang, X.H. (ed.) (1995) *Fundamentals of Traditional Chinese Medicine (Standard Textbook for Chinese Herbal Pharmacy Students).* Shanghai Science & Technology Press, Shanghai, China, p. 264.

Yin, H., *et al.* (1992) *Fundamentals of Traditional Chinese Medicine.* Foreign Languages Press, Beijing, China.

Zhang, Y.H. and Rose, K. (2001) *A Brief History of Qi.* Paradigm Publications, Brookline, Massachusetts.

Chapter 4

Problems and Challenges of Chinese Herbal Medicine

Chun Guang Li, Keith Moyle & Charlie Changli Xue

4.1 Introduction

Chinese herbal medicine is one of the most developed remedies in traditional Chinese medicine. It has been widely used by Chinese medicine practitioners for different diseases and conditions. Thousands of herbal prescriptions or formulae are used everyday in various clinics or hospitals around the world, with a tremendous commercial market worth billions. As a result, the issue of Chinese herbal medicine, especially in recent times, has become a hot topic. Positive and negative comments and debates on its use have been featured in various media around the world.

This chapter focuses on the problems and challenges of Chinese herbal medicine. Given the complexities of the issue involved, and the fact that the background, belief and way of thinking by the readers will affect their views on Chinese herbal medicine, we have taken a broad approach to provide readers with the current trends in the growth in its use and the critical issues concerned.

4.2 The Trends

The extent of use of Chinese herbal medicine varies in different countries or regions, but the impact of Chinese herbal medicine on the health care systems around the world cannot be ignored. In China, for example, Chinese medicine (with Chinese herbal medicine as a major component) has already become a part of an integrated health care system, comprising about 40% of the total expenditure on health care (Hesketh and Zhu, 1997). Similar situations exist in many other Asian countries/regions, such as Japan and South Korea, where traditional medicine has been a priority for health care or is becoming part of the integrated medical system (WHO, 2002). On the other hand, in most developed countries Chinese herbal medicine is still regarded as a complementary or alternative treatment option, even though, it is now widely recognised that about half the population of industrialised countries regularly use complementary medicine including Chinese herbal medicine. For example, studies in the United States, Australia and the United Kingdom found about 30–50% of the population uses complementary medicine (Eisenberg *et al.*, 1998; MacLennan *et al.*, 2002; Thomas *et al.*, 2001; Nilsson *et al.*, 2001). In Australia alone, the use of alternative therapies has increased 120% since 1993 (MacLennan *et al.*, 2002). A recent study conducted in South Australia in 2000 found that about 52% of the population has used alternative medicine (including acupuncture and Chinese herbal medicine). This translates into expenditure on alternative therapies of A$2.3 billion, nearly four times the public contribution to all pharmaceuticals (MacLennan *et al.*, 2002). In the U.S., a study found that about 42% of the population used alternative medicines in 1997 with an estimated out-of-pocket expenditure of US$27 billion, which is comparable with projected out-of-pocket expenditure for all U.S. physician services (Eisenberg *et al.*, 1998).

On the other hand, concurrently with the increasing demand on complementary therapies, reports of adverse reactions associated with herbal medicines have also increased. There have been serious recent cases of toxicities, even death, associated with the use of some natural herbal products, including Chinese herbal medicines. The belief that "natural is safe" by some consumers has been criticised. As a result, health authorities in many developed countries have introduced stricter regulation of herbal medicine or other natural health products.

It is important for Chinese medicine practitioners and consumers to be aware of these trends in order to establish to a better patient-doctor relationship and compliance with treatment. Such trends also demand the development of new policies and regulations on evaluation, supply and quality control of related services and products.

4.3 The Gaps

Despite the strong consumer demand on complementary and alternative therapies including Chinese herbal medicine, there are still significant gaps in knowledge and attitudes among consumers, medical and health care practitioners, manufacturers, suppliers and policy makers or regulators regarding the use and evaluations of Chinese herbal medicine, especially in developed countries.

Firstly, there is a gap between consumers and health care providers on the use of herbal medicines. For example, some consumers tend to ignore the potential adverse reactions or drug-herb interactions associated with certain herbal products. For example, studies conducted in developed countries have found that most patients or consumers who take herbal or other natural products including Chinese herbal medicines failed to inform their orthodox medical practitioners (Eisenberg *et al.*, 2001). On the other hand, the knowledge of medical doctors in the developed countries on herbal medicine is limited, as most have not received the adequate education to be familiar with this kind of therapy and to learn how to analyse and assess critically the content validity of its claims. Thus, many Western medical professionals still express strong reservations or disbelief about the benefit of Chinese herbal medicine. The situation is different in countries like China where the integration of Chinese and Western medicine has long been promoted. A recent study by Harmsworth and Lewith (2001) on the attitudes of Western-trained doctors to traditional Chinese medicine in China found that most doctors (98%) had some theoretical and practical Chinese medicine training. There is clear consensus in China that Chinese herbal medicine is useful and safe in treating patients with chronic or intractable illness. The study also found that 76% of doctors treated their patients with Chinese medicine, 90% treated their friends or family and 82% referred patients to Chinese medicine specialists.

It should also be pointed out that the training of Chinese herbal medicine practitioners on orthodox medicine in many countries is also not adequate. Many practitioners do not have adequate knowledge of conventional medicine or current therapeutic drugs. Thus, they do not appreciate the potential adverse reactions or drug-herb interactions of

Chinese herbal medicine. Some even failed to acknowledge the limitations of Chinese herbal medicine for certain diseases and conditions, and thus delayed the proper diagnosis and treatment of the patients.

Secondly, there is a gap between the demand for high quality Chinese herbal products and those available on the market due to inadequate legislations/regulations. Studies have frequently found that the composition of many popular herbal products on the market do not match their labels. Given the lack of evidence of efficacy and safety of some of these products, it is important to understand the potential risk associated with Chinese herbal medicine, as the poor quality products will eventually turn away consumers. Contamination, adulteration and the inclusion of undisclosed ingredients or Western drugs often damage the reputation of Chinese herbal medicine.

This situation has resulted in part from the lack of adequate regulation of the herbal products and services worldwide. Current international regulations on herbal products are inadequate. Most countries have not yet developed satisfactory policies or regulations on Chinese herbal medicine. For example, in countries such as China and Australia, the manufactured Chinese herbal medicines are regulated as medicines but with different requirements and standards. In the U.S., Chinese herbal medicines are generally regarded as food supplements, regulated through the Dietary Supplements Health and Education Act, although the FDA has recently published a draft guidance for industry to facilitate and encourage development of botanical new drugs. The situation is similar in Canada and many European countries, though this is starting to change. It is likely that there will be rapid development in policy and regulations related to natural health products in the next two to five years. In fact, certain countries/regions, apart from China, such as Australia, Hong Kong and Singapore have already introduced legislation to regulate the Chinese medicine profession and Chinese herbal products. For example, the State of Victoria in Australia has introduced the Chinese Medicine Registration Act 2000 to regulate Chinese medicine as a profession. The Act also provides amendments to the current Drugs and Controlled Substances Act to allow a list of certain toxic Chinese herbs to be accessed only by registered Chinese medicine practitioners. Hong Kong has also set up similar but more stringent legislation to regulate the Chinese medicine profession and herbal products. In this aspect, it is ironic that China, as the birthplace of Chinese herbal medicine, has not developed an internationally accepted standard on growing, farming, processing and manufacture of Chinese herbal medicines. In fact, the global market share of herbal products by China is small. Some internationally popular products based on Chinese herbal medicine are developed by countries like Germany, Japan and South Korea. However, the Chinese government has now initiated programmes to introduce a range of standards (see below) on Chinese herbal medicine. It is expected that these measures will improve the quality of Chinese herbal products and subsequently increase their market share internationally.

Thirdly, there is a gap between the expenditure on Chinese herbal medicine and its widespread use for health and the expenditure on research into Chinese herbal medicine. Currently, the funding for recognised research into the use of complementary and alternative medicine (CAM) including Chinese herbal medicine is miniscule, considering their widespread use and the problems identified. While low expenditure on research is expected in most developing countries, research funding for CAM in most developed countries, such as Australia, the U.K. and Canada, is only a fraction of that available for research into orthodox medical and health care. The situation is similar in many other developed countries. However, there are signs of change. In the U.S., for example, the research funding for CAM research from the National Institutes of Health (NIH) has increased from US$2.5 million in 1992 to about US$100 million in 2002.

It is important for Chinese medicine practitioners and suppliers, as well as policy-makers, to recognise these gaps when making decisions on using, marketing and regulating Chinese herbal products. For example, it is critical for the manufacturers to understand the current regulations in the region in order to successfully enter the targeted markets.

4.4 The Problems

4.4.1 *Efficacy — level of evidence*

The long history of use of Chinese herbal medicine does not automatically indicate that its efficacy and safety has been scientifically proven. It is often argued by some Chinese medicine practitioners that there is already a vast body of evidence (mostly published in Chinese) for the efficacy of Chinese herbal medicine, and much of it is not known to the Western world. Thus, those practitioners tend to ignore the critics of Chinese herbal medicine. However, it is important for them to recognise that the available evidence must be properly assessed. There is no doubt about the rich literature on Chinese herbal medicine; however, the level of evidence it represents and how to assess it is less clear. For example, when referring to classical literatures on Chinese herbal medicine, one should always be cautious, as there are significant differences in clinical settings and factors, such as changes in environment and lifestyle as well as placebo effects, let alone the variation in quality of products used. Quite often, the classical evidence is subject to strong personal views rather than critical evaluation by modern scientific methods. Thus, bias or wrong conclusions are inevitable (such as treating the spontaneous remission as herbal effects). Even with modern research, the improper research design and procedures can also lead to the wrong conclusions.

The general approach is to rate the evidence according to certain standards. For example, the National Health and Medical Research Council (NHMRC) of Australia recommends a four-level system to assess the clinical evidence (NHMRC, 1999). Level 1: Evidence obtained from a systematic review or meta-analysis of all relevant randomised controlled trials; Level II: Evidence obtained from at least one properly designed randomised controlled trial; Level III-1: Evidence obtained from well-designed pseudo-randomised controlled trials (alternate allocation or some other method); Level III-2: Evidence obtained from comparative studies with concurrent controls and allocation not randomised (cohort studies), case control studies or interrupted time series with a control group; Level III-3: Evidence obtained from comparative studies with historical control, two or more single-arm studies or interrupted time series without a parallel control group; and Level IV: Evidence obtained from case series (either post-test or pre-test and post-test). It should also be pointed out that the level of evidence only indicate the capacity to minimise bias, caution should always be taken to explain different results, as there may be other explanations. Although there are inherent problems with randomised controlled clinical trials, systematic reviews and meta-analysis, there are currently no other standards superior to these for evidence assessments.

So what is the level of evidence in Chinese herbal medicine? Tang *et al.* (1999) reviewed randomised controlled trials of traditional medicine published and estimated there were about 10,000 randomised controlled trials conducted in China before 1997. In analysing 2938 randomised controlled trials, they concluded that although the quality of trials has been improving over the years, many problems remain. Most common ones include poorly described randomisation method, non-blinding, small sample sizes or the use of another Chinese medicine treatment not properly evaluated as a control. In addition, there was a lack of long-term outcome studies and many trials did not report on compliance and completeness of follow-up. The description of baseline data and side effects were also inadequate. Since most studies were positive, publication bias may be common (Tang *et al.*, 1999). Similar conclusions have been found in various critical reviews regarding Chinese herbal medicine against certain diseases or conditions. This implies that many clinical trials carried out previously in China may have to be repeated if they are to be used as evidence acceptable to the international community.

However, it should also be pointed out that, in most clinical trials on Chinese medicine, disease is often defined and diagnosed according to Western medicine and trial outcomes are often assessed by orthodox medicine complemented by Chinese medicine methods. Some traditional Chinese medicine practitioners strongly argue that traditional Chinese medicine has its own theory and diagnostic system which guide clinical practice, and consequently, trials based on Western medicine may generate inaccurate findings. Thus, they prefer trials purely based on Chinese medicine diagnosis and treatments. The problem with this approach is that it is often hard to clearly define the Chinese medicine standard itself. The diagnosis and treatment in Chinese medicine is often personalised — even experts may not always agree with each other's diagnosis and treatment principles. This divergence is often cited by Western medical practitioners who fundamentally disagree with the scientific basis of "Chi" and "meridian", etc. The lack of quantitative measures in Chinese medicine has always presented a challenge for the development of standards of diagnosis and treatment. In fact, the study of the nature of "Zheng (syndrome)" in Chinese medicine has always been a widely debated topic in recent years. Earlier studies have focused on various biochemical markers, while more recently efforts have been made to use other techniques such as cDNA micro-array techniques to study the genes which are affected in certain "Zheng".

Nevertheless, a few studies have attempted to integrate different methodologies. For example, Hsieh (1996) studied the effect of Chinese herbal medicine on childhood bronchial asthma using both the Western and traditional Chinese medicine diagnosis in multi-centre, double-blind and placebo-controlled trials. In addition to measuring symptom and medication scores, changes of immunoregulatory function and various inflammatory markers, patients were also classified by Chinese doctors, according to a standardised questionnaire designed on the basis of the fundamental logic of Chinese medicine, into three groups of specific constitution (e.g. classified as deficiencies in kidney and spleen). Each group consisted of both herb and placebo-treated patients. More than 300 asthmatic children were included. The results indicated that both herb-treated and placebo groups showed an improvement in all clinical parameters. However, the improvement was usually greater in the herb-treated group than in the placebo group. Thus, the traditional Chinese medicines used showed a certain degree of clinical efficacy. Similar studies have been conducted for irritable bowel syndrome and atopic eczema (Bensoussan *et al.*, 1998; Sheehan *et al.*, 1992). It can be predicated that the view of the use Chinese herbal medicine will be changed as more evidence becomes available through proper clinical trials and critical reviews.

4.4.2 *Quality*

This is one of the most difficult issues encountered by the industry and the regulators. Unlike conventional drugs, the quality of herbal products can be influenced by a range of natural factors, such as climate changes, soil quality, as well as factors such as processing, harvesting, extracting procedures, etc. Additionally it is difficult to define the herbal quality due to the lack of internationally accepted standards and the fact that active ingredients may not be known.

An indication of the current quality of Chinese herbs on the market can be found from the data released by the State Drug Administration of Chinese Government from surveys of the major specialised herbal markets in China between 2000–2001, which found that about 50% of raw herbs are below the national standard (Chinese Pharmacopeia). This also raised a question of the quality of herbs exported from China to other countries. It should be pointed out that assurance of the control of quality of formulated proprietary medicines is even more difficult than raw herbs as the former are often made from a group of herbs in various ways The major quality control problems for Chinese herbal medicine are as follows.

Content of ingredients

Studies have found the content of herbal ingredients varies significantly in herbs collected from different locations and in different seasons. For example, the active components in *A. sieboldi* have been found to change up to 20-fold in ten different samples (Yuan and Lin, 2000). Thus, the quality control of herbal products is difficult. In this regard, the general message to the consumer is "do not always believe the labels" (or even if the label is accurate, the effect from one pack to the next sometime may be hugely variable). Studies have frequently found the most herbal products on the market failed to meet what their labels say. Importantly, if the Chinese herbal medicine contains potent ingredients such as toad venom, any changes of ingredients will significantly affect the actions and safety profiles of the products.

Standards

Unfortunately, there is still no internationally accepted standard on Chinese herbal medicine, even with raw herbs. Part of the reason is the lack of understanding of the chemical composition and active ingredients of each herb, let alone the formulated products. Most quality measures included in Chinese Pharmacopoeia still need to be improved to reflect the overall quality of the herb. To control the quality and proper use of Chinese herbal medicines effectively, a universal standard on the growing, harvesting, manufacturing, extracting and packaging and supplying of herbs need to be agreed upon. In this regard, the Chinese government has recently made significant progress with the introduction of standards on Good Agriculture Practice (GAP), Good Manufacturing Practice (GMP), Good Laboratory Practice (GLP), Good Clinical Practice (GCP) and Good Selling Practice (GSP) for Chinese herbs.

Misidentification, contamination and adulteration

The authenticity of Chinese herbs (Di Dao Yao Cai) has always been an important issue in Chinese herbal medicine. There have been numerous cases of misidentification, contamination and adulteration of Chinese herbs reported in the Chinese literature (Chan *et al.*, 1993a). Studies published in English also highlight the extent of the problem. An example is the well-documented kidney failure and urothelial carcinoma cases caused by an adulteration of *Stephania tetrandra* with more toxic *Aristolochia fangchi* (Vanherweghem *et al.*, 1993; Nortier and Vanherweghem, 2002) (see below).

One of the major problems for Chinese herbal products is contamination with conventional Western drugs, which quite often are not shown on the product labels (Ernst, 2002). A number of Chinese herbal products containing conventional drugs have been identified by the U.S. Food and Drug Administration (FDA) as well as by health authorities in other countries. The most common drugs found in Chinese herbal medicines are analgesic, anti-inflammatory and anti-allergy agents, steroids (especially in skin care products), antibiotics, vasodilators and caffeine. Quite often the nature of the drug contained also varies in different batches of the same product, even with the same manufacturer. For example, steroids have been detected in a number of Chinese herbal medicines (Keane *et al.*, 1999; Wood and Wishart, 1997). Another recent case occurred in the U.S. in relation to the dietary supplement/herbal products, SPES and PC-SPES. The latter is a popular and expensive product which is used for the treatment of prostate cancer and contains seven Chinese herbs and one American herb. Quality experimental and clinical trials have demonstrated the efficacy of PC-SPES. However, recent laboratory analysis of the products by the California Department of Health Services found PC-SPES contains warfarin and SPES contains alprazolam, and PC-SPES also contains diethylstilbestrol (Guns *et al.*, 2002). As a result, FDA has warned consumers to stop taking the products. There have also been reports from Hong Kong, the U.S. and Australia of proprietary medicines containing paracetamol, aspirin, antihistamines, theophylline, bromhexine and synthetic corticosteroids (Allen and Parkinson, 1990; Ernst, 2002). For example, there have been cases of serious adverse reactions even death associated with Chinese herbal medicine containing undeclared Western drugs (Ries and Sahud, 1975).

It is understood that some pharmaceutical manufacturers in China produce the drug-containing herbal products deliberately in order to make additional therapeutic claims or to ensure the efficacy of their products. It is likely that, in some cases, the mixture of Western and Chinese herbs may result in additional efficacy and reductions in unwanted side effects associated with Western drugs. However, this needs to be properly evaluated and reflected on the label, In many other cases, drugs in mislabelled herbal medicines will expose the consumers to a potential risk for overdose and drug-herb interactions. This practice may also damage the reputation of Chinese herbal medicine more generally since it may be blamed for any observed side effects or toxicities, even though the observed problems may not actually be caused by Chinese herbs.

Heavy metals and pesticides

Historically Chinese medicine also uses minerals to treat diseases/conditions. Some of them are heavy metals, and most of them are restricted to external use. The value of these therapies should be properly evaluated rather than discarded totally. A good example is the recent development of the use of arsenic trioxide to treat relapsed acute promyelocytic leukemia (APL) (Chen *et al.*, 2002; Mayorga *et al.*, 2002), multiple myeloma (MM) (Hayashi *et al.*, 2002) and possibly other cancers (Chen *et al.*, 2002). Arsenic-containing compounds have long been used for treating various cancers in Chinese medicine. Recent studies have found arsenic trioxide can affect intracellular signal transduction pathways causing alterations in cellular function which result in the induction of apoptosis, the inhibition of growth and angiogenesis, and the promotion of differentiation (Miller *et al.*, 2002).

However, frequent exposure to heavy metals such as cadmium, lead and arsenic or pesticides causes serious problems. For example, there have been many recent cases of lead and mercury poisoning due to Chinese herbal medicines (Chan *et al.*, 1993b; Cheng *et al.*, 1998; Wong *et al.*, 1993; Markowitz *et al.*, 1994; Wu *et al.*, 1996; Li *et al.*, 2000; Auyeung *et al.*, 2002; Koh and Woo, 2000). It is quite clear that contaminated herbal medicines are not acceptable according to international standards (Espinoza *et al.*, 1995; Ernst, 2002). To prevent this problem, herbs need to be grown in optimal soils and conditions and to avoid the use of fertilisers and pollutants. Recently, there have been significance advances on this issue with the Chinese government introducing GLP to minimise the use of fertilisers and pesticides in the farming of Chinese medicinal herbs.

4.4.3 *Adverse reactions*

Contrary to some Chinese medicine practitioners' view, reports of adverse reactions to Chinese herbal medicine have significantly increased in recent years. For example, studies carried out in China found that the reported cases of adverse reactions associated with Chinese herbal medicines (including extracts) have increased from 398 cases in the 1970s, to 2217 cases in the 1980s, and further to 2724 cases between 1990–1994. The reported adverse reactions cover 518 different kinds of herbal medicines (Wang *et al.*, 2001). In 1996 alone, there were 748 reported adverse reaction cases including 23 deaths, ranging from cardiovascular (28.9%), neural (32.6%), allergy (25.5%), gastrointestinal (20.7%), respiratory (15%), urogenital (7.6%), blood and endocrine system (5.7%), and addiction (0.13%), mainly caused by improper use, overdosing and allergies (Wang *et al.*, 2001). The most commonly reported herbs are Datura Flower, Aconite, *Tripterygium wilfordii* Hook., etc. It should be mentioned, however, that the reported cases in China also include non-traditional preparations such as concentrated or purified extracts, tablets and injections. Nevertheless, the actual cases can be much higher considering under-reporting is likely to be widespread.

In Hong Kong, a study found that out of 1701 patients admitted to a Hong Kong hospital, three were admitted because of adverse reactions to Chinese herbal medicines (Chan *et al.*, 1992). In Taiwan, herbal medicines ranked third among the categories of medicines responsible for causing adverse effects (4%, 108 of 2695 patients admitted to a Taiwanese hospital had drug-related problems) (Lin and Lin, 1993). Similarly, the London-based National Poisons Unit received a total of 1070 enquiries relating to herbal and other traditional medicines between January 1983 and March 1989 (Perharic *et al.*, 1994). Surveillance studies conducted in Australia also found that the adverse events associated with the use of complementary and alternative medicines in children (Shenfield *et al.*, 2002). In particular, an average of one adverse event for every 633 Chinese medicine consultation has been reported (Bensoussan *et al.*, 2000).

However, there is clear evidence that a raw herb is generally significantly less toxic than single "active ingredients" isolated from it. Despite the complexity of different ingredients, Chinese herbal medicine is generally safe when properly used. The apparent adverse reactions are mostly associated with relatively few toxic herbal ingredients (Tomlinson *et al.*, 2000), often related to toxic herbs previously recognised in Chinese medicine, e.g. those marked as toxic in Chinese Pharmacopoeia. On the other hand, some adverse reactions are caused by herbs commonly regarded as non-toxic. An example is Gancao (liquorice) which can cause mineralocorticoid excess syndrome, expressed as sodium retention, potassium loss and suppression of the renin-angiotensin-aldosterone system, in addition to clinical consequences such as raised blood pressure and oedema, if used in large doses or for a prolonged period (Olukoga and Donaldson, 2000). Traditionally, the toxicology aspect of Chinese herbal medicine focuses on acute toxicity, e.g. fatal when taking or overdosing. The chronic toxicity of herbs (e.g. toxic effects after taking herbs for months or years) is often not known. In addition, caution should always be exercised when using Chinese herbal medicine in certain populations, such as pregnant women or children. The following highlights some well-known cases of adverse reactions related with Chinese herbal medicine.

Kidney toxicity

It is known that a number of Chinese herbs can cause kidney damage as a result of overdose. There were numerous reports of kidney damage in China from 1980–1999, mostly caused by Lei Gong Teng, Yu Dan, Ban Chan and contaminated honey. However, one of the most well-known cases is that of the renal damage case reported in Belgium, now often referred to as Chinese herbs nephropathy. The case involves the use of Chinese herbal medicine as a slimming therapy in a weight-loss clinic. It was found that the patients developed end-stage renal failure and urothelial carcinoma (Vanherweghem *et al.*, 1993; Nortier and Vanherweghem, 2002; Arlt *et al.*, 2002). The subsequent studies found that the toxicity is likely to be caused by an adulteration of *Stephania tetrandra* with more toxic *Aristolochia fangchi* due to a manufacturing error (*Aristochia* spp. is known for its nephrotoxic and carcinogenic actions) (Vanherweghem *et al.*, 1993; Nortier and Venherweghem, 2002). After the initial report in Belgium in 1992, more similar cases were reported in other countries/regions in the U.K., France, Japan and Taiwan. For example, a recent study in Taiwan found that there is a strong correlation between rapidly progressive interstitial renal fibrosis and the consumption of Chinese herbs (Chang *et al.*, 2001). As a result, using herbs containing aristolochic acid (including a number of plants of the *Aristolochia* genus) have now been banned in many countries. In addition, the use of herbs considered to be substitutes for *Aristolochia* plants has also been questioned. Interestingly, the kidney damage caused by *Aristolochia* herbs had previously been reported in China in the 1970s and 1980s but the Chinese Pharmacopoeia did not mention its toxicity until after the Belgian case in 2000.

Liver toxicity

It is known that certain Chinese herbs, such as Lei Gong Teng and Huang Yao Zi, can cause liver damage following overdose or improper use. Another example is a Chinese herbal medicine, Jin Bu Huan Anodyne tablets, which can cause acute hepatitis (Woolf *et al.*, 1994). Studies found that the product contained different ingredients from those shown on the label. The mechanism of its toxicity had not been identified, though it appeared that the wrong herb was used in the product (Yuan Hu (Rhizoma Corydalis Yanhusuo) instead of Yuan Zhi (Radix Polygalae Tenuifoliae) (Woolf *et al.*, 1994). In other reported incidents, some children who took an overdose of Jin Bu Huan also developed rapid onset of life-threatening bradycardia and central nervous system and respiratory depression (Horowitz *et al.*, 1996). Thus the potential risk for herbal hepatotoxicity should be recognised and monitored.

Similarly, in a report from Guy's Hospital Medical Toxicology Unit (1991–1995), nine cases of toxicity from heavy metals were confirmed following exposure to traditional remedies from the Indian sub-continent. In the same report, 21 cases of liver toxicity, including two deaths, were associated with the use of Chinese herbal medicines, although no causal agent was identified (Shaw *et al.*, 1997).

Cardiovascular toxicity

There are frequent case reports of toxicity associated with aconitine-containing herbs. The unprepared forms of aconitum species used in Chinese medicine (e.g. *Wu Tou, Cao Wu, Chuan Wu*) are highly toxic and have been implicated in a number of deaths in China, Hong Kong and Australia (Chan *et al.*, 1994; Chan, 2002; Kelly, 1990). However, the prepared form (*Zhi Fu Zi*) is comparatively safe when correctly prescribed as clinical reports on Fu Zi's toxicity are not common. The important factors in determining aconite toxicity are processing procedures such as boiling that can cause hydroxylation of aconitine.

It should be pointed out that there are significant differences in adverse reactions reported with raw herbs in traditional use and those with herbal extracts in non-traditional use. For example, reports of adverse reactions to Ma Huang as the raw herb are rare in published literature of Chinese medicine in China in the last several decades. Only one reported adverse reaction was found with raw herb, although it is acknowledged that under-reporting is possible, while there were a number of reports with purified Ma Huang extracts between 1919 to 1994 (Wang and Zhang, 2001). In contrast, most documented cases of toxicity of Ma Huang in food supplements were reported in the U.S., often after long term use as a weight loss agent (e.g. 140 adverse reactions including ten deaths between June 1997 to March 1999) (Haller and Benowitz, 2000).

4.4.4 *Drug-herb interactions*

There are increasing concerns for both Chinese medicine and orthodox medicine practitioners on the possible interactions between medicinal herbs and conventional drugs. Such concern is valid especially for patients who take Chinese herbal medicines with multiple drugs for various conditions (particularly for chronic diseases/conditions in the elderly). For example, a number of herbs (including both Chinese and Western herbs) can interact with warfarin (and related drugs, such as heparin, aspirin and coumarin derivatives), the agents which decrease the platelet aggregation. Thus, they can cause blood disorders, such as bleeding, when taken together. Such herbs include Ginkgo, Ginseng, Danshen (*Salvia miltiorrhiza*), Dangqui, etc. (Heck *et al.*, 2000; Yu *et al.*, 1997; Vaes and Chyka, 2000).

Another example is Ma Huang which contains ephedrine. Traditionally, combinations of Ma Huang with various herbs can increase or decrease actions of other herbs, e.g. Ma Huang can decrease actions of Shu Di Huang (Bensky and Gamble, 1993). Certain Western drugs such as sympathomimetic agents, e.g. monoamine oxidase inhibitors and clonidine may increase the actions of Ma Huang or vice versa (Huang, 1996; Zhu, 1998). On the other hand, Ma Huang may decrease the actions of bethanidine and guanethidine. Similarly, licorice, plantain, hawthorn and ginseng may interfere with digoxin, and licorice with spironolactone (Miller, 1998).

The interactions between drugs and herbs can be due to various factors. It may result from chemical reactions between different ingredients, or from changes or modifications to specific pathways involved in the metabolism or actions of certain drugs or herbs. It has been known that certain Chinese herbs may interfere with the body's drug transport and metabolism enzymes, resulting in an increase or decrease of metabolism and therefore the actions of various drugs. Clearly, the drug-herb interaction is an important area requiring further research in order to eliminate potentially high-risk or fatal drug-herb interactions. On the other hand, elucidation of the mechanisms involved in drug-herb interaction may also promote the rational use of a combination of Chinese herbal medicine and conventional drugs for conditions such as chemotherapy or radiotherapy for cancer patients.

4.4.5 *Other issues*

The development of the Chinese herbal medicine market worldwide will put increasing pressure on the sources of supply of quality Chinese herbs.

There have already been signs of imbalanced supply of certain Chinese herbs in China. In some areas, the condition for herb farming is deteriorating due to the environmental and human problems. These trends are likely to continue.

Another aspect is rational use of Chinese herbal medicines. As stated in the WHO Traditional Medicine Strategy 2002–2005 document, rational use of Chinese herbal medicine may have many aspects including qualification and licensing of providers; proper use of products of assured quality; good communication between medical practitioners and patients; and provision of scientific information and guidance for the public. These highlight enormous tasks for achieving rational use of Chinese herbal medicine especially in developed countries.

Currently the communication between consumers and general medical practitioners is generally poor. Some consumers still hold the "natural is safe" attitude towards Chinese herbal medicine; thus they tend to ignore some potential risk associated with herbal medicine. Many countries and regions still lack adequate policies or regulations on Chinese herbal medicine. Thus, the standard of practice for Chinese herbal medicine practitioners varies considerably. In some regions, people can still practise Chinese herbal medicine without formal or recognised education or training. In those regions, the public is exposed to higher risks. On the other hand, the exchange of information on Chinese herbal medicine is not adequate and a significant amount of previous work has not been properly recognised or evaluated. In addition, for various reasons, there are numerous professional associations of Chinese herbal medicine practitioners around the world but the links between them is generally weak. There is still no recognised international society to represent Chinese medicine professionals worldwide. Thus, the voice to promote and raise public awareness of the proper use of Chinese herbal medicine is often not united.

In addition, there are problems with intellectual property rights on Chinese herbal medicine. Compared with the development of Western drugs, the intellectual property and patent rights for traditional herbal medicines have not been properly resolved. This in some way may have delayed the development of some Chinese herbal medicines into large-scale production. There have been various cases of intellectual properties issues in China in recent years. In some cases, there are difficulties for treating traditional remedies as commercial patents. On the other hand, there are loopholes for the implementation of protections for patent-related products.

4.5 The Challenges

4.5.1 *Policies and regulations*

With the increasing demand on herbal products worldwide, it is inevitable for health authorities to be confronted with the policy or regulation issues on Chinese herbal medicine. However, apart from few countries/regions such as China where the regulations on Chinese medicine has become a part of national health framework, many countries still lack adequate regulations on Chinese herbal medicine. One of the biggest challenges is to harmonise scopes of regulations and practice. The challenges can come in two fronts: regulations on Chinese medicine practitioners and Chinese medicine products. Different approaches or models of regulation should be developed to fit the culture or regional backgrounds. For example, it is unlikely for Western countries to adopt entirely the Chinese model due to cultural and political differences. Nevertheless, the current view in many developed countries is that the Chinese medicine practice and Chinese herbal medicine, as part of complementary medicine, should be properly regulated. This can best be tackled within a national policy framework including practice licensing and training, safety and quality of products, and priorities for research (WHO TM strategy 2002–2005). A good example is the pioneering work developed by the Victoria State of Government in Australia to legally regulate Chinese medicine practice as a primary health care profession (Chinese Medicine Registration Act 2000). In this Act, the title of Chinese Medicine Practitioners in Chinese herbal medicine, acupuncture and herbal dispense are protected through registration. Only recognised practitioners with proper trainings can be registered to use the proper title while others are not. This will protect the public interests and increase the standard of practice. Similar efforts have also been made or are in the process of development in other countries/regions, such as Hong Kong, Singapore, the U.K. and Canada. Such national policies will promote global development on this issue.

The regulation of Chinese herbal product is more complicated. There are barriers of mutual understanding and regulating (e.g. food verse medicine). The lack of knowledge of understanding the pharmacological basis of herbal products and efficacy evidence creates technical problems for regulating them as conventional therapeutical drugs. On one hand, there are views regarding the Chinese herbal products as low standards lacking of quality controlled products; on the other, there is argument that they should be regulated differently as conventional chemical drugs due to their nature of traditional use. Nevertheless, as mentioned above, certain countries or regions have developed or are in the process of development of related policies or regulations on herbal products as therapeutic medicines. In Hong Kong, for example, series of regulations on herbal products have been introduced to classify Chinese herbal medicine in different categories (e.g. toxic and non-toxic Chinese herbs in different "Schedules"). In the state of Victoria, Australia, a list of Schedule 1 poisons will be introduced to control potential Chinese herbs used only by registered practitioners.

4.5.2 *Assessment and research*

Efficacy

It is important to develop related methods and protocols to improve the quality of clinical research on Chinese herbal medicine to clearly demonstrate its efficacy and safety. The evidence-based approach is critical, although different approaches in Western and Chinese medicine should be properly balanced. For example, specially designed randomised controlled clinical trials to test standard Chinese herbal formula or individualised herbal treatments should be developed. The trials based on Chinese medicine theory should also be explored. The trial should be adequately designed with baseline data and detailed procedures on randomisation, blinding, placebo or proper controls, balanced sample sizes, outcome measures, compliance, follow-ups and descriptions of adverse reactions, etc. The trial should be focused on primary diseases or conditions which

Chinese herbal medicine may have a potential effect, such as chronic conditions, cancer, etc.

In addition, the existing evidence should be critically and systematically reviewed. In this regard, the effort to set up the first Cochrane Center for Chinese Medicine in China is encouraging. There have been various databases on Chinese herbal medicine worldwide but the one with integrated, quality controlled and evidence-based approaches is still lacking. Thus a united and combined international effort is needed to promote high quality information exchange in Chinese herbal medicine practice and research.

Standards

It is vital to establish a complete and internationally recognised standard for Chinese herbal medicine. This should include standardisations for naming, growing, harvesting, processing, identifying and manufacturing (including extracting, packaging, supplying, storing and assessing). The importance of standardisation and quality control in herbal medicine in order to protect the public interests and promote evidence-based medical practice can never be understimated. For example, differentiations in term of usage of some Chinese herbs from different plants/species, such as Mu Tong, should be recognised. The different toxicity properties of these plants indicate different safety profiles if used indiscriminately. This has been approved in recent kidney toxicity cases around the world (see the above). Ironically, current Pharmacopoeia of the People's Republic of China (PPRC) includes more toxic Guan Mu Tong rather than less toxic Mu Tong. It is noted that the Chinese government has at last intended to introduce a series of standards on Chinese herbal products after decades of deliberation. It is quite clear now that without the proper standards and quality control procedures in place, any attempt to promote Chinese herbal medicine will result in failure in the long run, as allowing low quality or contaminated herbal products into the market will damage the reputation of Chinese medicine as a whole. However, the difficulties facing the standardisation on Chinese herbal medicine are enormous. Currently, most feasible approaches seem to use certain analytical techniques or molecular/biochemical markers to map the fingerprint of the herbal product. Ideally, this should be in combination with functional or biochemical bioassays to monitor the actions of products. However, to adopt these procedures to the commonly used Chinese herbal medicines, which are often in formulas and may contain a number of individual herbs, is still a great challenge. Theoretically, since many herbal active ingredients are unknown, any standards introduced have yet to be confirmed.

Safety

Assessment

The view on the safety of Chinese herbal medicine should be improved, as there is generally a weakness in Chinese medicine in evaluating the toxicity and long-term safety of herbal products. The traditional view on the "herbal toxicity" should be modified from that largely emphasised on acute toxicity to those in recognising the importance of long-term safety evaluation in order to establish a clear benefit/risk ratio. The procedures for assessing potential adverse reactions and related mechanisms should also be developed. In addition, the guide for practicing Chinese herbs should be updated and progressed along with the scientific evidence rather than purely based on traditional or historical uses.

Monitoring

It is necessary to establish an efficient national/international system to monitor the potential adverse reactions associated with Chinese herbal medicine. In this regard, the existing system for Western drugs such as those used in the U.K. (Yellow Card System) and in Australia (Blue Card system) can be extended to Chinese herbal medicine. What is important is to educate Chinese medicine practitioners and other health care providers who use the Chinese herbal medicine to understand and use the system properly. There is a wrong impression by some Chinese medicine practitioners, i.e. reporting adverse reactions of Chinese herbal medicine used in their clinics will reflect their incompetence in practice. This should be corrected. If a patient has suffered an adverse reaction to an herbal product, this should be reported regardless how it occurs. It is important to design the reporting system to include necessary information on the prescription, including sources, ingredients, processing procedures and supplier of the product.

4.5.3 *Health economics and development issues*

In some countries/regions, the access of quality service of Chinese herbal medicine is still a challenge due to unbalanced ratio of practitioners to population. In addition, in countries like China where Chinese medicine is fully institutionalised, challenges for balanced and cost-effective growth are also increasing. For example, Bodeker (2001) pointed out that traditional Chinese medicine in China is largely an outpatient, low technology specialty; most of the income of traditional hospitals comes from the sale of traditional medicines. Even with the 25% mark-up allowed, it is hard to cover operational costs. Although government subsidies currently ensure survival, there is no surplus for improving services, and further market reforms may threaten this subsidy system. In contrast, in developed countries/regions, the rational use of Chinese herbal medicine needs to be properly addressed. The public attitudes on Chinese medicine need to be guided and monitored. The adequate research on health economics and trainings on practitioners should be promoted. In addition, solutions are needed for increasing pressures for supplying quality Chinese medicinal plants. With changes in natural and trade environments, the importance of sustainable growth or use of Chinese medicinal plants should be addressed. Furthermore, the development of an internationally recognised protection of intellectual knowledge on Chinese herbal medicine should be further discussed and properly implemented.

4.5.4 *Education*

The challenges come in two fronts: (1) how to educate the general public on the proper use of Chinese herbal medicine and (2) how to improve the education of Chinese herbal medicine practitioners. It is important to alert the public on the "natural" is "safe" attitude, and to provide them with the right information. On the other hand, people involved in the practice of Chinese herbal medicine in certain countries or regions are still lacking in formal training and proper education. Many of them only have limited training in private colleges or with private practitioners. Such low standard practices threaten the reputation of Chinese medicine. Thus, collaborations and discussions should be implemented in order to introduce an international standard on Chinese medicine education. In this regard, formal education at the university level with support from the government is critical. It is encouraging that today in some Western countries, apart from China, Chinese medicine is being offered as a degree course (such as a five-year full-time double degree in RMIT, Australia, and a three-year Masters degree in the U.K.).

4.6 Conclusion

There is a trend of increasing usage of Chinese herbal medicines in the general population, which is concurrently associated with certain problems and challenges, such as adverse reactions, quality assessment of herbal products and policies/regulations. There is also a growing body of evidence of the efficacy of Chinese herbal medicine, however the need for further imposing evidence-based research on efficacy and safety is warranted. It can be predicated that by overcoming the problems and meeting the challenges as discussed in this chapter, the Chinese herbal medicine will play a greater role in promoting the well-being of mankind in the 21st century.

References

Allen, B.R. and Parkinson, R. (1990) Chinese herbs for eczema. *Lancet* **336**(8708), 177.

Arlt, V.M., Stiborova, M. and Schmeiser, H.H. (2002) Aristolochic acid as a probable human cancer hazard in herbal remedies: A review. *Mutagenesis* **17**, 265–277.

Auyeung, T.W., Chang, K.K., To, C.H., Mak, A. and Szeto, M.L. (2002) Three patients with lead poisoning following use of a Chinese herbal pill. *Hong Kong Med. J.* **8**, 60–62.

Bensky, D. and Gamble, A. (1993) *Chinese Herbal Medicine Materia Media*, Revised Ed. Eastland Press, Washington, USA.

Bensoussan, A., Myers, S.P. and Carlton, A.L. (2000) Risks associated with the practice of traditional Chinese medicine: An Australian study. *Arch. Fam. Med.* **9**, 1071–1078.

Bensoussan, A., Talley, N.J., Hing, M., Menzies, R., Guo, A. and Ngu. M. (1998) Treatment of irritable bowel syndrome with Chinese herbal medicine: A randomized controlled trial. *J. Am. Med. Assoc.* **280**, 1585–1589.

Bodeker, G. (2001) Lessons on integration from the developing world's experience. *Br. Med. J.* **322**, 164–167.

Chan, T.Y., Chan, A.Y. and Critchley, J.A. (1992) Hospital admissions due to adverse reactions to Chinese herbal medicines. *J. Trop. Med. Hyg.* **95**, 296–298.

Chan, T.Y., Chan, J.C., Tomlinson, B. and Critchley, J.A. (1993a) Chinese herbal medicines revisited: A Hong Kong perspective. *Lancet* **342**, 1532–1534.

Chan, T.Y., Chan, J.C., Tomlinson, B. and Critchley, J.A. (1993b) Chinese herbal medicines revisited: A Hong Kong perspective. *Lancet* **342**, 1532–1534.

Chan, T.Y., Tomlinson, B., Tse, L.K., Chan, J.C., Chan, W.W. and Critchley, J.A. (1994) Aconitine poisoning due to Chinese herbal medicines: A review. *Vet. Hum. Toxicol.* **36**, 452–455.

Chan, T.Y. (2002) Incidence of herb-induced aconitine poisoning in Hong Kong: Impact of publicity measures to promote awareness among the herbalists and the public. *Drug Saf.* **25**, 823–828.

Chang, C.H., Wang, Y.M., Yang, A.H. and Chiang, S.S. (2001) Rapidly progressive interstitial renal fibrosis associated with Chinese herbal medications. *Am. J. Nephrol.* **21**, 441–448.

Chen, Z., Chen, G.Q., Shen, Z.X., Sun, G.L., Tong, J.H., Wang, Z.Y. and Chen, S.J. (2002) Expanding the use of arsenic trioxide: Aleukemias and beyond. *Semin. Hematol.* **39**(2 Suppl. 1), 22–26.

Cheng, T.J., Wong, R.H., Lin, Y.P., Hwang, Y.H., Horng, J.J. and Wang, J.D. (1998) Chinese herbal medicine, sibship, and blood lead in children. *Occup. Environ. Med.* **55**, 573–576.

Eisenberg, D.M., Davis, R.B., Ettner, S.L., Appel, S., Wilkey, S., Van Rompay, M. and Kessler, R.C. (1998) Trends in alternative medicine use in the United States, 1990–1997: Results of a follow-up national survey. *J. Am. Med. Assoc.* **280**, 1569–1575.

Eisenberg, D.M., Kessler, R.C., Van Rompay, M.I., Kaptchuk, T.J., Wilkey, S.A., Appel, S. and Davis, R.B. (2001) Perceptions about complementary therapies relative to conventional therapies among adults who use both: Results from a national survey. *Ann. Intern. Med.* **135**, 344–351.

Ernst, E. (2002) Adulteration of Chinese herbal medicines with synthetic drugs: A systematic review. *J. Intern. Med.* **252**, 107–113.

Espinoza, E.O., Mann, M.J. and Bleasdell, B. (1995) Arsenic and mercury in traditional Chinese herbal balls. *N. Engl. J. Med.* **333**, 803–804.

Guns, E.S., Goldenberg, S.L. and Brown, P.N. (2002) Mass spectral analysis of PC-SPES confirms the presence of diethylstilbestrol. *Can. J. Urol.* **9**, 1684–1688.

Haller, C.A. and Benowitz, N.L. (2000) Adverse cardiovascular and central nervous system events associated with dietary supplements containing ephedra alkaloids. *N. Engl. J. Med.* **343**, 1833–1838.

Harmsworth, K. and Lewith, G.T. (2001) Attitudes to traditional Chinese medicine among Western trained doctors in the People's Republic of China. *Soc. Sci. Med.* **52**, 149–153.

Hayashi, T., Hideshima, T., Akiyama, M., Richardson, P., Schlossman, R.L., Chauhan, D., Munshi, N.C., Waxman, S. and Anderson, K.C. (2002) Arsenic troxide inhibits growth of human multiple myeloma cells in the bone marrow microenvironment. *Mol. Cancer Ther.* **1**, 851–860.

Heck, A.M., DeWitt, B.A. and Lukes, A.L. (2000) Potential interactions between alternative therapies and warfarin. *Am. J. Health Syst. Pharm.* **57**, 1221–1227.

Hesketh, T. and Zhu, W.X. (1997) Health in China. Traditional Chinese medicine: One country, two systems. *Br. Med. J.* **315**, 115–117.

Horowitz, R.S., Feldhaus, K., Dart, R.C., Stermitz, F.R. and Beck, J.J. (1996) The clinical spectrum of Jin Bu Huan toxicity. *Arch. Intern. Med.* **156**, 899–903.

Hsieh, K.H. (1996) Evaluation of efficacy of traditional Chinese medicines in the treatment of childhood bronchial asthma: Clinical trial, immunological tests and animal study. Taiwan Asthma Study Group. *Pediatr. Allergy Immunol.* **7**, 130–140.

Huang, K.C. (1996) *The Pharmacology of Chinese Herbs*, 2nd Ed. CRC Press, USA.

Keane, F.M., Munn, S.E., du Vivier, A.W., Taylor, N.F. and Higgins, E.M. (1999) Analysis of Chinese herbal creams prescribed for dermatological conditions. *Br. Med. J.* **318**, 563–564.

Kelly, S.P. (1990) Aconite poisoning. *Med. J. Aust.* **153**, 499.

Koh, H.L. and Woo, S.O. (2000) Chinese proprietary medicine in Singapore: Regulatory control of toxic heavy metals and undeclared drugs. *Drug Saf.* **23**, 351–362.

Li, A.M., Chan, M.H., Leung, T.F., Cheung, R.C., Lam, C.W. and Fok, T.F. (2000) Mercury intoxication presenting with tics. *Arch. Dis. Child.* **83**, 174–175.

Lin, S.H. and Lin, M.S. (1993) A survey on drug-related hospitalization in a community teaching hospital. *Int. J. Clin. Pharmacol. Ther. Toxicol.* **31**, 66–69.

MacLennan, A.H., Wilson, D.H. and Taylor, A.W. (2002) The escalating cost and prevalence of alternative medicine. *Prev. Med.* **35**, 166–173.

Markowitz, S.B., Nunez, C.M., Klitzman, S., Munshi, A.A., Kim, W.S., Eisinger, J. and Landrigan, P.J. (1994) Lead poisoning due to hai ge fen. The porphyrin content of individual erythrocytes. *J. Am. Med. Assoc.* **271**, 932–934.

Mayorga, J., Richardson-Hardin, C. and Dicke, K.A. (2002) Arsenic trioxide as effective therapy for relapsed acute promyelocytic leukemia. *Clin. J. Oncol. Nurs.* **6**, 341–346.

Miller, L.G. (1998) Herbal medicinals: Selected clinical considerations focusing on known or potential drug-herb interactions. *Arch. Intern. Med.* **158**, 2200–2211.

Miller, W.H. Jr, Schipper, H.M., Lee, J.S., Singer, J. and Waxman, S. (2002) Mechanisms of action of arsenic trioxide. *Cancer Res.* **62**, 3893–3903.

National Health and Medical Research Council (NHMRC) (1999) *A Guide to the Development, Implementation and Evaluation of Clinical Practice Guidelines*. Commonwealth of Australia, Canberra.

Nilsson, M., Trehn, G. and Asplund, K. (2001) Use of complementary and alternative medicine remedies in Sweden. A population-based longitudinal study within the northern Sweden MONICA Project. Multinational monitoring of trends and determinants of cardiovascular disease. *J. Intern. Med.* **250**, 225–233.

Nortier, J.L. and Vanherweghem, J.L. (2002) Renal interstitial fibrosis and urothelial carcinoma associated with the use of a Chinese herb (*Aristolochia fangchi*). *Toxicology* 181–182, 577–580.

Olukoga, A. and Donaldson, D. (2000) Liquorice and its health implications. *J. R. Soc. Health* **120**, 83–89.

Perharic, L., Shaw, D., Colbridge, M., House, I., Leon, C. and Murray, V. (1994) Toxicological problems resulting from exposure to traditional remedies and food supplements. *Drug Saf.* **11**, 284–294.

Ries, C.A. and Sahud, M.A. (1975). Agranulocytosis caused by Chinese herbal medicines. Dangers of medications containing aminopyrine and phenylbutazone. *J. Am. Med. Assoc.* **231**, 352–355.

Shaw, D., Leon, C., Kolev, S. and Murray, V. (1997) Traditional remedies and food supplements. A 5-year toxicological study (1991–1995). *Drug Saf.* **17**, 342–356.

Sheehan, M.P., Rustin, M.H., Atherton, D.J., Buckley, C., Harris, D.W., Brostoff, J., Ostlere, L., Dawson, A. and Harris, D.J. (1992) Efficacy of traditional Chinese herbal therapy in adult atopic dermatitis. *Lancet* **340**, 13–17.

Shenfield, G., Lim, E. and Allen, H. (2002) Survey of the use of complementary medicines and therapies in children with asthma. *J. Paediatr. Child. Health* **38**, 252–257.

Tang, J.-L., Zhan, S.-Y. and Ernst, E. (1999) Review of randomised controlled trials of traditional Chinese medicine. *Br. Med. J.* **319**, 160–161.

Thomas, K.J., Nicholl, J.P. and Coleman, P. (2001) Use and expenditure on complementary medicine in England: A population based survey. *Complement. Ther. Med.* **9**, 2–11.

Tomlinson, B., Chan, T.Y., Chan, J.C., Critchley, J.A. and But, P.P. (2000) Toxicity of complementary therapies: An eastern perspective. *J. Clin. Pharmacol.* **40**, 451–456.

Vaes, L.P. and Chyka, P.A. (2000) Interactions of warfarin with garlic, ginger, ginkgo, or ginseng: Nature of the evidence. *Ann. Pharmacother.* **34**, 1478–1482.

Vanherweghem, J.L., Depierreux, M., Tielemans, C., Abramowicz, D., Dratwa, M., Jadoul, M., Richard, C., Vandervelde, D., Verbeelen, D., Vanhaelen-Fastre, R., *et al.* (1993) Rapidly progressive interstitial renal fibrosis in young women: Association with slimming regimen including Chinese herbs. *Lancet* **341**, 387–391.

Wang, Q., Li, H. and Zhang, Z. (2001) Causes and countermeasures about adverse reaction of traditional Chinese medicine. *Zhong Yao Cai* **24**, 430–433 (in Chinese).

WHO (2002). *WHO Traditional Medicine Strategy 2002–2005.* World Health Organization, Geneva.

Wong, M.K., Tan, P. and Wee, Y.C. (1993) Heavy metals in some Chinese herbal plants. *Biol. Trace Elem. Res.* **36**, 135–142.

Wood, B. and Wishart, J. (1997) Potent topical steroid in a Chinese herbal cream. *N. Z. Med. J.* **110**, 420–421.

Woolf, G.M., Petrovic, L.M., Rojter, S.E., Wainwright, S., Villamil, F.G., Katkov, W.N., Michieletti, P., Wanless, I.R., Stermitz, F.R., Beck, J.J., *et al.* (1994) Acute hepatitis associated with the Chinese herbal product jin bu huan. *Ann. Intern. Med.* **121**, 729–735.

Wu, M.S., Hong, J.J., Lin, J.L., Yang, C.W. and Chien, H.C. (1996) Multiple tubular dysfunction induced by mixed Chinese herbal medicines containing cadmium. *Nephrol. Dial. Transplant.* **11**, 867–870.

Yu, C.M., Chan, J.C. and Sanderson, J.E. (1997) Chinese herbs and warfarin potentiation by "danshen". *J. Intern. Med.* **241**, 337–339.

Yuan, R. and Lin, Y. (2000) Traditional Chinese medicine: An approach to scientific proof and clinical validation. *Pharmacol. Ther.* **86**, 191–198.

Zhu, Y.P. (1998) *Chinese Materia Medica Chemistry, Pharmacology and Applications.* Harwood Academic Publishers, The Netherlands.

Chapter 5

Biochemistry and Herbs

Simon Ming Yuen Lee, Kit Man Lau, Johnny Chi Man Koon,
Judy Yuet Wa Chan & Kwok Pui Fung

5.1 Introduction

Under the U.S. Food and Drug Administration (FDA), most of the commercial herbal products in the United States are categorised as a type of dietary supplement. By law, products can be claimed as dietary supplements if these products claim to be beneficial to a nutrient deficiency disease or particular structure or functioning of the human body. Products can be deemed as drug products with approval from the FDA if these products can treat, cure or prevent disease. Recently, there is an increasing amount of plant-based drugs registered under the FDA. In order to obtain registration via filing under the Investigational New Drug (IND) and New Drug Application (NDA), the sponsor is required to thoroughly document evidences for pre-clinical research, clinical trial investigation and good manufacture process to ensure the safety, quality and efficacy of the products. This chapter gives a brief outline on those essential laboratory tests and pre-clinical research methods that can meet the application of IND and NDA registered under the FDA. This chapter also highlights on how modern biochemistry, genomic and molecular biology, helps the authentication, quality control and identification of pre-clinical pharmacological efficacy of herbal complex components.

5.2 Purity Test for Herbs and Herbal Products

5.2.1 *Heavy metal*

Examination of chemical impurities involves the detection of a variety of heavy metals (e.g. Arsenic, Mercury, Lead, Cadmium Chromium, Tin and Antimony). Generally speaking, the maximum daily intake of lead (Pb), cadmium (Cd), mercury (Hg) and arsenic (As) ranges from 0.043 mg/day to 0.21 mg/day (WHO, 1998). The Elemental Analysis Manual (EAM) (*http://www.cfsan.fda.gov/~dms/eam-toc.html*) developed by the FDA laboratories provides methods for detection of cadmium and mercury using atomic absorption spectrometry. The amount of arsenic in herbs and herbal products can be determined by a colorimetric detection method (WHO, 1998).

5.2.2 *Pesticides*

The United States Environmental Protection Agency (EPA) sets the tolerance limit for pesticide residual on food products. Tolerance established by the EPA is set in Title 40 of the Code of Federal Regulations (CFR); Part 180 for raw agricultural commodities and Part 185 for processed food. Aldrin, Dieldrin, Chlordane, DDT, Heptachlor, Hexachlorobenzene, BHCs/Lindane and Pentachloronitrobenzene (PCNBs) are common pesticides used in agriculture, which together with their parent pesticides, these pesticides are essentially subjected to testing. Generally, the maximum pesticide residue limit should not be more than 0.05 mh/kg according to the recommendation of the World Health Organization (WHO) (WHO, 1997). Pesticides have a diverse classification based on their chemical compositions or structures. Most pesticides are chlorinated hydrocarbon and organophosphorus. Thus, common methods to detect pesticides are based on the detection of organically bound chlorine and phosphorus with Gas Chromatography and High Performance Liquid Chromatography. The Pesticide Analytical Manual (PAM) (*http://www.cfsan.fda.gov/~frf/pami1.html*) is a repository of the analytical methods currently used in the FDA laboratories to examine food with pesticide residues for regulatory purposes.

5.2.3 *Microbiology*

Examination of biological impurities involves monitoring of microbial contamination, namely yeast, mould and bacteria; for example *Escherichia coli*, *Salmonellae* and *Staphylococcus aureus*. Generally, the limit of total aerobic bacterial count should be less than 10^5/gram, and total yeast and mould count should be less than 500/gram in herbal product. *Escherichia coli*, *Salmonellae* and *Staphylococcus aureus* must be absent in each gram of the herbal product. Most microorganism detection methods are based on cultivating testing articles in selective nutrition medium. After incubation, further identification of the enriched microorganism with biochemical tests (Downes and Ito, 2001). FDA Microbiological Analytical Manual (*http://www.cfsan.fda.gov/~comm/microbio.html*) is one of the essential references for microorganism detection.

5.3 Safety Test for Herbs and Herbal Products

Since FDA recognises that some of the traditional herbs and herbal products are in use for a long time, herbal products that were sold in the market as food or diet supplement without any report of adverse effect may not require to undergo all toxicity tests to obtain FDA's recognition. New herbs and herbal products without a well-documented history of traditional usage are strictly subjected to systematic toxicological evaluation. Sponsors must have sufficient toxicological evaluation to ensure the safety of herbal products before any clinical studies. The systematic toxicological evaluation includes the assessment of general toxicity, teratogenicity, mutagenicity and carcinogenicity in the finished herbal products. Identification of teratogenicity, mutagenicity and carcinogenicity in the products are important, as these adverse effects are difficult to be detected in human clinical studies.

5.3.1 *Acute and chronic toxicity tests*

Acute toxicity test is designed to observe acute toxic signs. In acute toxicity, testing animals are dosed once or more than once within a range of dosages in a 24-hour time period. Chronic toxicity test is used to define the toxicity of using repeated doses in animal models from two weeks to 12 months. Generally, toxic signs induced by cumulative biological effects are accessed by the animals' weight measurement, behaviour observation, haematological examination, renal and hepatic function tests, macroscopic and histopathological examination of relevant organs (ICH, 1997; WHO, 1993).

5.3.2 *Genotoxicity and carcinogenesis tests*

A genotoxicity test is used to assess drugs that can potentially cause damage to the genetic material of a higher organism (ICH, 1997b). On the other hand, a carcinogenicity test evaluates the potential of carcinogensis of a certain test substance. After a relatively high exposure level and a considerably long time period, test animals are observed for any signs of tumour development in the relevant organs and tissues (ICH, 1997c and 1998).

5.3.3 *Developmental and reproductive toxicity tests*

The International Conference on Harmonisation (ICH) guideline established three basic types of studies — Segments I, II and III — based on dosing test animals during different stages of the reproductive cycle. In Segment I, the test substance is administrated prior to pregnancy. Adult fertility and early embryonic development to implantation are evaluated. In Segment II, the test substance is administrated during the period of organogenesis of the foetuses. Foetuses are examined one day prior to parturition. In Segment III, the test substance is administrated during prenatal and lactation periods. Development of relevant organs and tissues, learning ability and memory of the litters are some of the evaluation parameters (ICH, 1994a and b).

5.4 Tests for Quality Control of Herbs and Herbal Products

The chemical composition of raw plant material and finished herbal product may vary due to the different agricultural conditions and manufacture processes. In order to minimise the batch-to-batch variation, the plant used for product preparation should be cultured according to the instruction of Good Agricultural Practice (GAP) and manufactured according to Good Manufacturing Practice (GMP). Besides, it is essential to establish the physical, chemical and biological activity profiles of the raw plant and finished product as a reference for quality control. A monograph is required for each herb, so that one can reference to the pharmacopoeial monograph when performing the quality assessment test. A monograph is a comprehensive summary that describes the biological activity, physical and chemical property of the herb. It is intended to provide quality assurance and safety information for the widely used medicinal plants.

5.4.1 *Chemical markers*

Chemical composition in herbs and herbal products are very complicated. The therapeutic action is always attributed to one or more active ingredients in the herbs. The ideal situation is to identify all active ingredients in the herbal products for authentication, quality control in the manufacture process, and calculation of the quantity of the plant material in the finished product. If the active ingredient is unknown at the initial stage of IND application, it is essential to identify one or more chemically defined constituents from the herbs to serve as markers for quality control and quantitative standardisation. Generally, High Performance Liquid Chromatography (HPLC) or Thin Layer Chromatography (TLC) can be used to generate chromatographic fingerprintings for the purpose of quality control.

5.4.2 *High performance liquid chromatography (HPLC)*

HPLC is a general term of liquid chromatography and its separation modes include size exclusion (Dudkiewics-Wilczynska *et al.*, 2002), ion exchange (Lahousen *et al.*, 2002), hydrophobic interaction and reversed phase (Montgomery *et al.*, 2001). Different separation modes employ different separation mechanisms, which exhibit different applications in separating biomolecules (Table 5.1). Among the different chromatographic

Table 5.1. Chromatographic modes of HPLC used in biomolecule separations.

Mode	Mechanism of separation	Application
Size exclusion	Molecular size	Peptides and proteins Polysaccharides
Ion exchange	Electrostatic interaction	Peptides and proteins Nucleic acids
Hydrophobic interaction	Dispersive interaction using salt gradient	Proteins Polysaccharides
Reverse phase	Dispersive interaction using aqueous/organic solvents	Proteins, peptides Amino acids Nucleic acids Proteins

modes (Table 5.1), the excellent resolving and separation power of reverse-phase chromatography (RPC), along with the availability of volatile mobile phases, has made PRC a favourable method for both analytical and preparative separations of herbal active components. Herbal active components can be simply classified as biomolecules, including peptide, protein and polysaccharide and metabolites. HPLC is originated from classical liquid chromatography. It employs a high-pressure and super-packing gel matrix system to provide a high performance (rapid) and high-resolution (good separation) separation process.

HPLC fingerprinting has been adopted as a rapid and reliable method for authentication of herb and herbal product. This method depends on the chemical constituents (chemical markers) in the herb and herbal product to generate a fingerprint (chromatographic map). Due to the complicated chemical composition of the herb, only a few chemical markers have been identified in the fingerprinting. Some of the markers are herb-specific and this can be an effective way to identify the herb and herbal product. Besides authentication, isolation of chemical markers in herbs is another important aspect for the herbal product industry to meet the GMP standard. However, the unavailability and unstability of the chemical markers always hinder the use of HPLC for quality control in the herbal manufacturing industry. Therefore, isolation and purification of chemical markers are the main task before any chemical or biological assays can be performed. Versatile HPLC chromatography can help to solve this problem. If only a small amount of marker is needed for testing its abundance, an analytical HPLC mode can be performed to obtain an adequate amount of marker. If a relatively large amount is needed, a preparative HPLC mode can be used instead. The latter employs a relatively more expensive HPLC column than the former, as preparative HPLC column needs higher capacity, and therefore more packing materials. Even if, an analytical HPLC column is overloaded, provided that special and tailor-made conditions have been setup, a small amount of chemical marker can be purified. Otherwise, other compounds can be mixed up in the purified marker, resulting in under-estimation of the marker content. Not only can HPLC be used in quantification of chemical markers, it can also be used in identification of the purified chemical markers. Using the combination of HPLC and ultra-violet photo-diode array detector as an example, an online check-up of the purity of resolved chromatographic peak can be accomplished by comparing the spectrophotometric spectrum with the identified marker. This method originates from the internal property of the single chemical marker that has an unique and comparable spectral characteristic. HPLC can also be coupled with a mass spectrometer to calculate the molecular weight and determine the structure of the chemical marker.

5.4.3 *DNA fingerprinting technology*

Identification of genetic markers is becoming an important tool for quick authentication of herb. Since most DNA fingerprinting techniques require high quality of genomic DNA, which can only be extracted from raw herbal material with minimum processing, this technology is always used to authenticate fresh or dried raw herbal materials besides the finished product. Randomly amplified polymorphic DNA (RAPD) fragment is the most simple and quick fingerprinting method. Briefly, RAPD analysis is based on random Polymerase Chain Reaction (PCR) amplification on the genomic DNA with one or more random primers (Shaw and But,

1995; Tochika-Komatsu *et al.*, 2001). However, the RAPD has poor reproducibility, as a lot of factors can affect the fingerprinting pattern generated from the RAPD. The factors include the PCR condition, concentration and quality of testing genomic DNA. Amplified fragment length polymorphisms (AFLP) technique is based on selective PCR amplification of restricted fragments from the total digested genomic DNA (Ha *et al.*, 2002). In AFLP, the genomic DNA is digested by two different restriction enzymes and two different endings (5' and 3') of the restricted fragments are ligated with different adaptors. The AFLP is better than RAPD in terms of reproducibility and consistency. Unique sequences in the rDNA internal transcribed spacer (ITS) region, *trnK* gene and *maK* gene identified by DNA sequencing is also a reliable approach in differentiating plants' taxonomic levels from family to species (Lau *et al.*, 2001). The DNA sequence of RAPD/RELP/rDNA-ITS fragments can be used for designing the Sequence Characterised Amplified Region (SCAR) markers, and these primers were successfully used in herb authentication (Wang *et al.*, 2001). Among these methods, simple sequence repeat (SSR) markers are efficient in the detection of a significantly higher degree of polymorphism in plant (Nagaraju *et al.*, 2002). However, it requires prior information on sequences of microsatellite loci.

5.4.4 *DNA microarray*

Currently, gene expression microarray is one of the important technologies to simultaneously and quickly identify the change of expression among large numbers of genes. Many drug targets are components of complex signalling pathways; and activation of these signaling pathways leads to changes in multiple mRNA expression. Thus, microarray technology can be used to provide a detailed quantitative assessment on the consequences of these activations and helps identify the target of drug action efficiently (Lee *et al.*, 2002; Waring *et al.*, 2001). In the near future, gene expression microarray will become a powerful and reliable platform to standardise the drug efficacy and predict the toxicity effect of complex components in herbal products. Development of Lab-on-chip technology and biosensor by integration of molecular DNA detection and electronic system is a popular area of research. A silicon-based polymerase chain reaction microreactor is developed for DNA sequence-based identification of toxic medicinal plants (Carles *et al.*, 2001).

5.4.5 *Stability test*

The quality of finished herbal products may change due to exposure to fluctuated environmental conditions during transportation, storage and sale on the market. The sponsor needs to test the stability of the product under different environmental conditions (e.g. 40°C and 75% relative humidity are conditions of accelerating stability test). Generally, the herbal product is considered to be stable for two years under ambient condition if it is stable when stored under accelerated condition for three months. In a stability test, the physical properties (e.g. appearance, water content and disintegration), chemical properties (e.g. active components or chemical markers), microbiological properties (e.g. aerobic microbial count, *Escherichia coli* and total combined mould and yeast count) and biological properties (e.g. specific bioassay for each herbal component) of the product are monitored when testing under a variety of environmental factors, such as temperature, humidity and light (ICH, 1996, Chinese Pharmacopedia, 2000). Then, the manufacturer can choose an appropriate package and storage condition to ensure that the product is within an acceptable limit of the quality and efficacy during a specific period of time.

5.5 Biochemical Assay of Active Components in Herbs and Herbal Products

Sufficient amount of evidence of drug efficacy in pre-clinical biological assay should be provided when applying for initial clinical trials. In addition, the proof of efficacy is required in order to support the therapeutic potential of herbal products. Moreover, biological assay is one of the quality control tests for monitoring the consistency of the herbal product manufacturing process. Generally speaking, the biological assay can be performed in the test tube or cell line model (*in vitro*), and an animal model (*in vivo*). *In vivo* and *in vitro* models of threatening diseases, including cancer, diabetes mellitus, inflammation, cardiac attacks, osteoporosis and severe acute respiratory syndrome (SARS) are reviewed as follows.

5.5.1 *Antioxidant*

Oxidants are generated in human bodies under normal physiological processes. They are so reactive that they can react with a wide variety of biomolecules, including DNA, protein and lipid that eventually cause cell damages. It is recognised that herbs with antioxidant effect may have the potential to prevent or ameliorate oxidant-related disorders, such as myocardial ischaemia-reperfusion injury, atherosclerosis, cancer and ageing. To evaluate the antioxidant activity in potential herbs, several assays can be employed. Phenazin methosulfate-nicotinamide adenine dinucleotide (reduced form) (PMS-NADH) system (van Noorden and Butcher, 1989; Liu *et al.*, 1997) and 1,1-diphenyl-2-picrylhydrazyl (DPPH) radical-scavenging assay (Jung *et al.*, 2002; Santosh Kumar *et al.*, 2002; Shimoji *et al.*, 2002) are two simple test-tube methods for fast radical-scavenging drug screening and activity-guided isolation of active components. The antioxidant activities of some Chinese medicines such as *Paeonia suffruticosa*, *Polygonum multiflorum*, *Coptis chinensis*, *Prunella vulgaris* and *Senecio scandens* have been explored by these two methods (Liu and Ng, 2000; Ryu *et al.*, 2002; Yoshikawa *et al.*, 2000). On the other hand, metal ion-induced lipid peroxidation and radical-induced red blood cell haemolysis are two well-established *in vitro* models using biomolecules as protective targets (Miki *et al.*, 1987; Kikugawa *et al.*, 1992; Lau *et al.*, 2002; Sugiyama *et al.*, 1993; Teng *et al.*, 1996). For *in vivo* models, levels of endogenous antioxidant enzymes such as superoxide dismutase (SOD), glutathione peroxidase (GSH-Px), catalase and glucose-6-phosphate dehydrogenase (G6PDH) can reflect the antioxidant status of animals (Eder *et al.*, 2002). *Herba Epimedii*, a traditional Yang invigorating Chinese herb, has been demonstrated to significantly increase superoxide dismutase (SOD) and glutathione peroxidase (GSH-Px) activities in aged mice (Zeng *et al.*, 1997). In the previous decade, there have been a number of projects to develop genetically-modified animals for relevant investigation between oxidative stress and diseases, and the mechanistic studies of the antioxidant effect of potential drugs. For examples, the nematode *Caenorhabditis elegans* with single gene mutant — *aga-1* and the transgenic *Drosophila melanogaster* on both cytosolic and mitochondrial forms of SOD can, more or less, demonstrate the free radical theory of ageing (Larsen, 1993; Parkes *et al.*, 1998; Sun *et al.*, 2002; Sun and Tower, 1999; Vanfleteren, 1993). On the other hand, superoxide dismutase-2 (SOD-2) nullizygous mouse can act as a model to screen the efficacy of potential herbs. Due to the absence of the gene for SOD-2, this strain of mice normally die at the age of about one week. If the herb is effective, it may extent the lifespan of the mice (Melov *et al.*, 1998; Melov *et al.*, 2001).

5.5.2 *Anti-hyperlipidaemia and anti-atherosclerosis*

Hyperlipidaemia is a common problem for people who are adopting to the Western style of living. It can initiate a series of vascular events that results in atherosclerosis (Lusis, 2000). Hyperlipidemia generally refers to high level of blood lipids such as triglyceride (TG) and cholesterol. In the serum, cholesterol is carried by very low-density lipoprotein (VLDL), low-density lipoprotein (LDL) and high-density lipoprotein (HDL). The content of serum LDL and HDL are crucial factors in determining the atherosclerosis index. LDL is termed as "bad" cholesterol while HDL is termed as "good" cholesterol. The atherosclerosis index (Mertz, 1980), expressed as the LDL-cholesterol : HDL-cholesterol ratio, is used to determine whether a patient is susceptible to heart disease. For serious cases where a patient has high LDL-cholesterol : HDL-cholesterol ratio, a controlled low-fat diet or medical treatment will be prescribed in preventing the development of other diseases such as myocardial infarction and unstable angina.

High LDL-cholesterol in the bloodstream can induce an inflammatory response, which causes a series of vascular events and results in the development of atheroma in the main blood vessel, e.g. the aorta.

Enlargement of atheroma size can lead to partial or complete blockage in the blood vessels. If the blood supply is obstructed by atheroma in the essential organs of the body, it may be lethal to the patient. Stroke, myocardial infarction and angina are the obvious clinical syndromes.

The inflammatory response includes the accumulation of modified lipid, mainly the oxidised low-density lipoprotein (oxLDL). oxLDL can exert oxidative stress to the blood vessel, thus leading to vascular endothelial cell dysfunction and activation. oxLDL seems to play an essential role in the development of atherosclerosis. Activation of endothelial cell by oxLDL can lead to an increased expression of adhesion molecules. Adhesion molecules can initiate inflammatory cells such as macrophages migration and activation that in turn, cause smooth muscle cells recruitment and proliferation (Ozer *et al.*, 1993). This inflammatory response can result in the development of atheroma/atherosclerosis. Furthermore, dysfunction of endothelial cell can lower the expression and activity of nitric oxide synthase (NOS), which results in depletion of nitric oxide (NO) in regulating vascular tone (Liao *et al.*, 1995). Anti-oxidants isolated from natural plant, herbs or traditional Chinese medicine, such as *Rhus verniciflua* and green tea have been found to prevent LDL oxidation (Ryu, 2000; Luo *et al.*, 1997). They are claimed to have anti-atherosclerosis properties.

The most important effector cell involved in the development of atherosclerosis is vascular endothelial cell. Circulating LDL or oxLDL can increase the expression of intracellular adhesion molecule-1 (ICAM-1), vascular cell adhesion molecule-1 (VCAM-1), monocyte chemoattractant protein-1 (MCP-1), macrophage colony stimulating factor (M-CSF), etc. ICAM-1 and VCAM-1 are endothelial expression molecules (Takei *et al.*, 2001; Verma *et al.*, 2002) used to recruit monocytes into the vascular intimal layer. MCP-1 and M-CSF are responsible for the differentiation from monocyte into macrophage, and proliferation of macrophage. Cytokines and growth factors secreted by macrophage and T-cells are important for smooth muscle cell (SMC) migration, proliferation and extracelluar matrix production. Foam cell formation through engulfing of oxLDL by macrophage plus migrated SMC to intimal site causes formation of atheroma and results in acute thrombosis and clinical syndrome such as myocardial infarction. Some active components in

Chinese medicine have been found to alleviate the expression of adhesion molecule such as baicalein from *Scutellaria baicalensis Radix* (Kimura *et al.*, 2001).

Anti-hyperlipidaemia or anti-atherosclerosis animal models are induced by diet supplement with fat or/and cholesterol. Golden Syrian hamster is chosen for these models because of its similar lipoprotein profile to human. However, some researchers prefer to use rat, as it is easier and more common to handle. For study of vascular biology, New Zealand rabbit is more suitable because its blood vessel is larger for visualisation after staining with Sudan III dye. Chinese medicine extract such as *Puerariae Radix* has been found to lower the triglyceride and cholesterol content in plasma as compared to the control group (Lee *et al.*, 1999).

5.3.3 *Cardio-tonic*

Heart disease is the leading cause of death around the world. In the U.S., it caused 710,760 deaths in 2000 (*http://www.cdc.gov/nchs/fastats/heart.htm*). In Hong Kong, 5087 people died from this disease in 2002 (*http://www.info.gov.hk/censtatd/eng/hkstat/hkinf/health/health_2_index.html*). For a patient with coronary artery disease, percutaneous transluminal coronary angioplasty (PTCA) or balloon inflation is always applied to tackle the problem. However, free radicals will be generated when the blood vessel is re-opened for blood flow restoration, resulting in the so-called ischaemia-reperfusion (IR) injury. Therefore, it is vital to screen herbal preparation or compound that can prevent IR-induced cardiac damage. In order to mimic the situation of PTCA in laboratory, Langendorff apparatus can be employed. It is a well-designed apparatus for *ex vivo* heart experiments. Heart excised from cervical-dislocated rat is immediately attached onto the Langendorff apparatus. As usual, Kreb's solution is applied to provide normal physiological environment for the heart. After a period of equilibration time, ischaemia can be induced by cutting off the flow of Kreb's solution and reperfusion can be introduced by restoring the buffer flow. Generally speaking, 30-minute ischaemia and 40-minute reperfusion is sufficient for injury induction and parameter monitoring. Coronary flow rate, contractile force, level of creatine kinase (CK) and lactate dehydrogenase (LD) in perfusate are usually measured (Ko and Yiu, 2001; Li *et al.*, 1000; Margreiter *et al.*, 2002). It has been reported that some Chinese medicines, formulae and/or their active components can protect isolated rat heart from ischaemia-reperfusion injury. For example, *Radix Stephaniae* tetrandrae, its compound tetrandrine, and magnolol extracted from *Magnolia officinalis* exhibited ameliorating effects on arrhythmia and infarct induced by ischaemia and reperfusion (Lee *et al.*, 2001; Yu *et al.*, 2001). On the other hand, Sheng-Mei-San, a traditional Chinese prescription consisting of *Radix Ginseng*, *Radix Ophiopogonis* and *Fructus Schisandrae*, can improve post-ischaemic myocardial dysfunction through the opening of the mitochondrial K^+-ATP channels (Wang *et al.*, 2002).

Apart from anti-IR efficacy, herbs' vasodilation and anti-hypertension effects in preventing/treating cardiac diseases are also of interest to many scientists. For the vasodilation model, the aorta is a good target site for investigation. Incubated in an organ bath with 95% O_2 and 5% CO_2 gassing, the aorta segment can be pre-contracted by noradrenaline (NA), 5-hydroxytryptamine (5-HT), phenylephrine or by the thromboxane mimetic U46619 (Amerini *et al.*, 1997; Wylam *et al.*, 2001). Relaxation of the aorta after adding the sample can be recorded in the computer system through force-displacement transducers. Dehydroevodiamine isolated from *Evodia rutaecarpa*, tetrandrine from *Stephania tetrandra*, tetramethylpyrazine from *Ligusticum chuanxiong*, and leonurine from *Leonurus* species have been demonstrated to possess vasodilation effects (Chen and Kwan, 2001; Chiou *et al.*, 1996; Kwan *et al.*, 1999; Tsai *et al.*, 2002). On the other hand, spontaneously hypertensive rats (SHR) are usually employed in an anti-hypertension assay. Change in blood pressure is a simple and direct index for evaluating the potency of target herbs. The extract of *Clerodendron trichotomum* can lower the blood pressure of SHR after an acute or chronic treatment (Lu *et al.*, 1994). Also, cell growth, proliferation, and the Ca^{2+} influx of cultured smooth muscle cells can be investigated (Lee *et al.*, 2001; Zhao *et al.*, 2001).

5.5.4 *Anti-diabetics*

Diabetes mellitus can be divided into two types. Type 1 diabetes is primarily due to autoimmune-mediated destruction of pancreatic β-cell islets, resulting in an absolute insulin deficiency. Patients with type 1 diabetes must take exogenous insulin for survival. Therefore, type 1 diabetes is also called insulin-dependent diabetes mellitus (IDDM). On the other hand, type 2 diabetes is characterised by insulin resistance or secretion deficiency developed in different kinds of cell. Exogenous insulin administration is not essential for treatment. Thus, type 2 diabetes is named as non-insulin-dependent diabetes mellitus (NIDDM). Research on anti-diabetic drugs mainly focuses on NIDDM because it accounts for over 90% of the diabetics cases globally (Zimmet et al., 2001). Neonatal-streptozotocin (STZ) model is a well-established animal model for anti-diabetic drug screening. Wistar rats at zero, two or five days old are intraperitoneally injected with STZ at the dosage of 100 mg/kg, 90 mg/kg and 70 mg/kg, respectively. When they become matured, NIDDM can be developed which is reflected by the elevation of basal plasma glucose, glucose intolerance and insufficient insulin release in response to glucose (Blondel *et al.*, 1989; Portha and Serradas, 1991). In 1998, Masiello and colleagues developed a new experimental NIDDM model. Intraperitoneal administration of nicotinamide 15 minutes before intravenous injection of STZ can induce NIDDM in adult rats (Masiello *et al.*, 1998). Basal glycaemia test and anti-hyperglycaemia test (such as oral glucose tolerance test, OGTT) can be carried out in these two animal models to investigate the anti-diabetic effects of potential herbs (Murali and Goyal, 2001). *Aloe vera* and *Andrographis paniculata* were shown to possess an anti-diabetic effect in rats (Okyar *et al.*, 2001; Zhang and Tan, 2000). Also, liuwei dihuang decoction and its compositions including *Radix Rehmanniae*, *Fructus Corni*, *Cortex Moutan*, *Rhizoma Dioscoreae*, *Poria* and *Rhizoma Alismatis* can reduce blood sugar level in mice (Liu *et al.*, 1991). To evaluate blood glucose lowering mechanisms in detail, several assays can be employed. Glucose transport and level of glucose transporter in red blood cells and adipocytes can be determined (Enrique-Tarancon *et al.*, 1998; Whitehead *et al.*, 2001). Glucose metabolism such as gluconeogenesis can also be studied by using H4IIE cell lines (Lochhead *et al.*, 2000; Wang *et al.*, 2000). Lastly, glucose uptake from the gut can be shown from the brush border membrane vesicle (BBMV) assay (Hopfer *et al.*, 1973; Semenza *et al.*, 1984).

5.5.5 *Anti-tumour*

Nowadays, many people are aware of the possibility of herbs in treating cancers. Their anti-tumour effects can be examined both *in vitro* and *in vivo*. Human cancer cell lines have the advantage of maintaining its biological stability and rapidly reproducing a large quantity of cells; therefore, it has been widely used for studying cancer biology. American Tissue Culture Collection (ATCC) holds over 950 cancer cell lines from different organs and species. The most challenging and difficult step is to generate normal cell line models to compare with cancer cells. Normal human cell lines are generated from specific cell types that are isolated from a primary fresh tissue. At the same time, the primary culture has limited cycles of cell division. The successful immortalisation of primary cells with telomerase is a breakthrough. These primary cells stably express exogenous human telomerase reverse transcriptase (hTERT), which allow the cells to divide indefinitely while retaining their normal phenotype and function (Bodnar *et al.*, 1998; Jiang *et al.*, 1999; Morales *et al.*, 1999). The *in vitro* effect of herbal products can be assessed by inhibition of the proliferation of human cancer cell lines with growth inhibition assay (Siu *et al.*, 2002) or ^{3}H-thymidine incorporation assay (Mak *et al.*, 1996). For example, 15 Tanshinone analogues isolated from the chloroform extract of Danshen roots (*Salviae Miltiorrhizae Radix*) by chromatographic procedures have been tested for their cytotoxic activities against KB, Hela, Colo-205 and Hep-2 carcinoma cell lines. Several of them were effective at concentrations below 1 g/ml (Wu *et al.*, 1991). *In vivo* studies involved the study of anti-tumour effect of the herbal formula on the mouse tumour bearing Balb/c mice via stimulation of the immune system. *In vivo* studies also direct cytotoxic effect of herbal products on human tumour-bearing athymic nude mice. Size, weight or number of tumour cells (e.g. sarcoma SC-181 or Ehrlich Ascites Tumour (EAT) cell), subcutaneously inoculated into Balb/c mice, can be measured before and after treatment of herbal products (Kim *et al.*, 2003). Modulation in immune system can be studied in plasma or splenocytes (Wong *et al.*, 1994). In nude mice model, direct cytoxicity effect on human tumour cells, e.g. human hepatoma HepG2 cells, bearing in nude mice was studied (Wang *et al.*, 2003). Recently, genetically engineered mouse models introduce a new source of tumour model. Transgenic mice expressing oncogene or mice with tumour suppressor gene knockout develop tumour autonomously. A collection of these genetically engineered mouse tumour models is available in The Jackson Laboratory (*http://www.jax.org/*).

5.5.6 *Immuno-modulatory*

Herbal products that possess immune-stimulation properties may be useful in preventing and reducing the risk of cancer. Several biochemical parameters are available to measure the immune response of the mice after treating with herbal products. These parameters included proliferation of T-lymphocytes and macrophage (Nose *et al.*, 1998), detection of lymphocyte surface antigen, nitric oxide (NO) production (Yamaoka *et al.*, 1996), and secretion of different types of cytokines (Choi *et al.*, 2001). T-cell proliferation can be measured by tritiated thymidine uptake assay (George *et al.*, 2003). To detect CD antigen (such as CD3, CD4, CD8, etc.), flow cytometry technology was applied (van Overtvelt *et al.*, 2002). The level of cytokine secretion by splenocytes is a good indicator in monitoring the immune response against the herbal product (Yang *et al.*, 2002). For example, Chang and colleagues studied the stimulating effect of *Radix aconiti* extracts on cytokine secretion (Chang *et al.*, 1994).

5.5.7 *Anti-inflammation*

Nitric oxide (NO) is released during inflammation and it serves as a marker for inflammatory responses. Lipopolysaccharide (LPS)-stimulated macrophage cell line with detection of NO production is one of the *in vitro* models used to identify anti-inflammatory potential substances (Ismaili *et al.*, 2002; Kim *et al.*, 2000). There are several inflammatory animal models for different degrees and types of inflammatory responses. Carrageenan-induced paw oedema represents an acute *in vitro* model. A suspension of carrageenan is injected subcutaneously into the hind-paw of rat, and the volume of the hind-paw is measured in order to assess the degree of inflammatory response. Formation of cotton pellet induced-granuloma is a sub-acute *in vitro* model. A sterile cotton pellet is implanted subcutaneously into the shoulder of rats. Then, together with the granuloma, the cotton pellet was removed for measurement of granuloma formation. Acetic acid-induced writhing test can also be used where a 0.7% dilution of acetic acid (v/v) is injected intraperitoneally, and the number of writhes induced by acetic acid solution is counted. Freund's adjuvant induced-arthritis can be used as a chronic model of inflammation (Khanna and Sharma 2001; Ozaki *et al.*, 1997; Shimizu *et al.*, 1986). Besides the route of induction mentioned above, inflammation can be artificially caused by topical application of croton oil on mice ear (Segura *et al.*, 1998; Tubaro *et al.*, 1985). At the end of the experiment, standard size ear plugs are removed with stainless steel punch for weight measurement and comparison. All of these models are commonly used to evaluate the anti-inflammatory activity of experimental substances.

5.5.8 *Anti-osteoporosis*

Osteoporosis is the second most important health problem for women after breast cancer. It happens as a result of an imbalance between bone resorption and formation. The most current therapies for bone disease treatment target the bone-resorption systems. The anti-resorbing agents, including bisphosphonates, oestrogen, selective oestrogen receptor modulators (SERMs) and calcitonin are the mainstream. However, all these agents are associated with side effects, such as increased rate of breast cancer, vaginal bleeding, endometrial hyperplasia, endometrial carcinoma or vasomotor symptoms. This has led to more patients turning towards specific drugs and alternative medicine. Ovariectomised (OVX) ten-month-old SD rats are used as the standard post-menopausal osteoporosis model (Fung and Wang, 1998). This model was used to study the efficacy of herbal medicine on the treatment or prevention of osteoporosis (Chae *et al.*, 2001; Hidaka *et al.*, 1999; Noguchi *et al.*, 2003; Prabhakara Reddy and Lakshmana, 2003; Xu and Prince, 2003). Bone mineral density, histomorphometry and biomechanical strength of femur, tibia and spine are usually used to indicate the severity of osteoporosis. Bone mineral density can be non-invasively detected by X-ray absorptiometry or quantitative computed tomography (pQCT). When working with pQCT, specific sites at tibia and the vertebrate of mature OVX rat are suitable for bone mineral density analysis in terms of consistent reproducibility of measurement. For tibia, measurement line is set at 5 mm, 5.5 mm, 13 mm and 15 mm from the knee joint. For vertebrate, measurement line is set at 3 mm and 4 mm from the proximal of L4 vertebrate. Bone formation markers, such as bone-specific alkaline phosphatase and osteocalcin; and bone resorption markers, such as urine deoxypyridine and deoxypyridinoline, are often used to indicate the bone turnover in rat.

5.5.9 *Anti-SARS associated coronavirus*

Recently, Severe Acute Respiratory Syndrome (SARS) has become a global health hazard. Since there is no effective prevention and treatment of SARS, agents against this disease is urgently needed. Developing a Western drug to inhibit the SARS coronavirus with established safety data may take many years. Yet, herbal medicine may provide a good form of prevention and treatment, since herbal products have been used for a long time to prevent infectious diseases like influenza. Hence, a possible quick strategy to fight against SARS is to consider the development of herbal formulae. Screening potential herbal extract to test for direct growth-inhibiting effect on the coronavirus *in vitro* may provide sound preliminary of scientific evidence for further herbal formula development. Recently, Glycyrrhizin, an active component of liquorice roots was found to have an inhibitory effect on the replication of the SARS-associated virus in cell culture (Cinatl *et al.*, 2003). Yet, *in vitro* assay in inhibiting the growth of SARS virus in monkeys' kidney cell culture can only be carried out in laboratory with biosafety level 3. *In vitro* assay to inhibit SARS coronaviral 3CL-^{Pro} proteinase (Anand *et al.*, 2003) and RNA-dependent RNA polymerases Ackermann and Padmanabhan (2001) should be two quick and safe models for screening potential herbs that exhibit anti-SARS coronavirus effect.

5.6 Conclusion

Since the chemical components in herbs are very complicated, the study of quality control methods and drug actions in herbs is a challenging area. This chapter not only provides an outline of those essential purity and toxicity tests for herbs; it also provides a review of current modern techniques for studying herbs. HPLC, DNA fingerprint and DNA microarray technologies can be used to identify and control the quality of raw herbs and/or herbal finished product. Many *in vitro*/*in vivo* disease models had been used to study the therapeutic efficacies and drug actions of herbs. The modern biochemistry technologies are indispensable for finding out scientific evidences for the development of herbal medicine.

References

Ackermann, M. and Padmanabhan, R. (2001) *De novo* synthesis of RNA by the dengue virus RNA-dependent RNA polymerase exhibits temperature dependence at the initiation but not elongation phase. *J. Biol Chem.* **276**, 39926–39937.

Amerini, S., Filippi, S., Parenti, A., Ledda, F. and Ziche, M. (1997) Vasorelaxant effects induced by the antiangiogenic drug linomide in aortic and saphenous vein preparations of the rabbit. *Br. J. Pharmacol.* **122**, 1739–1745.

Anand, K., Ziebuhr, J., Wadhwani, P., Mesters, J.R. and Hilgenfeld, R. (2003) Coronavirus main proteinase (3CLpro) structure: basis for design of anti-SARS drugs. *Science* **13**, 13.

Blondel, O., Bailbe, D. and Portha, B. (1989) Relation of insulin deficiency to impaired insulin action in NIDDM adult rats given streptozocin as neonates. *Diabetes* **38**, 610–617.

Bodnar, A.G., Ouellette, M., Frolkis, M., Holt, S.E., Chiu, C.P., Morin, G.B., Harley, C.B., Shay, J.W., Lichtsteiner, S. and Wright, W.E. (1998) Extension of life-span by introduction of telomerase into normal human cells. *Science* **279**, 349–352.

Carles, M., Lee, T., Moganti, S., Lenigk, R., Tsim, K.W., Ip, N.Y., Hsing, I.M. and Sucher, N.J. (2001) Chips and Qi: microcomponent-based analysis in traditional Chinese medicine. Fresenius. *J. Anal. Chem.* **371**, 190–194.

Chae, H.J., Kang, J.S., Kim, J.H., Kim, C.W., Yoo, S.K., Shin, T.Y., Choi, B., Kim, H.M. and Kim, H.R. (2001) Antiosteoporotic activity of Dae-Bo-Won-Chun in ovariectomized rats. *Phytother Res.* **15**, 53–57.

Chang, J.G., Shih, P.P., Chang, C.P., Chang, J.Y., Wang, F.Y. and Tseng, J. (1994) The stimulating effect of *Radix aconiti* extract on cytokines secretion by human mononuclear cells. *Planta Med.* **60**, 576–578.

Chen, C.X. and Kwan, C.Y. (2001) Endothelium-independent vasorelaxation by leonurine, a plant alkaloid purified from Chinese motherwort. *Life Sci.* **68**, 953–960.

Chiou, W.F., Liao, J.F., Shum, A.Y. and Chen, C.F. (1996) Mechanisms of vasorelaxant effect of dehydroevodiamine: a bioactive isoquinazolinocarboline alkaloid of plant origin. *J. Cardiovasc. Pharmacol.* **27**, 845–853.

Choi, C.Y., Kim, J.Y., Kim, Y.S., Chung, Y.C., Hahm, K. and Jeong, H.G. (2001) Augmentation of macrophage functions by an aqueous extract isolated from Platycodon grandiflorum. *Cancer Lett.* **166**, 17–25.

Cinatl, J., Morgenstern, B., Bauer, G., Chandra, P., Rabenau, H. and Doerr, H.W. (2003) Glycyrrhizin, an active component of liquorice roots, and replication of SARS-associated coronavirus. *Lancet* **361**, 2045–2046.

Downes, F.P. and Ito, K. (eds.) (2001) *Compendium of Methods for the Microbiological Examination of Foods*, 4th Ed. American Public Health Association, Washington, D.C.

Dudkiewicz-Wilczynska, J., Snycerski, A. and Tautt, J. (2002) Application of high-performance size exclusion chromatography to the determination of erythropoietin in pharmaceutical preparations. *Acta Pol. Pharm.* **59**, 83–86.

Eder, K., Flader, D., Hirche, F. and Brandsch, C. (2002) Excess dietary vitamin E lowers the activities of antioxidative enzymes in erythrocytes of rats fed salmon oil. *J. Nutr.* **132**, 3400–3404.

Enrique-Tarancon, G., Marti, L., Morin, N., Lizcano, J.M., Unzeta, M., Sevilla, L., Camps, M., Palacin, M., Testar, X., Carpene, C. and Zorzano, A. (1998) Role of Semicarbazide-sensitive amine oxidase on glucose transport and GLUT4 recruitment to the cell surface in adipose cells. *J. Biol. Chem.* **273**(14), 8025–8032.

Fung, K. and Wang, J.Z. (1998) *Osteoporotic Animal Experimental Models.* (Eds.) Liu. Science Publisher, Beijing, China,.pp. 501–511.

George, J., Greenberg, S., Barshack, I., Goldberg, I., Keren, G. and Roth, A. (2003) Immunity to heat shock protein 65-an additional determinant in intimal thickening. *Atherosclerosis* **168**, 33–38.

Ha, W.Y., Shaw, P.C., Liu, J., Yau, F.C. and Wang, J. (2002) Authentication of *Panax ginseng* and *Panax quinquefolius* using amplified fragment length polymorphism (AFLP) and directed amplification of minisatellite region DNA (DAMD). *J. Agric. Food Chem.* **50**, 1871–1875.

Hidaka, S., Okamoto, Y., Yamada, Y., Kon, Y. and Kimura, T. (1999) A Japanese herbal medicine, Chujo-to, has a beneficial effect on osteoporosis in rats. *Phytother Res.* **13**, 14–19.

Hopfer, U., Nelson, K., Perrotto, J. and Isselbacher, K.J. (1973) Glucose transport in isolated brush border membrane from rat small intestine. *J. Biol. Chem.* **248**, 25–32.

International Conference on Harmonisation of Technical Requirements for Registration of Pharmaceuticals for Human Use (ICH) (1994) *S5A Detection of Toxicity to Reproduction for Medicinal Products* (issued 9/1994, posted 4/23/1997).

International Conference on Harmonisation of Technical Requirements for Registration of Pharmaceuticals for Human Use (ICH) (1997) *S5B Detection of Toxicity to Reproduction for Medicinal Products: Addendum on Toxicity to Male Fertility.*

International Conference on Harmonisation of Technical Requirements for Registration of Pharmaceuticals for Human Use (ICH) (1996) *ICH Topic Q1B Stability Testing of New Drug Substances and Products.*

International Conference on Harmonisation of Technical Requirements for Registration of Pharmaceuticals for Human Use (ICH) (1997) *M3 Nonclinical Safety Studies for the Conduct of Human Clinical Trials for Pharmaceuticals* (issued 11/1997, posted 11/25/1997).

International Conference on Harmonisation of Technical Requirements for Registration of Pharmaceuticals for Human Use (ICH) (1997) *S2B Genotoxicity: A Standard Battery for Genotoxicity Testing of Pharmaceuticals* (issued 11/21/1997, posted 5/4/1998).

International Conference on Harmonisation of Technical Requirements for Registration of Pharmaceuticals for Human Use (ICH) (1997) *S1C(R) Guidance on Dose Selection for Carcinogenicity Studies of Pharmaceuticals: Addendum on a Limit Dose and Related Notes* (issued 12/4/1997, posted 12/11/1997).

International Conference on Harmonisation of Technical Requirements for Registration of Pharmaceuticals for Human Use (ICH) (1998) *S1B Testing for Carcinogenicity of Pharmaceuticals* (issued 2/28/1998, posted 3/24/1998).

Ismaili, H., Sosa, S., Brkic, D., Fkih-Tetouani, S., Ilidrissi, A., Touati, D., Aquino, R.P. and Tubaro, A. (2002) Topical anti-inflammatory activity of extracts and compounds from *Thymus broussonettii*. *J. Pharm. Pharmacol.* **54**, 1137–1140.

Jiang, X.R., Jimenez, G., Chang, E., Frolkis, M., Kusler, B., Sage, M., Beeche, M., Bodnar, A.G., Wahl, G.M., Tlsty, T.D. and Chiu, C.P. (1999) Telomerase expression in human somatic cells does not induce changes associated with a transformed phenotype. *Nat. Genet.* **21**, 111–114.

Jung, Y.S., Kang, T.S., Yoon, J.H., Joe, B.Y., Lim, H.J., Seong, C.M., Park, W.K., Kong, J.Y., Cho, J. and Park, N.S. (2002) Synthesis and evaluation of 4-hydroxyphenylacetic acid amides and 4-hydroxycinnamamides as antioxidants. *Bioorg. Med. Chem. Lett.* **12**, 2599–2602.

Khanna, N. and Sharma, S.B. (2001) Anti-inflammatory and analgesic effect of herbal preparation: septilin. *Indian J. Med. Sci.* **55**, 195–202.

Kikugawa, K., Kojima, T., Yamaki, S. and Kosugi, H. (1992) Interpretation of the thiobarbituric acid reactivity of rat liver and brain homogenates in the presence of ferric ion and ethylenediaminetetraacetic acid. *Anal. Biochem.* **202**, 249–255.

Kim, H.J., Mun, J.Y., Chun, Y.J., Choi, K.H., Ham, S.W. and Kim, M.Y. (2003) Effects of a naphthoquinone analogue on tumour growth and apoptosis induction. *Arch. Pharm. Res.* **26**, 405–410.

Kim, Y.H., Ko, W.S., Ha, M.S., Lee, C.H., Choi, B.T., Kang, H.S. and Kim, H.D. (2000) The production of nitric oxide and TNF-alpha in peritoneal macrophages is inhibited by *Dichroa febrifuga* Lour. *J. Ethnopharmacol.* **69**, 35–43.

Kimura, Y., Matsushita, N., Yokoi-Hayashi, K. and Okuda, H. (2001) Effects of baicalein isolated from Scutellaria baicalensis Radix on adhesion molecule expression induced by thrombin and thrombin receptor agonist peptide in cultured human umbilical vein endothelial cells. *Planta Med.* **67**(4), 331–334.

Ko, K.M. and Yiu, H.Y. (2001) Schisandrin B modulates the ischaemia-reperfusion induced changes in non-enzymatic antioxidant levels in isolated-perfused rat hearts. *Mol. Cell. Biochem.* **220**, 141–147.

Kwan, C.Y., Ma, F.M. and Hui, S.C.G. (1999) Inhibition of endothelium-dependent vascular relaxation by tetrandrine. *Life Sci.* **64**, 2391–2400.

Lahousen, T., Roller, R.E., Lipp, R.W. and Schnedl, W.J. (2002) Silent haemoglobin variants and determination of HbA(1c) with the HPLC Bio-Rad Variant II. *J. Clin. Pathol.* **55**, 699–703.

Larsen, P.L. (1993) Aging and resistance to oxidative damage in *Caenorhabditis elegans*. *Proc. Natl. Acad. Sci. U.S.A.* **90**, 8905–8909.

Lau, D.T., Shaw, P.C., Wang, J. and But, P.P. (2001) Authentication of medicinal *Dendrobium* species by the internal transcribed spacer of ribosomal DNA. *Planta Med.* **67**, 456–460.

Lau, K.M., He, Z.D., Dong, H., Fung, K.P. and But, P.P. (2002) Anti-oxidative, anti-inflammatory and hepato-protective effects of *Ligustrum robustum*. *J. Ethnopharmacol.* **83**, 63–71.

Lee, C.N., Wong, K.L., Liu, J.C., Chen, Y.J., Cheng, J.T. and Chan, P. (2001) Inhibitory effect of stevioside on calcium influx to produce antihypertension. *Planta Med.* **67**, 796–799.

Lee, J.S., Lee, K.H. and Jeong, J.H. (1999) Effects of extract of *Puerariae radix* on lipid metabolism in rats fed high rat diet. *J. Korean Soc. Food Sci. Nutr.* **28**(1), 218–224.

Lee, S.M., Li, M.L., Tse, Y.C., Leung, S.C., Lee, M.M., Tsui, S.K., Fung, K.P., Lee, C.Y. and Waye, M.M. (2002) *Paeoniae Radix*, a Chinese herbal extract, inhibit hepatoma cells growth by inducing apoptosis in a p53 independent pathway. *Life Sci.* **71**, 2267–2277.

Lee, Y.M., Hsiao, G., Chen, H.R., Chen, Y.C., Sheu, J.R. and Yen, M.H. (2001) Magnolol reduces myocardial ischaemia/reperfusion injury via neutrophil inhibition in rats. *Eur. J. Pharmacol.* **422**, 159–167.

Li, F., Hayes, J.K., Wong, K.C. and Szakacs, J. (2000) Administration of sevoflurane and isoflurane prior to prolonged global ischaemia improves heart function in isolated rat heart. *Acta Anaesthesiol. Sinica* **38**, 113–121.

Liao, J.K., Shin, W.S., Lee, W.Y. and Clark, S.L. (1995) Oxidized low-density lipoprotein decreased the expression of endothelial nitric oxide synthase. *J. Biol. Chem.* **270**, 319–324.

Liu, B., Wen, W., Zhu, D. and Jiang, Y. (1991) Effects of liuwei dihuang decoction and its compositions on blood sugar and glycogen in mice. *Zhongguo Zhong Yao Za Zhi* **16**, 437–438, 448 (in Chinese).

Liu, F. and Ng, T.B. (2000) Antioxidative and free radical scavenging activities of selected medicinal herbs. *Life Sci.* **66**, 725–735.

Liu, F., Ooi, V.E.C. and Chang, S.T. (1997) Free radical scavenging activities of mushroom polysaccharide extracts. *Life Sci.* **60**, 763–771.

Lochhead, P.A., Salt, I.P., Walker, K.S., Hardie, D.G. and Sutherland, C. (2000) 5-aminoimidazole-4-carboxamide riboside mimics the effects of insulin on the expression of the 2 key gluconeogenic genes PEPCK and glucose-6-phosphatase. *Diabetes* **49**, 896–903.

Lu, G.W., Miura, K., Yukimura, T. and Yamamoto, K. (1994) Effects of extract from Clerodendron trichotomum on blood pressure and renal function in rats and dogs. *J. Ethnopharmacol.* **42**, 77–82.

Luo, M., Kannar, K., Wahlqvist, M.L. and O'Brien, R.C. (1997) Inhibition of LDL oxidation by green tea extract. *Lancet* **349**(9048), 360–361.

Lusis, A.J. (2000) Atherosclerosis. *Nature* **407**(6801), 233–241.

Mak, N.K., Wong-Leung, Y.L., Chan, S.C., Wen, J., Leung, K.N. and Fung, M.C. (1996) Isolation of anti-leukemia compounds from *Citrus reticulata*. *Life Sci.* **58**, 1269–1276.

Margreiter, J., Mittermayr, M., Mair, J., Hammerer-Lercher, A., Kountchev, J., Klingler, A. and Schobersberger, W. (2002) Influence of antithrombin on ischaemia/reperfusion injury in the isolated blood-free perfused rat heart. *Throm. Res.* **108**, 249–255.

Masiello, P., Broca, C., Gross, R., Roye, M., Manteghetti, M., Hillaire-Buys, D., Novelli, M. and Ribes, G. (1998) Experimental NIDDM. Development of a new model in adult rats administered streptozotocin and nicotinamide. *Diabetes* **47**, 224–229.

Melov, S., Doctrow, S.R., Schneider, J.A., Haberson, J., Patel, M., Coskun, P.E., Huffman, K., Wallace, D.C. and Malfroy, B. (2001) Lifespan extension and rescue of spongiform encephalopathy in superoxide dismutase-2 nullizygous mice treated with superoxide dismutase-catalase mimetics. *J. Neurosci.* **21**, 8348–8353.

Melov, S., Schneider, J.A., Day, B.J., Hinerfeld, D., Coskun, P., Mirra, S.S., Crapo, J.D. and Wallace, D.C. (1998) A novel neurological phenotype in mice lacking mitochondrial manganese superoxide dismutase. *Nat. Genet.* **18**, 159–163.

Mertz, D.P. (1980) "Atherosclerosis-index" (LDL/HDL): risk indicator in lipid metabolism disorders. *Med. Klin.* **75**(4), 159–161.

Miki, M., Tamai, H., Mino, M., Yamamoto, Y. and Niki, E. (1987) Free-radical chain oxidation of rat red blood cells by molecular oxygen and its inhibition by a-tocopherol. *Arch. Biochem. Biophy.* **258**, 373–380.

Montgomery, E.R., Edmanson, A.L., Cook, S.C. and Hovsepian, P.K. (2001) Development and validation of a reverse-phase HPLC method for analysis of efavirenz and its related substances in the drug substance and in a capsule formulation. *J. Pharm. Biomed. Anal.* **25**, 267–284.

Morales, C.P., Holt, S.E., Ouellette, M., Kaur, K.J., Yan, Y., Wilson, K.S., White, M.A., Wright, W.E. and Shay, J.W. (1999) Absence of cancer-associated changes in human fibroblasts immortalized with telomerase. *Nat. Genet.* **21**, 115–118.

Murali, B. and Goyal, R.K. (2001) Improvement in insulin sensitivity by losartan in non-insulin-dependent diabetic (NIDDM) rats. *Pharmacol. Res.* **44**, 385–389.

Nagaraju, J., Kathirvel, M., Kumar, R.R., Siddiq, E.A. and Hasnain, S.E. (2002) Genetic analysis of traditional and evolved Basmati and non-Basmati rice varieties by using fluorescence-based ISSR-PCR and SSR markers. *Proc. Natl. Acad. Sci. U.S.A.* **99**, 5836–5841.

Noguchi, M., Ikarashi, Y., Yuzurihara, M., Kase, Y., Chen, J.T., Takeda, S., Aburada, M. and Ishige, A. (2003) Effects of the Japanese herbal medicine

Keishi-bukuryo-gan and 17β-estradiol on calcitonin gene-related peptide-induced elevation of skin temperature in ovariectomized rats. *J. Endocrinol.* **176**, 359–366.

Nose, M., Terawaki, K., Oguri, K., Ogihara, Y., Yoshimatsu, K. and Shimomura, K. (1998) Activation of macrophages by crude polysaccharide fractions obtained from shoots of *Glycyrrhiza glabra* and hairy roots of *Glycyrrhiza uralensis in vitro. Biol. Pharm. Bull.* **21**, 1110–1112.

Okyar, A., Can, A., Akev, N., Baktir, G. and Sutlupinar, N. (2001) Effect of *Aloe vera* leaves on blood glucose level in type I and type II diabetic rat models. *Phyto. Res.* **15**, 157–161.

Ozaki, Y., Rui, J., Tang, Y. and Satake, M. (1997) Anti-inflammatory effect of *Forsythia suspensa* Vahl and its active fraction. *Biol. Pharm. Bull.* **20**, 861–864.

Ozer, N.K., Palozza, P., Boscoboinik, D. and Azzi, A. (1993) d-a-Tocopherol inhibits low density lipoprotein induced proliferation and protein kinase C activity in vascular smooth muscle cell. *FEBS Lett.* **322**(3), 307–310.

Parkes, T.L., Elia, A.J., Dickinson, D., Hilliker, A.J., Phillips, J.P. and Boulianne, G.L. (1998) Extension of Drosophila lifespan by overexpression of human SOD1 in motorneurons. *Nat. Genet.* **19**, 171–174.

Portha, B. and Serradas, P. (1991) Improvement in glucose-induced insulin secretion in diabetic rats after long-term gliclazide treatment: a comparative study using different models of non-insulin-dependent diabetes mellitus induced by neonatal streptozotocin. *Am. J. Med.* **90**, 15S–21S.

Prabhakara Reddy, N. and Lakshmana, M. (2003) Prevention of bone loss in calcium deficient ovariectonized rats by OST-6, a herbal preparation. *J. Ethnopharmacol.* **84**, 259–264.

Ryu, B.H. (2000) Inhibition of human low density lipoprotein oxidation by extracts from *Rhus verniciflua* strokes. *Food Sci. Biotechnol.* **9**(4), 204–208.

Ryu, G., Ju, J.H., Park, Y.J., Ryu, S.Y., Choi, B.W. and Lee, B.H. (2002) The radical scavenging effects of stilbene glucosides from *Polygonum multiflorum. Arch. Pharm. Res.* **25**, 636–639.

Santosh Kumar, S., Priyadarsini, K.I. and Sainis, K.B. (2002) Free radical scavenging activity of vanillin and o-vanillin using 1,1-diphenyl-2-picrylhydrazyl (DPPH) radical. *Redox Report* **7**, 35–40.

Segura, L., Vila, R., Gupta, M.P., Espósito-Avella, M., Adzet, T. and Canigueral, S. (1998) Anti-inflammatory activity of *Anthurium cerrocampanense* Croat in rats and mice. *J. Ethnopharmacol.* **61**, 243–248.

Semenza, G., Kessler, M., Hosang, M., Weber, J. and Schmidt, U. (1984) Biochemistry of the Na^+, D-glucose cotransporter of the small-intestinal brush-border membrane. The state of the art in 1984. *Biochim. Biophys. Acta* **779**, 343–379.

Shaw, P.C. and But, P.P. (1995) Authentication of *Panax* species and their adulterants by random-primed polymerase chain reaction. *Planta Med.* **61**, 466–469.

Shimizu, M., Fukumura, H., Tsuji, H., Tanaami, S., Hayashi, T. and Morita, N. (1986) Anti-inflammatory constituents of topically applied crude drugs. I. Constituents and anti-inflammatory effect of *Eriobotrya japonica* LINDL. *Chem. Pharm. Bull. (Tokyo)* **34**, 2614–2617.

Shimoji, Y., Tamura, Y., Nakamura, Y., Nanda, K., Nishidai, S., Nishikawa, Y., Ishihara, N., Uenakai, K. and Ohigashi, H. (2002) Isolation and identification of DPPH radical scavenging compounds in Kurosu (Japanese unpolished rice vinegar). *J. Agric. Food Chem.* **50**, 6501–6503.

Siu, K.P.Y., Chan, J.Y.W. and Fung, K.P. (2002) Effect of arsenic trioxide on human hepatocellular carcinoma HepG2 cells: inhibition of proliferation and induction of apoptosis. *Life Sci.* **71**, 275–285.

Sugiyama, H., Fung, K.P. and Wu, T.W. (1993) Purpurogallin as an antioxidant protector of human erythrocytes against lysis by peroxyl radicals. *Life Sci.* **53**, PL39–43.

Sun, J. and Tower, J. (1999) FLP recombinase-mediated induction of Cu/Zn-superoxide dismutase transgene expression can extend the life span of adult *Drosophila melanogaster* flies. *Mol. Cell Biol.* **19**, 216–228.

Sun, J., Folk, D., Bradley, T.J. and Tower, J. (2002) Induced overexpression of mitochondrial Mn-superoxide dismutase extends the life span of adult *Drosophila melanogaster. Genet.* **161**, 661–672.

Takei, A., Huang, Y. and Lopes-Virella, M.F. (2001) Expression of adhesion molecules by human endothelial cells exposed to oxidized low density lipoprotein. Influences of degree of oxidation and location of oxidized LDL. *Atherosclerosis* **154**, 79–86.

Teng, C.M., Hsiao, G.., Ko, F.N., Lin, D.T. and Lee, S.S. (1996) N-allylsecoboldine as a novel antioxidant against peroxidative damage. *Euro. J. Pharmacol.* **303**, 129–139.

Tochika-Komatsu, Y., Asaka, I. and Ii, I. (2001) A random amplified polymorphic DNA (RAPD) primer to assist the identification of a selected strain, aizu K-111 of *Panax ginseng* and the sequence amplified. *Biol. Pharm. Bull.* **24**, 1210–1213.

Tsai, C.C., Lai, T.Y., Huang, W.C., Liu, I.M. and Cheng, J.T. (2002) Inhibitory effects of potassium channel blockers on tetramethylpyrazine-induced relaxation of rat aortic strip *in vitro*. *Life Sci.* **71**, 1321–1330.

Tubaro, A., Dri, P., Delbello, G., Zilli, C. and Loggia, R.D. (1985) The croton oil ear test revisited. *Agents Actions* **17**, 347–349.

van Noorden, C.J.F. and Butcher, R.G. (1989) The involvement of superoxide anions in the nitro blue tetrazolium chloride reduction mediated by NADH and phenazine methosulfate. *Anal. Biochem.* **176**, 170–174.

van Overtvelt, L., Andrieu, M., Verhasselt, V., Connan, F., Choppin, J., Vercruysse, V., Goldman, M., Hosmalin, A. and Vray, B. (2002) *Trypanosoma cruzi* down-regulates lipopolysaccharide-induced MHC class I on human dendritic cells and impairs antigen presentation to specific CD8(+) T lymphocytes. *Int. Immunol.* **14**, 1135–1144.

Vanfleteren, J.R. (1993) Oxidative stress and ageing in *Caenorhabditis elegans*. *Biochem. J.* **292**, 605–608.

Verma, S., Li, S.H., Badiwala, M.V., Weisel, R.D., Fedak, P.W., Li, R.K., Dhillon, B. and Mickle, D.A. (2002) Endothelin antagonism and interleukin-6 inhibition attenuate the proatherogenic effects of C-reactive protein. *Circulation* **105**(16), 1890–1896.

Wang, J., Ha, W.Y., Ngan, F.N., But, P.P. and Shaw, P.C. (2001) Application of sequence characterized amplified region (SCAR) analysis to authenticate *Panax* species and their adulterants. *Planta Med.* 67, 781–783.

Wang, J.C., Stafford, J.M., Scott, D.K., Sutherland, C. and Granner, D.K. (2000) The molecular physiology of hepatic nuclear factor 3 in the regulation of gluconeogenesis. *J. Biol. Chem.* **275**, 14717–14721.

Wang, N., Minatoguchi, S., Arai, M., Uno, Y., Nishida, Y., Hashimoto, K., Xue-Hai, C., Fukuda, K., Akao, S., Takemura, G. and Fujiwara, H. (2002) Sheng-Mai-San is protective against post-ischaemic myocardial dysfunction in rats through its opening of the mitochondrial KATP channels. *Circul. J.* **66**, 763–768.

Wang, Y.Q., Ugai, S., Shimozato, O., Yu, L., Kawamura, K., Yamamoto, H., Yamaguchi, T., Saisho, H. and Tagawa, M. (2003) Induction of systemic immunity by expression of interleukin-23 in murine colon carcinoma cells. *Int. J. Cancer* **105**, 820–824.

Waring, J.F., Ciurlionis, R., Jolly, R.A., Heindel, M. and Ulrich, R.G. (2001) Microarray analysis of hepatotoxins *in vitro* reveals a correlation between gene expression profiles and mechanisms of toxicity. *Toxicol. Lett.* **120**, 359–368.

Whitehead, J.P., Molero, J.C., Clark, S., Martin, S., Meneilly, G. and James, D.E. (2001) The role of Ca^{2+} in insulin-stimulated glucose transport in 3T3-L1 cells. *J. Biol. Chem.* **276**(30), 27816–27824.

WHO (1993) *Research Guidelines for Evaluating the Safety and Efficacy of the Herbal Medicine.* WHO Regional Office for the Western Pacific, Manila (ISBN-92 9061-110-3).

WHO (1997) *Guideline for Predicting Dietary Intake of Pesticide Residues*, 2nd Revised Ed. World Health Organization, Geneva.

WHO (1998) *Quality Control Methods for Medicinal Plant Materials.* World Health Organization, Geneva.

Wong, C.K., Leung, K.N., Fung, K.P. and Choy, Y.M. (1994) Immunomodulatory and anti-tumour polysaccharides from medicinal plants. *J. Int. Med. Res.* **22**, 299–312.

Wu, W.L., Chang, W.L. and Chen, C.F. (1991) Cytotoxic activities of tanshinones against human carcinoma cell lines. *Am. J. Chin. Med.* **19**, 207–216.

Wylam, M.E., Metkus, A.P. and Umans, J.G. (2001) Nitric oxide dependent and independent effects of *in vitro* incubation or endotoxin on vascular reactivity in rat aorta. *Life Sci.* **69**, 455–467.

Xu, M. and Prince, R.L. (2003) Effects of a herbal extract on the bone density, strength and markers of bone turnover of mature ovariectomized rats. *Am. J. Chin. Med.* **31**, 87–101.

Yamaoka, Y., Kawakita, T., Kaneko, M. and Nomoto, K. (1996) A polysaccharide fraction of *Zizyphi fructus* in augmenting natural killer activity by oral administration. *Biol. Pharm. Bull.* **19**, 936–939.

Yang, S.H., Hong, C.Y. and Yu, C.L. (2002) The stimulatory effects of nasal discharge from patients with perennial allergic rhinitis on normal human neutrophils are normalized after treatment with a new mixed formula of Chinese herbs. *Int. Immunopharmacol.* **2**, 1627–1639.

Yoshikawa, M., Ohta, T., Kawaguchi, A. and Matsuda, H. (2000) Bioactive constituents of Chinese natural medicines. V. Radical scavenging effect of Moutan Cortex. (1): Absolute stereostructures of two monoterpenes, paeonisuffrone and paeonisuffral. *Chem. Pharm. Bull.* **48**, 1327–1331.

Yu, X.C., Wu, S., Wang, G.Y., Shan, J., Wong, T.M., Chen, C.F. and Pang, K.T. (2001) Cardiac effects of the extract and active components of radix stephaniae tetrandrae. II. Myocardial infarct, arrhythmias, coronary arterial flow and heart rate in the isolated perfused rat heart. *Life Sci.* **68**, 2863–2872.

Zeng, N., Meng, X., Zhang, Y., Lai, X., Zheng, J., Chen, L. and Ren, C. (1997) Antioxidative effect of constituents of *herba Epimedii* (ESPS). *Zhongguo Zhong Yao Za Zhi* **22**, 46–48, 63 (in Chinese).

Zhang, X.F. and Tan, B.K.H. (2000) Anti-diabetic property of ethanolic extract of *Andrographis paniculata* in streptozotocin-diabetic rats. *Acta Pharmacol. Sin.* **21**, 1157–1164.

Zhao, G., Li, Z. and Gu, T. (2001) Antihypertension and anti-cardiovascular remodeling by phenylalanine in spontaneously hypertensive rats: effectiveness and mechanisms. *Chin. Med. J.* **114**, 270–274.

Zimmet, P., Alberti, K.G.M.M. and Shaw, J. (2001) Global and societal implications of the diabetes epidemic. *Nature* **414**, 782–787.

Chapter 6

How Does Acupuncture Work?

Zhen Zheng

6.1 Introduction

The mechanisms of the therapeutic effect of acupuncture have been written about by many authors, and most of the writings are focused on its neurophysiological and neurohumoral mechanisms. In this chapter, I will focus on how to use these theories to explain clinical features of acupuncture with a brief introduction to the above theories. For people who would like to know the details of how these theories are developed, please refer to the cited researches. The content of this chapter includes explanations of:

- why placebo, suggestibility and stress are not the suitable mechanisms underlying acupuncture analgesia;
- the combined use of local and remote points with segmental and descending inhibition and neurohumoral theories;
- the therapeutic effect of acupuncture on viscera with the theory of somatovisceral reflexes;
- the calming effect of acupuncture with studies on the limbic systems;
- the specificity of acupuncture points and the rationale for utilising Chinese medicine diagnosis with results from functional magnetic resonance imaging (fMRI) and position emission tomography (PET) studies in the human brain;
- the time course of acupuncture effect; and
- the individual variations of responses to acupuncture with results from genetic studies.

Finally, I will discuss the future work that will enhance our understanding of how acupuncture works and how human bodies work.

6.2 Prevalent Theories on Acupuncture

Textbooks about acupuncture indicate that many health conditions can be treated with this therapy, such as pains, vertigo, cough, asthma, palpitation, diarrhea, constipation, impotency, irregular periods, etc. World Health Organization (WHO) lists six categories of 36 health conditions that acupuncture is recommended to treat. They are problems of upper respiratory tract, respiratory system, gastrointestinal disorders, neurological and musculoskeletal disorders, and mouth and eye conditions (Bannerman, 1979). A Consensus Development Panel on Acupuncture of the National Institutes of Health (NIH) in the United States identifies 11 conditions that can be effectively helped (NIH, 1998).

Western medicine practitioners and patients often wonder why inserting needles as thin as sewing needles into the human body can treat so many problems. A Chinese medicine practitioner will have no problems answering this question by explaining the concept of body Qi. The free flow of Qi is the foundation of a balanced mind and body, i.e. a healthy person. Diseases are the products or indications of the interrupted flow of Qi or the weakness of Qi. The main function of acupuncture is to restore its free flow.

The above explanation is not easily accepted by practitioners or patients influenced by Western medical science. What is Qi? Where does it flow? Can we measure or see it? What does free flow mean? Is there any certain speed to indicate the freeness? Indeed, so far we do not know what Qi consists of and what it looks like. As a consequence, we do not have any instrument with which we can measure the level of Qi. Thus, Qi is considered by some to be a metaphysical understanding of the human body and its functions, and the therapeutic effects of acupuncture have been thought to be those of placebo, suggestion (and hypnosis) and stress. Research suggests that these explanations of acupuncture are inadequate.

6.3 Placebo

Placebo is "an epithet given to any medicine adapted more to please than to benefit the patient" (Oxford English Dictionary, 1982; p. 2192). The fact that the patient is getting treatment for their problems can itself bring some therapeutic outcome. Other placebo factors are the care expressed by the practitioner, the social contact during the consultation, and suggestions from the practitioner that certain treatments will be good for the patient. Placebo effect is powerful, and this is why evidence-based medicine requires that all therapies should be measured against placebo control. Basically, placebo effect exists in every therapy, and acupuncture is not immune from this.

Placebo is, however, not the only mechanism to explain the actions of acupuncture. There are several lines of clinical evidence to support this notion: (1) Acupuncture analgesia (AA) is commonly seen in animals; (2) AA can be achieved in children; and (3) results from a review of clinical trials on acupuncture and chronic pain suggest that placebo effect involved in AA may be seen in 30% of patients with chronic pain, while AA can help up to 70% of patients (Pomeranz, 1989).

6.4 Suggestibility (Hypnosis)

Acupuncture procedure has been thought to be due to some form of suggestibility (or hypnosis) performed by the practitioner. This view is discarded for the following reasons: (1) AA is achieved while the patients are wide awake and are engaging in active conversation which is not seen in hypnosis patients (Melzack, 1975); (2) AA is also commonly seen in animals; and (3) psychophysical studies in humans have demonstrated that both good and poor hypnotic subjects (assessed by Harvard Group Scale for Hypnotic Suggestibility) achieved equal AA, and a similar effect was also shown in chronic pain patients (Ulett, 1989).

6.5 Stress

When people are in stressful conditions, for example, when running for their lives or fighting to win, their pain threshold is increased. This is called stress-induced analgesia (SIA). AA is not mediated via stress analgesia although some stress may be produced by the needling procedure. A psychophysical study has shown that subjects who achieved good AA are not more anxious than those who did not have AA (Zaretsky *et al.*, 1976). The anxiety level cannot account for AA, at least as seen in the study.

6.6 Neurophysiology of Acupuncture Effects

The acupuncture effects are better explained by the reactions of the nervous system to potential noxious stimulation to the musculoskeletal system. Some features of acupuncture are associated with pain and injury. Manual acupuncture consists of penetration of skin and De Qi sensation, which can be heaviness, distention, numbness, deep aching, warmth, tingling and soreness. De Qi sensation indicates the activation of nerve endings. The close association between acupuncture and pain allows the theories of pain induction and modulation to become the basis of the neurophysiology of the acupuncture effects. In the following sections, I shall use three cases to illustrate how theories like segmental inhibition, descending inhibition, counter-irritation, i.e. diffuse noxious inhibition controls (DNICs), somatovisceral reflexes and endogenous opioid peptides are used to explain the selection of local and remote points and the local and general effects of acupuncture.

6.7 Clinical Cases

6.7.1 *Case 1*

Peter, 65 years old, retiree, painful knees for eight years

The knee pain is diagnosed as osteoarthritis. Pain is mainly in both knees. The Chinese medicine diagnosis is Kidney deficient with blood stagnation. Acupoints selected are SP10 (Xuehai), ST35 (Wai Dubi), extra (Nei Dubi), ST34 (Liangqiu), BL23 (Shenshu) and BL26 (Guanyuangshu) (Fig. 6.1).

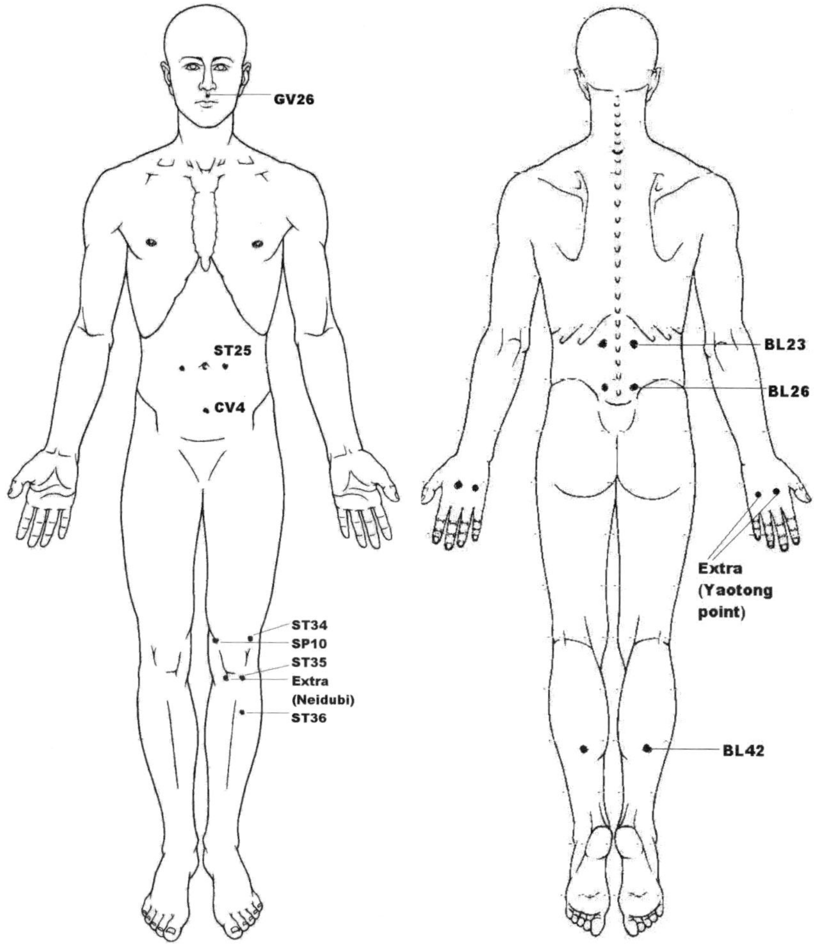

Figure 6.1. A diagram of the location of the acupuncture points used in the three cases.

6.7.2 *Case 2*

Jane, 24 years old, student, chronic diarrhea for three years

Jane suffers from watery diarrhea in the early morning. No pathological changes have been identified. Pattern of Chinese medicine diagnosis is Kidney Yang deficient. Points are ST25 (Tianshu), ST36 (Zusangli), BL23 (Shenshu) and CV4 (Guanyuan).

6.7.3 *Case 3*

John, 35 years old, carpenter, lower back pain for one hour

He experienced severe pain and cramps in the lower back when he stood up after putting down a piece of heavy wood. He could hardly walk, nor could he bend forward. It is diagnosed as acute back pain. Points are GV26 (Renzhong), Extra (Yaotong Point) and/or BL42 (Chengshang).

6.8 The Points Selection Explained by Chinese Medicine Theory

In the above cases, the selection of most points is explained by guidelines of Chinese acupuncture.

- Using the specificity of points. ST25 is the Mu point of Large Intestine, and the essential point for diarrhea.
- Selecting points according to the differentiation diagnosis. BL23 and 26 are the Shu point of Kidney and Guanyuan, and are important points for knee pain due to Kidney deficiency.
- Utilising the local functions of the points. Wai Dubi is a local point for relieving knee pain.
- Selecting points according to the traveling route of meridians. In Case 3, GV26 is used for lower back pain in the middle line because the Governor Vessel (GV), one of the 14 main meridians, travels along the posterior midline of the body.

There are, however, some points that are not explained by any Chinese medicine theory, such as Yaotong point, which is located in the 2nd and 4th dorsal interosseous muscles in the hand. Such points are called "Jing Wai Qi Xue", that are extra points located outside of the meridians.

How does neurophysiology explain the selection of local and remote points and the impact of needling?

6.9 Which Types of Afferent Fibres Transmit De Qi Sensation?

Needle insertion stimulates nerve endings in the skin, subcutaneous tissues, fascia and muscles. The understanding of afferent fibres stimulated by needle insertion is through measuring conduction velocity of impulses, and using nerve block and interneural microstimulation (INMS). "De Qi" sensation is the result of the activation of Aβ and Aδ fibres in the skeletal muscles. Intramuscular procaine, but not subcutaneous procaine, blocked De Qi sensation (Chiang *et al.*, 1973). When De Qi is blocked, acupuncture analgesia cannot be induced. Furthermore, patients with brachial plexus and spinal transactional lesions do not experience De Qi sensation (Department of Physiology and Acupuncture Research Group, 1973). These studies suggest that intact afferent pathways, in particular the ones in the muscles, are essential for the acupuncture effects. Table 6.1 is a summary of afferent fibres involved.

Table 6.1. A summary of afferent fibres in acupuncture needling sensation.

Sensory fibres (ABC system)	Sensory fibres (I–IV system)	Function	Needling sensation
	Group Ia	Muscle spindle: Monitoring muscle length and joint movement	
Aβ	Group II	Skin: Touch, vibration Muscle spindle: Monitoring muscle length and joint movement	Touch Numbness
Aδ	Group III	Skin/fascia: First pain,* pricking, cold Muscle ergoreceptors	Pricking, sharp Heaviness, distension, aching
C	Group IV	Skin: Second pain,† warmth, itchiness Muscle: Deep pain, dull aching	Warmth Soreness

Source: Adapted from White (1999).

*First pain: Painful sensation is experienced immediately after stimulation and prior to the second pain. It is conducted by Aδ afferent fibres, and the pain is localised and usually sharp and pricking in quality. First pain is associated with withdrawal reflex upon noxious stimulation to the body.

†Second pain: Painful sensation is experienced a few seconds after the stimulation. It is conducted via C afferent fibres, and the pain is diffused and is warm and soreness in quality. Second pain is associated with the emotional reaction to noxious stimulation.

Table 6.2. Nerves and tissues at some acupuncture points.

	Spinal segment of innervated tissue (Chen, 1995)	Organs innervated by the nerves at the same spinal segment (Head, 1893; Hamill, 1996)
SP10 Xuehai	Skin: Anterior femoral nerve L3 Vastus medialis muscle: L2–L4	L2 → Pelvic colon, rectum, genitourinary tract
ST34 Liangqiu	Skin: L2 Between rectus femoris and vastus lateralis muscles: L2–L4 Lateral collateral tendon of knee joint: L2–L4	L2 → Pelvic colon, rectum, genitourinary tract
ST35 Dubi	Skin: L3 Knee bursa → Lateral meniscus or medial bursa	Not mapped
BL23 Shenshu	Skin: L2 Superficial layer of thoracolumbar fascia: C6–C8 and lumbar nerve Deeper layer of the fascia: L1–L3 Sacrospinalis muscle: L2–L3	C6–C8: Not mapped L1–L2 → Pelvic colon, rectum, KI, ureter, uterus, UB, epididymis
BL26 Guanyuanshu	Skin: L4, L5 dorsal division Sacrospinalis: Dorsal division L5	L5 → Prostate, uterus
BL42 Chenshan	Skin: L4 Gastrocnemius muscle: S1, S2 Soleus muscle: S1, S2	S1 → Prostate, uterus S2 → Lower colon, rectum, UB, prostate, uterus
GV26 Renszhong	Skin: CN V Orbicularis oris muscle: CN VII	CN VII → Lacrimal and palatine glands
Yaotongxue	Skin: C6–C7 2nd and 4th dorsal interosseous muscle: C8–T1	T1 → HT, LU
CV4 Guanyuan	Skin: 12th intercostals nerve Linae alba and abdominis muscles: T6–T12	T6–T9 → ST T10 → LI, GB, upper colon, KI, ureter, prostate, tests, ovaries, uterus T11–T12: Upper colon, KI, ureter, UB, uterus, epididymis LI → GB, upper colon

Table 6.2. (*Continued*)

	Spinal segment of innervated tissue (Chen, 1995)	Organs innervated by the nerves at the same spinal segment (Head, 1893; Hamill, 1996)
ST25 Tianshu	Skin: 10th intercostals nerve Rectus abdominal muscle, inferior epigastric artery and vein: T7–T12 intercostal nerve Point: 10th intercostals nerve	T10 → LI, GB, upper colon, KI, ureter, prostate, tests, ovaries, uterus T7–T12 → ST, SI, adrenal medulla, colon
ST36 Zusangli	Skin: L5 Tibialis anterior muscle: L4–L5, S1 Interosseous membrane and tibialis posterior: L5–S1	S1: Prostate, uterus

*C: Cervical, T: thoracic, L: lumbar, S: sacral, HT: heart, LU: lung, KI: kidney, ST: stomach, SI: small intestine, UB: urinary bladder and GB: gall bladder.

6.10 Local and Remote Points

6.10.1 *How do local points work — Segmental inhibition and descending inhibition*

Chinese acupuncture emphasises the use of local points and the "A Shi" points. In Case 1, points like SP10, ST34 and ST35 are all located in the muscles that control the movement of knees (Table 6.2). These muscles are innervated by spinal nerves L2–S1. Acupuncture analgesia in this case is explained by the segmental inhibition.

Segmental inhibition suggests that inhibition on pain signals occurs at the local spinal level. The main source of the inhibition comes from the inputs from large myelinated afferent fibres ($A\beta$). First, the input activates the inhibition interneurons that secret γ-amino butyric acid (GABA), which then produce pre-synaptic inhibition on spinal transmission interneurons (T). T neurons are also activated by inputs from unmyelinated afferent fibres (C) and transmit nociceptive information (Fig. 6.2). Second, $A\beta$ input is transmitted to the supraspinal level via dorsal column (DC). When DC is stimulated, it again activates inhibitory neurons. Thus, at the segmental level, activation of large myelinated afferent fibres inhibits the

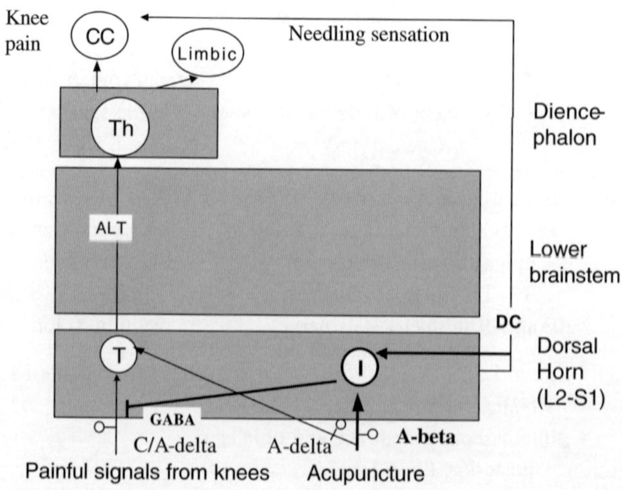

Figure 6.2. A simplified diagram of the segmental inhibition of acupuncture (T: Transmission interneuron, I: inhibition interneuron, Th: thalamus, CC: cerebral cortex, DC: dorsal column, ---/ inhibitory effect, and → excitatory effect).

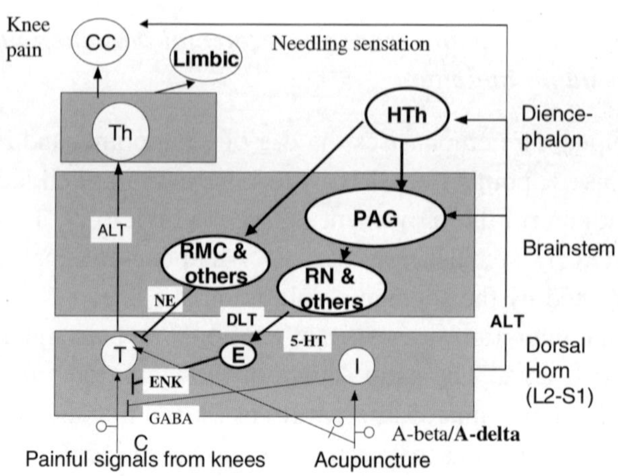

Figure 6.3. A simplified diagram of the descending pathway of acupuncture (T: Transmission interneuron, I: inhibition interneuron, E: enkephalinergic neurons, ENK: enkephalins, NE: nonepinephrin, 5-HT: serotonin, RN: raphe nuclei, RMC: reticular magnocellar nuclei, PAG: periaqueductal grey, Th: thalamus, HTh: hypothalamus, CC: cerebral cortex, ALT: anterolateral tract, DLT: dorsolateral tract, ---/ inhibitory effect, and → excitatory effect). Adapted from Cheng (1989), Han (1989) and Pomeranz (1989).

input from C fibres directly and indirectly via DC. This is part of the gate control theory (Melzack and Wall, 1996). Acupuncture activates Aβ fibres, therefore likely produces the analgesic effect.

The other source of segmental inhibition comes from supraspinal levels, i.e. descending inhibition. Needling procedure activates Aδ fibres. Figure 6.3 illustrates the pathway of Aδ afferent inputs which travel along the anterolateral tract (ALT) and activate structures involved in pain modulation along the way, such as reticular formation (RF), periaqueductal grey (PAG), thalamus and hypothalamus. Two descending pathways have been hypothesised: Serotonin (5-HT) and non-epinephrine (NE). The serotonin pathway is activated by the descending information from the PAG, then activates enkephalin-neurons which then produces pre-synaptic inhibition on transmission neurons at the segment where the painful stimulation comes. The non-epinephrine pathway descends from the hypothalamus and induces inhibition on transmission neurons at the dorsal horn via the dorsal lateral tract as the serotonin pathway (Cheng, 1989; White, 1999).

In Case 1, painful signals from knees are transmitted by C fibres in the lumbar spinal nerves. As shown in Table 6.2, needling the local

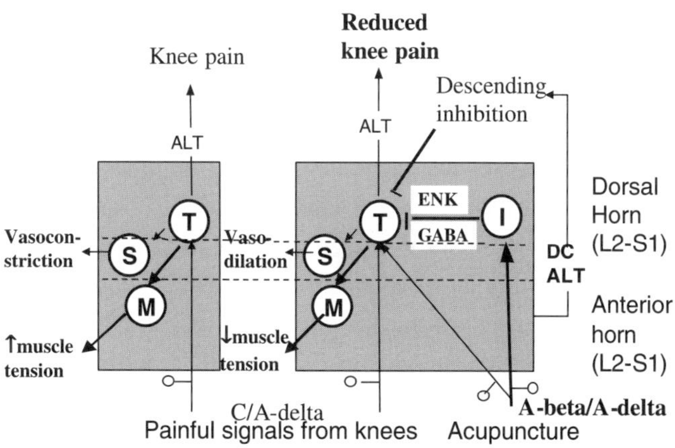

Figure 6.4. A diagram of the nocifensive reflex and inhibition on the reflex with acupuncture (T: Transmission interneuron, I: inhibition interneuron, M: motor neurons, S: sympathetic neurons, ALT: anterolateral tract, ---/ inhibitory effect, and → excitatory effect.

points around knee and lumbar points activate Aβ and Aδ fibres in the L2–S1 spinal nerves. Together the two pathways produce inhibition on the painful signals from knees at the lumbar segment.

One must remember that noxious stimulation from the knee, such as inflammation, not only induces painful sensation, but also induces muscle contraction and vasoconstriction in the muscles around the knee, which is called nocifensive reflex (Fig. 6.4). Muscle contraction further worsens ischaemia, thereby inducing painful sensation and limited movement of the knee. A vicious circle is thus formed. Segmental and descending inhibitions reduce the activity of transmission neurons, and as a consequence, suppress the nocifensive reflex. Pain as well as muscle tension are therefore reduced.

6.10.2 *How do remote points work — Diffuse noxious inhibition control and neuroiumoral theory*

In Chinese acupuncture, remote points are selected based on the Chinese medicine diagnosis (e.g. Cases 1 and 2) or empirical observation (e.g. Case 3). In Case 1, BL23 and BL26 are distal to knee, however they are actually innervated by spinal nerves L4–L5 (Table 6.2), similar to local points of ST34, 35 and SP10. The action of BL23 and BL26 is explained by segmental inhibition.

In Case 3, remote points like GV26 and Yaotong points are innervated by cranial and cervical nerves, respectively. Their action of reducing lumbar pain is therefore not explained by segmental theory, but by the diffuse noxious inhibition controls (DNICs). DNICs are the underlying mechanism for counter-irritation, which means that painful sensation at one part of the body can be suppressed by pain at other parts of the body. For instance, hammering on the finger can relieve headache. DNICs are likely evoked by input from Aδ and C fibres. The analgesic effect is not somatotopically organised, instead it spreads over the body. The strength of the analgesia is proportional to the intensity of noxious stimulation (Le Bars *et al.*, 1979). That is to say, needling any part of the body can reduce pain in any other part. The stronger the needling sensation, the greater the pain relief is. This is why although there is no neural network connecting the lumbar area and GV26 or Yaotgong points, stimulation of such points can relieve lumbar pain. By the same token, one should be able to successfully relieve acute lower back pain by stimulating Shi Xuan, extra points that are located on the fingertips.

DNICs do not explain the whole effects of acupuncture. Firstly, most acupuncture procedure does not induce very strong painful sensation; secondly, the effect of acupuncture often outlasts the stimulation. Analgesia produced by the DNICs is immediate, but short-lasting for a few minutes only.

The neurohumoral theory offers an explanation for the general and long-lasting effect of acupuncture. The theory was first hypothesised in the 1970s. Han and colleagues found that infusion of the cerebrospinal fluid (CSF) from a rabbit that presented analgesia after acupuncture to a second rabbit that was not treated with acupuncture induced analgesia in the second rabbit. The result indicates that some analgesic substance is released into the CSF upon acupuncture. Later, several main neurotransmitters and neuropeptides have been identified to be involved in acupuncture action; opioid peptides, 5-HT, NE, GABA, dopamine, somatostatin, cholecystokinin (CCK) and substance P (SP) (Han, 1989).

Among neurotransmitters and neuropeptides mentioned above, endogenous opioid peptides (EOP) are best studied in relation to acupuncture. Three types of EOP have been identified upon acupuncture (in particular EA): dynorphins, enkephalins and β-endorphins. Table 6.3 is a summary of the locations of action and preferable EA frequency for each peptide.

Acupuncture may activate the pituitary-hypothalamic complex. β-endorphin in the hypothalamus activates PAG, therefore activating the

Table 6.3. A summary of endogenous opioid peptides after electroacupuncture.

Types	Location	Type of opioid receptors	EA frequency
β-endorphin	Hypothalamus to PAG, blood, not in spinal cord	μ: Can be blocked by naloxone	2 and 15 Hz
Enkephalins	Hypothalamus, spinal cord	δ: Can be blocked by naloxone	2 Hz
Dynorphins	Spinal cord, not in PAG	κ: Relatively resistant to naloxone	100 Hz

Source: Han (1989).

descending inhibition. β-endorphin released from the pituitary may also go to CSF or through the blood-brain barrier to blood circulation, and produce analgesia by binding to opioid receptors at the spinal cord, brain and in the periphery.

The opioid peptides theory of acupuncture has been used to reduce the withdrawal symptoms of drug addiction (Severson *et al.*, 1977; Ulett *et al.*, 1998) and to reduce the intake of exogenous opioids for post-operative pain control (Wang *et al.*, 1997).

6.11 How Does Acupuncture Regulate Viscera — Somatovisceral Reflex

Somatovisceral reflexes mean that stimulating somatic structures, such as skin, subcutaneous tissue, fascia or skeletal muscles, can elicit visceral response. The afferent arm of the reflex are Aβ, Aδ and C afferent fibres in the skin or muscles. The integrative centres lie in the intermediolateral part of the spinal cord between T1–T12 and S2–S4, brain stem (medulla) and hypothalamus. The efferent arm is the postganglionic fibres to the target organs.

In case 2, ST25, CV4 and ST36 are used to reduce diarrhea. As indicated in Table 6.2, ST25 and CV4 are innervated by T6–T12 spinal nerves, which also innervate small intestines and colon. Stimulating the abdominal area has been shown to inhibit the motility of the gastro-intestinal tract via segmentally increasing the activity of the gastric sympathetic nerves (Sato *et al.*, 1993). ST36 is innervated by L3–L5 spinal nerves, at which segment no sympathetic or parasympathetic preganglionic neuron is located. A study has shown that stimulating hind paws induces facilitation of mobility via a supraspinal centre (Sato *et al.*, 1993). Thus, acupuncture's effect on reducing diarrhea can be explained by the segmental and supraspinal somatovisceral reflexes.

Recently, EOPs have been indicated in the autonomic activities. Morphine can regulate blood pressure in human subjects who have either lower or higher BP (Rubin, 1984). Naloxone, an opioid antagonist, increases blood pressure in hypotension rats (Blake *et al.*, 1984), and reverses the inhibition effect of EA on bradykinin-induced myocardial infarction (Chao *et al.*, 1999). The most likely pathway is that acupuncture regulates the vasomotor centre in the brainstem via stimulating the release of β-endorphin.

Together, somatovisceral reflexes and the release of β-endorphin in the hypothalamus by acupuncture needling may underline the regulating effect of acupuncture on the immune system, cardiovascular system, respiratory system, gastrointestinal system and genitourinotary system (Andersson and Lundberg, 1995; Lundberg, 1999).

6.12 Calming Effect — Effect on the Limbic System

Acupuncture treatment often produces calming, relaxed feelings or even euphoria in both healthy people and patients. Campbell (1999) hypothesised that the unusual feeling during or after acupuncture is related to the limbic system, which is associated with emotions like fear, anger and anxiety. The limbic system has been shown to be highly active in chronic pain patients (Apkarian *et al.*, 2001), and this may explain why these patients are often depressed and easily anxious.

Three fMRI studies (Wu *et al.*, 1999; Hui *et al.*, 2000; Wu *et al.*, 2002) have suggested that acupuncture regulates the limbic system. When De Qi sensation is achieved with manual needling of LI4 or ST36, the activation of the limbic system was reduced in anterior cingular cortex, amygdala formation and hippocampus. Superficial needling without De Qi sensation does not deactivate the limbic system. These studies were conducted in healthy humans, and further studies must investigate the inhibition effect on the limbic systems in patients with chronic pain or chronic diseases.

In conclusion, acupuncture works with four aspects: segmental, descending regulation, general and emotional (Fig. 6.5). Firstly, at the same spinal segment of the noxious input, stimulating local points or points at the same segment inhibits the transmission of noxious stimulation, thus reducing pain and relaxing tensed muscles. It also initiates somatovisceral reflex to regulate the visceral functions. Secondly, acupuncture stimulates the supraspinal structures to produce descending inhibition, thereby reducing pain. At the supraspinal level, it may also regulate the vasomotor centre so that it influences the sympathetic tone. Thirdly, the DNICs explain the immediate and general analgesia induced by acupuncture.

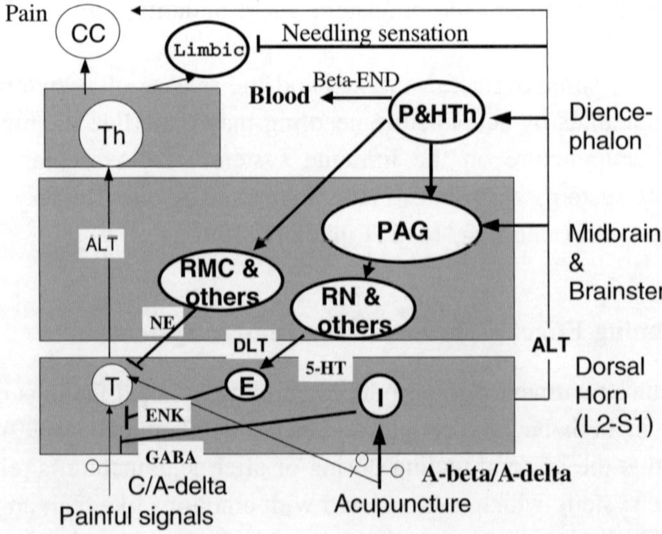

Figure 6.5. A simplified diagram of the actions of acupuncture (T: Transmission interneuron, I: inhibition interneuron, E: enkephalinergic neurons, ENK: enkephalins, Beta-END: β-endorphin, NE: nonepinephrin, 5-HT: serotonin, RN: raphe nuclei, RMC: reticular magnocellar nuclei, PAG: periaqueductal grey, Th: thalamus, HTh: hypothalamus, P: pituitary, CC: cerebral cortex, ALT: anterolateral tract, DLT: dorsolateral tract, ---/ inhibitory effect, and → excitatory effect). Adapted from Han (1989), Cheng (1989) and Pomeranz (1995).

The DNICs may play an unimportant role in acupuncture as the intensity of needling may not often be strong enough to induce a strong counter-irritation effect. The neurohumoral theory provides the biochemical mechanisms for the descending regulations and general effects on pain and visceral functions, and also explains the prolonged effect of acupuncture. Finally, acupuncture deactivates the limbic systems and tunes down the emotional stress associated with pain or discomfort brought about by illness.

6.13 Specific Effect of Acupuncture Points

One of the main debates in acupuncture research is whether acupuncture points have their specific effects as indicated by classic literatures. The segmental theory of acupuncture effect explains why stimulating ST25 or BL23 can regulate colon or relieve pain in the knees, but it could not explain why ST36 is considered to be the essential point for stomach function or why ST44 (on the web between the 2nd and 3rd toes) indicates for epistaxis as suggested by many acupuncture textbooks. If the effects of ST36 and ST44 are due to the general effect of acupuncture, then any point can be used to treat stomach pain or epistaxis, which is neither true nor practiced clinically.

If there is no evidence to support the special functions of acupuncture points, then traditional Chinese acupuncture and its theory about point selection should and will give way to medical acupuncture, which is practiced based on current knowledge of neuroanatomy and neurophysiology.

A morphological study on rats reveals the neuroanatomic connection between ST36 and stomach with a standard transneuronal viral labelling method (Lee *et al.*, 2001). The authors injected two different viruses into the stomach and ST36, respectively, so that the viruses can self-replicate in the neurons associated with these two structures. After five days, the authors found that the commonly labelled spinal areas are in the thoracic, lumbar and sacral segments. The common brain areas are those controlling the autonomic functions, such as epinephrine cells, nonepinephrine cells, hypothalamus, etc. That is to say that a group of brain cells control both the stomach and ST36.

A recent study with fMRI has also shed some light on the special functions of acupoints (Cho *et al.*, 1998). BL60, 65, 66 and 67 (VA8, 3,2,1) are indicative for vision-related problems in Korean acupuncture. Stimulating the VA points, in particular VA1, activate the visual cortex. On the contrary, stimulating the non-acupoint 2 cm medial to VA1 does not produce the same effect. Cho and colleagues later investigated Guangming (GB37) and Jiaxi (GB43), points for blindness and deafness, respectively, and they found visual and auditory cortexes were activated (Shen, 2001). They are the first two studies to show some physiological basis for the specificity of acupuncture points. The significance of the study lies beyond acupuncture. So far, there is no knowledge of the physical or biochemical connection between BL67, GB37 or GB43 and visual or auditory cortexes. Future research should replicate the study, establish the correlation between other acupoints and viscera/organs, and explore the possible pathway for these acupoints to the brain.

6.14 Time Course of Acupuncture Effect

The length of the effect of acupuncture varies from person to person. Some people have a miracle cure after one session of acupuncture, while others need more than six sessions of treatment before any sustained effect is indicated. In general, each acupuncture treatment induces at least two stages of effect: one quick-onset, short-lasting stage and a slow-onset and long-lasting stage (Fig. 6.6). Most patients say that their pain or other conditions, such as cough or nausea disappear or reduce dramatically after the insertion of needles. This effect is likely to reduce within a few hours of the treatment. Over the next 72–96 hours, patients often experience a gradual improvement in their symptoms, followed by a gradual reduction.

The two stages may be related to the different mechanisms of acupuncture. The effects of the DNICs and segmental inhibition are often of short duration. On the contrary, humoral effect is slow onset because of the synthesis of neuropeptides.

Neuropeptides are derived from precursor polypeptides. The time course of the humoral effect can therefore be indicated by measuring the

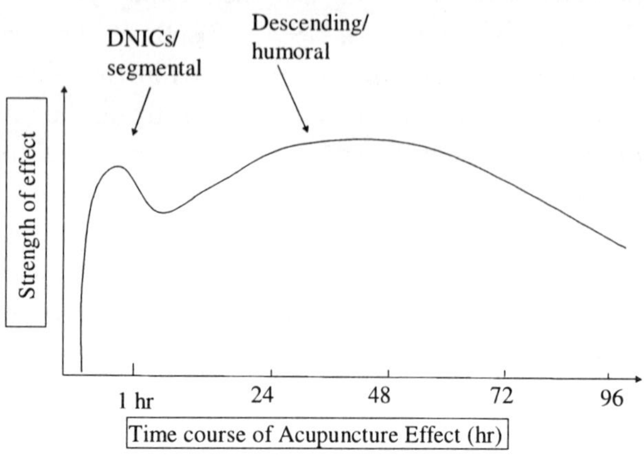

Figure 6.6. A simplified diagram of the possible time course of acupuncture effect.

change of precursor polypeptides over time. Studies in rats have shown that EA increases the expression of preproenkephalin (PPE) mRNA and preproopiomelanocortin (POMC) mRNA in hypothalamus and PAG. This increase lasts from 24 to 96 hours (He, 1987; Zheng *et al.*, 1987; Yu *et al.*, 1994).

Electroacupuncture also increases the numbers of opioid receptors binding sites in rats, in particular those of μ receptors in the brain (Gao *et al.*, 1997), so that it enhances the efficacy of exogenous or endogenous opioid peptides. Future studies must answer whether the effect is accumulative with repeated acupuncture. This may explain why acupuncture effect increases with repeated treatment.

6.15 Individual Response to Acupuncture

It is commonly accepted that everyone responds to acupuncture differently. The *Miraculous Pivot* (item 67) (Anonymous, 475–221 BC) discussed four types of people based on their response to acupuncture: very quickly, normally, delayed or slowly. The book attributed the differences to the Yin-Yang variation of each individual. Basically, quick responders are of high active Yang, while slow responders are of high proportion of Yin.

The study by Cho *et al.* (1998) reported that the brain reaction to acupuncture differs in subjects with different Yin-Yang constitution. Yin subjects have increased activity upon acupuncture, while Yang ones show decreased activity.

Mann (2000) categorises people into four types: very strong, strong, normal and non-reactors to acupuncture. Han has also documented that about 20–30% humans and animals do not respond to electrical acupuncture (Han, 1989). A similar percentage of non-responders has also been noted in morphine tests (Lasagna and Beecher, 1954). One of the factors of low-responder is anti-opioid peptides cholecystkinin-8 CCK. Reducing the amount of CCK in the central nervous system successfully converts the low-responder rats to responders to acupuncture (Tang *et al.*, 1997).

Individual variation can be due to genetic disposition towards acupuncture. A recent study investigated the genotypes and electroacupuncture analgesia directly, and found that two of ten inbred strains of mice were most sensitive to EA. The study also indicated the interaction between genetics and environmental factors in acupuncture analgesia (Wan *et al.*, 2001). This genetic disposition may be associated with sensitivity to morphine. Rats with β-endorphin gene knockout did not show any analgesia after electroacupuncture with low frequency (Wan *et al.*, 1999). It will be of great value to acupuncture if the "acupuncture gene" is identified.

6.16 Work in the Future — What We Do Not Know

In this chapter, neurophysiological theories on acupuncture are used to explain some common clinical features. There are still many questions that remain unanswered. Four questions considered to be of most importance are (1) the evidence on the effectiveness of acupuncture; (2) the special functions of points and their clinical relevance; (3) the special function of points and their relation to human biology; (4) and the individual variation.

The great forward step in modern health care is the practice of evidence-based medicine. When we attempt to answer why acupuncture has multiple therapeutic effects, we must also investigate whether acupuncture does have the claimed effects. If it does, how strong is the effect. A series of systematic reviews point out the common problems with acupuncture research, that is most existing clinical trials are of poor quality so that no conclusion can be drawn (ter Riet *et al.*, 1990; Ernst, 1997; White and Ernst, 1999; Ezzo *et al.*, 2000; Park *et al.*, 2000; Tulder *et al.*, 2000; Park *et al.*, 2001; Smith and Crowther, 2001). High quality clinical trials are needed. Researchers in the areas of Chinese medicine must be equipped with strong knowledge of scientific research methods.

Whether each acupuncture point has claimed special functions is a question directly concerned with the clinical practice. If yes, selecting points according to Chinese medicine diagnosis becomes highly relevant. Most controlled clinical trials neglect Chinese medicine theories and used a standard formula for all the subjects in the trials. These trials reflect little of the clinical practice of acupuncture, and their conclusions cannot indicate the efficacy of acupuncture.

There are two approaches by which the above question may be answered. One is by conducting clinical trials so that the special functions of acupuncture points can be evaluated on certain diseases or conditions. The other is by conducting laboratory studies. Recently, there are increased amount of studies with a focus on the autonomic regulation and impact on brain function achieved by acupuncture. The results of such studies will also help to understand the therapeutic effects of acupuncture other than analgesia, such as regulating blood flow or the immune system. Moreover, these studies will advance our understanding on how the body works.

Finally, searching for the markers responsible for the individual responses is necessary for identifying suitable patients. Individualised treatment will be derived from both the manifestation and the individual suitability. Equipped with the above knowledge, acupuncture will exert better and more specific functions on maintaining health and combating against illness.

Acknowledgements

I would like to extend my gratitude to Drs. Ian Weeks and Robert Webb for their valuable comments on the manuscript.

References

Andersson, S. and Lundberg, T. (1995) Acupuncture — from empiricism to science: functional background to acupuncture effects in pain and disease. *Med. Hypotheses* **45**, 271–281.

Anonymous (475–221 BC) *The Yellow Emperor's Canon of Internal Medicine: Miraulous Pivot.*

Apkarian, A.V., Thomas, P.S., *et al.* (2001) Prefrontal cortical hyperactivity in patients with sympathetically mediated chronic pain. *Neurosci. Lett.* **311**(3), 193–197.

Bannerman, R.H. (1979) *Acupuncture: The World Health Organisation View*, World Health Organization.

Blake, M.J., Stein, E.A., *et al.* (1984) Effects of exercise-training on brain opioid peptides and serum LM in female rats. *Peptides* **5**, 953–938.

Campbell, A. (1999) The limbic system and emotion in relation to acupuncture. *Acupunct. Med.* **17**(2), 124–130.

Chao, D.M., Shen, L.L., *et al.* (1999) Naloxone reverses inhibitory effect of electroacupuncture on sympathetic cardiovascular reflex responses. *Am. J. Physiol.* **276**(6), 2127–2134.

Chen, E. (1995) *Cross-sectional Anatomy of Acupoints.* Churchill Livingstone, Edinburgh.

Cheng, R.S.S. (1989) Neurophysiology of electroacupuncture analgesia. In: *Scientific Bases of Acupuncture* (eds.) Pomeranze, B. and Stux, G. Springer-Verlag, Berlin, pp. 119–136.

Chiang, C.Y., Chang, C.T., *et al.* (1973) Peripheral afferent pathway for AA. *Scientia Sinica* **16**, 210–217.

Cho, Z.H., Chung, S.C., *et al.* (1998) New findings of the correlation between acupoints and corresponding brain cortices using functional MRI. *Proc. Natl. Acad. Sci. USA* **276**, 2670–2673.

Department of Physiology and Acupuncture Research Group, H.S.H., Shanghai First Medical College (1973) Observations on the absence of acupuncture effect in certain neurologic patients. *Ke Xue Tong Bao* **18**, 90–93.

Ernst, E. (1997) Acupuncture as a symptomatic treatment of osteoarthritis. A systematic review. *Scand. J. Rheumatol.* **26**(6), 444–447.

Ezzo, J., Berman, B., *et al.* (2000) Is acupuncture effective for the treatment of chronic pain? A systematic review. *Pain* **86**, 217–225.

Gao, M., Wang, M., *et al.* (1997) Changes of μ opioid receptor binding sites in rats brain following electroacupuncture. *Acupunct. Electrother. Res.* **22**(3–4), 161–166.

Hamill, R.W. (1996) Peripheral autonomic nervous system. In: *Primer on the Autonomic Nervous System.* (eds.) Robertson, D., Low P.A. and Polinsky, R.J. Academic Press, San Diego, pp. 12–25.

Han, J.S. (1989) Central neurotransmitters and acupuncture analgesia. In: *Scientific Bases of Acupuncture* (eds.) Pomeranz, B. and Stux, G. Springer-Verlag, Berlin, pp. 7–34.

He, L.F. (1987) Involvement of endogenous opioid peptide in AA. *Pain* **31**, 99–121.

Head, H. (1893) On disturbances of sensation with special reference to the pain of visceral disease. *Brain* **16**, 1–133.

Hui, K.K., Liu, J., *et al.* (2000) Acupuncture modulates the limbic system and subcortical gray structures of the human brain: evidence from fMRI studies in normal subjects. *Hum. Brain Mapp.* **9**(1), 13–25.

Lasagna, L. and Beecher, H.K. (1954) The optimal dose of morphine. *J. Am. Med. Assoc.* **156**, 230–234.

Le Bars, D., Dickenson, A.H., *et al.* (1979) Diffuse noxious inhibitory controls (DNIC). Effect on dorsal horn convergent neurons in the rat. *Pain* **6**, 283–304.

Lee, C.H., Jung, H.S., *et al.* (2001) Studies of the central pathways to the stomach and Zusanli (St36). *Am. J. Chin. Med.* **29**, 211–220.

Lundberg, T. (1999) Effects of sensory stimulation (acupuncture) on circulatory and immune systems. In: *Acupuncture: A Scientific Appraisal*. (eds.) Ernst, E. and White, A. Butterworth-Heinemann, Oxford, pp. 93–106.

Mann, F. (2000) *Reinventing Acupuncture: A New Concept of Ancient Acupuncture*. Butterworth-Heinemann, Oxford.

Melzack, R. (1975) How acupuncture can block pain. In: *Pain Clinical and Experimental Perspectives*. (ed.) Weisenberg, M. Mosby Company, Saint Louis.

Melzack, R. and Wall, P. (1996) Peripheral nerve and spinal mechanisms. In: *The Challenge of Pain*. Penguin Books, London, pp. 81–107.

NIH, C.D.P.O.A. (1998) Acupuncture. *JAMA* **280**(17), 1518–1524.

Oxford English Dictionary (1982) London.

Park, J., Hopwood, V., *et al.* (2001) Effectiveness of acupuncture for stroke: a systematic review. *J. Neurol.* **248**(7), 558–563.

Park, J., White, A.R., *et al.* (2000) Efficacy of acupuncture as a treatment for tinnitus: a systematic review. *Arch. Otolaryngol. Head Neck Surg.* **126**(4), 489–492.

Pomeranz, B. (1989) Acupuncture analgesia for chronic pain: brief survey of clinical trial. In: *Scientific Bases of Acupuncture*. (eds.) Pomeranz, B. and Stux, G. Springer-Verlag, Berlin, pp. 197–199.

Rubin, P.C. (1984) Opioid peptides in blood pressure regulation in man. *Clin. Sci.* **66**, 625–630.

Sato, A., Sato, Y., *et al.* (1993) Neural mechanisms of the reflex inhibition and excitation of gastric motility elicited by acupuncture-like stimulation in anesthetized rats. *Neurosci. Res.* **18**, 53–62.

Severson, L., Merkoff, R.A., *et al.* (1977) Heroin detoxification with acupuncture and electrical stimulation. *Int. J. Addict.* **132**, 911–922.

Shen, J. (2001) Research on the neurophysiological mechanisms of acupuncture: review of selected studies and methodological issues. *J. Altern. Complement. Med.* **7**(Suppl. 1), S121–S127.

Smith, C.A. and Crowther, C.A. (2001) Acupuncture for induction of labour. *Cochrane Database Syst. Rev.* (1), CD002962.

Tang, N.M., Dong, H.W., *et al.* (1997) Cholecystokinin antisense RNA increases the analgesic effect induced by electroacupuncture or low dose morphine: conversion of low responders rats into higher responders. *Pain* **71**, 71–80.

ter Riet, G., Kleijnen, J., *et al.* (1990) Acupuncture and chronic pain: a criteria-based meta-analysis. *J. Clin. Epidemiol.* **43**(11), 1191–1199.

Tulder, M.V., Cherkin, D.C., *et al.* (2000) Acupuncture for low back pain. *Cochrane Database Syst. Rev.* (2), CD001351.

Ulett, G. (1989) Studies supporting the concept of physiological acupuncture. In: *Scientific Bases of Acupuncture*. (eds.) Pomeranz, B. and Stux, G. Springer-Verlag, Berlin, pp. 177–196.

Ulett, G.A., Han, S.-P., *et al.* (1998) Electroacupuncture: mechanisms and clinical application. *Biol. Psychiatry* **44**, 121–128.

Wan, Y., Jeffrey, S.M., *et al.* (1999) Decrease of low frequency (2Hz) EA analgesia in mice lacking beta-endorphin. *Chin. J. Pain Med.* **5**, 161-167.

Wan, Y., Wilson, S.G., *et al.* (2001) The effect of genotype on sensitivity to electroacupuncture analgesia. *Pain* **91**, 5–13.

Wang, B.-G., Tang, J., *et al.* (1997) Effect of the intensity of transcutaneous acupoint electrical stimulation on the postoperative analgesic requirement. *Anesth. Analg.* **85**, 406–413.

White, A. (1999) Neurophysiology of acupuncture analgesia. In: *Acupuncture: A Scientific Appraisal*. (eds.) Ernst, E. and White, A. Butterworth Heinemann, Oxford, pp. 60–92.

White, A.R. and Ernst, E. (1999) A systematic review of randomized controlled trials of acupuncture for neck pain. *Rheumatology (Oxford)* **38**(2), 143–147.

Wu, M.T., Hsieh, J.C., *et al.* (1999) Central nervous pathway for acupuncture stimulation: localisation of processing with functional MRI imaging of the brain — preliminary experience. *Radiology* **212**, 133–141.

Wu, M.T., Sheen, J.M., *et al.* (2002) Neuronal specificity of acupuncture response: a fMRI study with electroacupuncture. *Neuroimage* **16**(4), 1028–1037.

Yu, Y.H., Gao, M., *et al.* (1994) Time course of alteration of propiomelanocortin mRNA level in rat hypothalamic arcuate nuscleus following electroacupuncture. *Acta Acad. Med. Shanghai* **21**(suppl.), 59–62.

Zaretsky, H.H., Lee, M.H., *et al.* (1976) Psychological factors and clinical observations in acupuncture analgesia and pain abatement. *J. Psychol.* **93**(1st Half), 113–120.

Zheng, M., Wang, L.J., *et al.* (1987) Electroacupuncture increases proopiomelanocotin mRNA in the pituitary and the proenkephalin mRNA in the adrenal gland in the rat. *Chin. J. Physiol. Sci.* **3**, 106.

Chapter 7

More Theories About Acupuncture

Baoyu Xin

7.1 Introduction

As a traditional healing modality, acupuncture originated in China more than 2500 years ago. Now it is still an important component of the health care system of China. It was brought to Japan, Korea and Southeast Asia in the sixth century, and then to Europe and the United States of America in the 17th and 19th centuries (Cao, 1999). Nevertheless, acupuncture was only widely used and studied until the recent 30 years, mainly on the relief of pain or acupuncture analgesia (AA). Developed from AA, acupuncture anaesthesia was once the extremely interesting medical focus throughout China in the 1960s and early 1970s. A lot of work has been done, but the mechanism of acupuncture was still unclear. Meanwhile, different approaches were applied to study how acupuncture works in Western countries, such as neuroanatomy, neuropharmacology, neurobiochemistry and neuromorphology. In order to regulate and standardise the methodologies in clinical research on acupuncture, the World Health Organization (WHO) issued a guideline in 1995 (WHO, 1995). To provide clinicians, patients and the general public with a responsible assessment of the use and effectiveness of acupuncture to treat a variety of conditions, the National Institutes of Health (NIH) held a consensus conference in 1997. The panels concluded that although many studies provide equivocal results because of design, sample size, appropriate controls, etc. Acupuncture is promising in treating such diseases as nausea and vomiting associated with chemotherapy, post-operative dental pain and on other situations. As to basic research, the possible mechanisms of action of acupuncture were put forward through human and animal experiments, including the release of opioids and other peptides in the central and peripheral nervous system (Acupuncture-NIH Consensus, 1998).

This chapter will review the past and present studies on AA, and the methodological problems and difficulties in clinical trials. Possible mechanism of action of acupuncture will be discussed as we go along.

7.2 Neurological Reasoning Theory

To fully understand how AA works, we should be very clear about the physiology of pain. Unlike other senses such as touch, taste, smell, hearing and vision, pain perception is a complex experience involving emotional feelings. Pain may also serve as one kind of defense mechanism to prevent or escape from injury or other harmful forms of stimulation (Huang, 1996).

In 1965, Melzack and Wall suggested a hypothesis to explain how the sensation of pain is regulated in the body. They thought that the dorsal horn of the spinal cord and the caudal trigeminal complex serve as a gate to control or filter the flow of impulses entering the central nervous system (Melzack and Wall, 1965). This modulation mechanism is known as "gate control theory", which can be presented in Fig. 7.1.

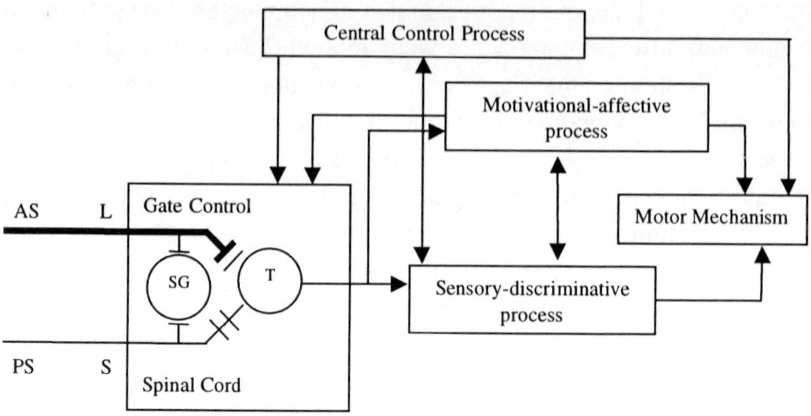

Figure 7.1. Conceptual model of the sensory, motivational and central determinations of pain. L: Large-diameter afferent fibres, S: small-diameter afferent fibres, SG: *Substantia gelatinosa*, T: central transmission cells, AS: acupuncture stimulus, PS: painful stimulus, +: facilitation, and −: inhibition (source: Melzack and Wall).

There are two kinds of fibres involved in this theory, namely large- and small-diameter afferent fibres. Pain impulses are transmitted to the higher levels through small-diameter afferent fibres, while acupuncture impulses are transmitted through large-diameter ones. Stimulation from large-diameter afferent fibres can inhibit the *substantia gelatinosa* (SG) cells and maintain them in a "close" condition, thus preventing the pain message transmission. In the case where the noxious stimuli is too strong, the pain signal is passed through the SG cells thus activating the central transmission (T) cells which transfer the pain message to higher brain centres for perception occurring at the thalamic and cortical levels (Klide and Kung, 1977). So the balance between these two kinds of transmission is an important "Gate" for controlling pain. It is also recognised that before entering the dorsal horn gray matter, the afferent fibres are transmitted cranially and caudally for several segments within the dorsolateral fasciculus. This explains why the regional analgesia can be induced (Latshaw, 1975).

7.3 Peripheral Pain Receptors and Afferent Fibres

Beneath the skin, free nerve endings and specific receptors are widely distributed. Today, all the specific receptors for pressure detection and thermoreceptors have been identified. But for pain perception, it is generally believed that free nerve endings mostly serve as pain receptors.

Inside the sensory nervous system, A-delta and C-fibres are thought to be closely related to pain transmission. A-delta fibres are thin and poorly myelinated while C-fibres are unmyelinated with only one-tenth the diameter of A-delta fibres. Since C-fibres transmit impulses ten times slower than A-delta fibres and have a higher threshold for stimulation, a more unpleasant pain sensation would be involved (Hyman and Cassem, 1989). There are two other kinds of pain fibres: A-alpha and A-beta. Located in the muscles and joints, A-alpha fibres are important for proprioception, and A-beta fibres are mainly responsible for mechanical stimulation, such as light touch and the blending of hairs. Both of them transmit information much faster than A-delta and C-fibres because of their large diameter. These fibres may play a role in some mechanisms of acupuncture (Gellman, 2002). There is another classification of afferent nerves according to their sizes and locations. A-beta (skin) or type I (muscle) are large-diameter myelinated nerves which transmit "touch" and proprioception, respectively. Small-diameter myelinated A-delta (skin) and unmyelinated C (skin), or types II and III (muscle), carry pain messages, and type IV is located within muscles (Stux and Hammerschlag, 2000).

7.4 Pain and Acupuncture Signals Pathway

Pain perception is a complicated process in which different tissues and structures are involved. Figure 7.2 shows a simple pathway for easy understanding, though it may not explain all the phenomena associated with pain. Painful injury stimulates the sensory receptors, mainly A-delta and C-fibres on the skin. Through the spinothalamic tract (STT) within the spinal cord, it further enters the thalamus and cortex to finally form the pain perception. From the spinal cord to the cortex, several other pathways are studied.

In clinic, acupuncture practitioners regard the "De Qi" sensation as the most important factor affecting the therapeutic effects. "De Qi" commonly

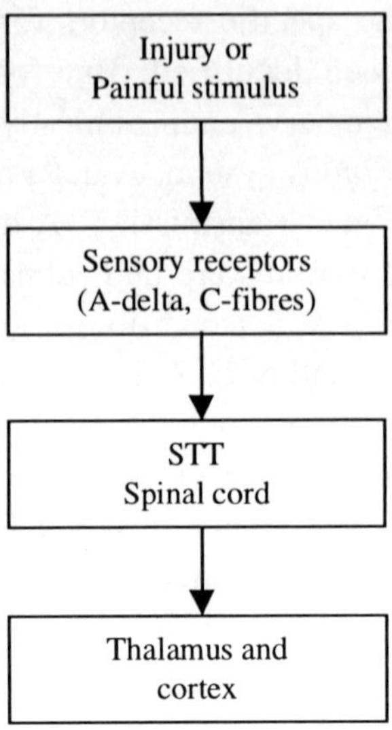

Figure 7.2. Simple pain transmission pathway.

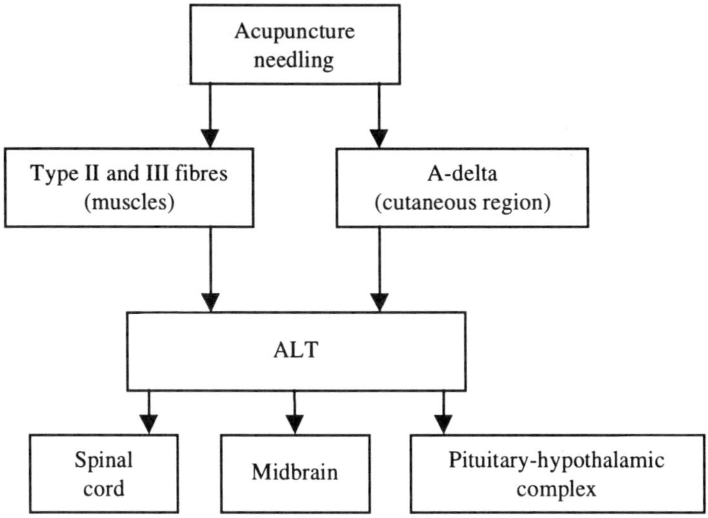

Figure 7.3. Acupuncture message transmission pathway.

means the sensation of numbness, fullness, heaviness and soreness. Neurophysiological studies have shown that the relationship between "De Qi" and the afferent nerves is that type II fibres are responsible for numbness, type III for fullness and type IV for soreness. When the needles are inserted into the body, the sensory receptors located inside the muscles (types II and III) and inside the cutaneous region (A-delta) are stimulated and the information is transferred to three centres (spinal cord, midbrain and pituitary-hypothalamic complex) via the anterolateral tract (ALT). The needling pathways are described in Fig. 7.3.

7.5 Acupuncture Analgesia Mechanism Inside the Three Centres

Three centres involved in AA are: the spinal cord, midbrain and hypothalamus/pituitary. Two different approaches have been studied. When low frequency, high intensity stimulation by electro-acupuncture (EA) was applied to activate the neurons within the spinal cord, these neurons will then control the release of enkephalin or dynorphin. Only enkephalin is released in the midbrain. At the higher level, hypothalamus-pituitary complex, the pituitary releases β-endorphins into the blood and cerebrospinal fluid (CSF) to block pain from a long distance. The hypothalamus also communicates with the midbrain via β-endorphins to activate the descending system and release adrenocorticotropic hormones (ACTH), which in turn promote the release of steroids from the adrenal cortex which can reduce inflammation. Another approach is high frequency with low intensity by EA. The impulses from this kind of stimulation act at two neural sites. Inside the spinal cord, they activate non-endorphinergic transmitters (such as gamma aminobutyric acid, GABA). In the midbrain, they stimulate the raphe nucleus to release serotonin and norepinephrine which can block pain (Birch, 1999). What is the importance of the three centres in clinic? It is found that needling local segment may attain more intensive analgesia than distal needling because the former activates all three centres. That is to say, it not only maximises the segmental circuits within the spinal cord, but also sends messages to the midbrain and the hypothalamus-pituitary complex. Furthermore, the findings of studies show that low frequency, high intensity stimulation have some kind of different effect from that of high frequency, low intensity stimulation. The effect of the former is slower onset, longer duration and is cumulative; on the contrary, that of the latter is faster onset, shorter duration with no cumulative effect. The low frequency, high intensity stimulation can also easily develop tolerance compared to stimulation with high frequency and low intensity.

7.6 Acupuncture Analgesia and Opioid and Antiopioid Peptides

In 1975, Hughes *et al.* discovered enkephalins, the first family of endogenous opioids (Hughes *et al.*, 1975). After that, two other opioid peptides, endorphins and dynorphins were discussed (Cox *et al.*, 1976; Goldstein *et al.*, 1979). The involvement of opiate in AA has three levels: opiate receptors, opioid peptides and neural pathways mediating opioid effects.

7.6.1 *Opiate receptors*

In 1976, Pomeranz and Chiu conducted an experiment in which mice were divided into seven groups: EA alone at LI4, EA plus saline, EA plus naloxone, sham EA at a non-acupuncture point, naloxone alone, saline alone, and no treatment at all. Naloxone was initially reported as an antagonist in this experiment. Mouse squeak latency paradigm was observed. The results showed that naloxone can completely block AA, naloxone produced little hyperalgesia, and sham EA produced no AA effect, which means EA does not have a psychological effect (Pomeranz and Chiu, 1976). One year later, Mayer *et al.* performed another experiment on human volunteers with acute laboratory-induced tooth pain. The subjects were given either acupuncture plus naloxone or acupuncture plus saline. It was found that naloxone blocked AA, but in those subjects who took acupuncture plus saline, AA was achieved after 30 minutes and it lasted for over an hour (Mayer *et al.*, 1977).

Further cross-tolerance studies found that both 100 Hz and 2 Hz can develop tolerance if either is singly applied for a long time (Han *et al.*, 1991). The tolerance disappeared when applying these two frequencies alternately, which implied that different mechanisms were involved. There are three categories of opioid receptors: μ, δ and η. It was recognised that 2 Hz and 15 Hz can activate μ and δ receptors and are sensitive to naloxone; 100 Hz was medicated by the η receptor. In many cases, the subjects may not have a response to EA. The reason is that they may genetically lack opiate receptors (Peets and Pomeranz, 1978) or endorphin molecules (Murai *et al.*, 1986).

7.6.2 *Opioid peptides*

Two approaches have been used to study the mechanism of opioid peptides in AA. Han *et al.* developed the technique of antibody microinjection which is used to identify the chemical nature of the mediators (He and Han, 1990; Wang *et al.*, 1990c). Each antibody used should recognise and bind to its specific target peptide preventing the interaction between peptide receptors. Their findings strongly support the hypothesis that 2 Hz EA uses β-endorphins in the midbrain and enkephalins in the spinal cord to produce AA, while 100 Hz EA uses dynorphins in the spinal cord. Another opioid peptide, endorphin, was discovered in the mid-1970s. The induction of AA by endorphins can be blocked by naxolone (Mayer *et al.*, 1977; Pomeranz and Chiu, 1976). Experiments on rats show that endorphins are involved in 2 Hz EA but not in 100 Hz, at least in the level of the spinal cord. Similar results were achieved by another approach, radioimmunoassay of spinal perfusate. The level of a particular peptide in CSF is determined by its release from the spinal cord. Through the radioimmunological technique, more enkephalins and dynorphins were found in CSF by 2 Hz EA and 100 Hz, respectively (Fei *et al.*, 1987). Han *et al.* also found the consistent results from human experiments (Han *et al.*, 1991).

7.6.3 *Neural pathways for opioid peptides*

Opioid peptides can only exert their action through some specific neural structure. There are different mechanisms for low frequency and high frequency EA analgesia. It has been known that in the arcuate nucleus of the hypothalamus (ARH), neurons containing β-endorphins aggregate there. But enkephalins and dynorphins are widely distributed in both the brain and spinal cord. Since low frequency analgesia is mediated through β-endorphins, the ARH should be the responsible structure. Several lesions were applied in the nuclei of the thalamus and hypothalamus in order to find the possible neural substrate within the midbrain (Wang *et al.*, 1990b). Kainic acid, which can selectively destroy neural cell bodies by microinjection into ARH, will reduce the effect of EA analgesia induced by 2 Hz, but not by 100 Hz. Cross-tolerance between 2 Hz EA analgesia and ARH stimulation-produced analgesia also offers further proof of the importance of ARH in mediating low frequency EA analgesia (Wang *et al.*, 1990a).

So what is the possible mechanism for 100 Hz EA analgesia? The results of a study found that the parabrachial nucleus (PBN) is the neural structure involved. The analgesic effect induced by 100 Hz but not 2 Hz can be selectively reduced by electrolytic or kainate lesions within the PBN. On the contrary, intra-PBN injection of glutamate can produce profound analgesia (Wang *et al.*, 1991).

Another study found that there is a common pathway for low and high frequency EA analgesia, i.e. the ventral portion of the periaqueductal gray (PAG). The analgesia effect induced by either 2 Hz or 100 Hz can be almost completely abolished if the ventral portion of PAG is destroyed by electrolytic and kainate lesion (Wang *et al.*, 1991).

7.6.3 *Antiopioid peptide-CCK-8*

As it is the most potent of antiopioid substances, CCK-8 has been thoroughly reported and studied (Han *et al.*, 1985). Han *et al.* found in these studies that the effect of EA has been gradually weakened with prolonged stimulation for more than three hours, but the content of opiate-like substances still remained at a high level. So the decline of analgesia effect cannot be caused by depletion of endogenous opiate-like substances. There must be a negative feedback mechanism with which to inhibit the release of opiate-like substances. After a lot of works, they finally determined that CCK-8 can be a potent antiopioid peptide (Han, 1992; Han, 1995a and b).

Animal studies conducted by Han *et al.* also showed a dose-dependent blockade of EA analgesia by CCK-8. Furthermore, CCK-8 appeared to be more potently active in the brain than in the spinal cord (Han *et al.*, 1985). Electrophysiological studies were then carried out in order to confirm their findings and similar results were obtained (Bian *et al.*, 1993).

Several neural structures have been found to be the possible acting sites of CCK-8 in the CNS. Microinjection techniques were applied in this kind of study and the results showed a 50% decrease of morphine analgesia when a proper dose of CCK-8 was microinjected into the rat PAG (Li and Han, 1989). Further studies implied that amygdala and nucleus accumbens were also involved as the acting sites (Zhou *et al.*, 1981 and 1984).

It has been mentioned that there are three subtypes of opiate receptors: μ, δ and η. All of them mediate the analgesic effects, but CCK-8 suppresses only the analgesia mediated by the μ and η, not by δ receptors which are specifically bound to enkephalins (Wang *et al.*, 1990d; Dickinson *et al.*, 1992).

7.7 What is the Nature of the Acupuncture Point and Meridian?

The studies on the nature of acupuncture points began a long time ago. Despite its clinical efficacy, Western doctors are still doubtful of the existence of these acupuncture points. Is there really a specific spot on the human body? Several methods have been used; including comparison between true points and sham points, the unique anatomical structures at acupuncture points, the electrical properties of skin at acupuncture points, and the nerves being activated by acupuncture.

In experiments of acute laboratory-induced pain in human subjects, needling at true points produced markedly analgesic effect while sham points produced only weak effect (Brockhaus and Elger, 1990; Chapman *et al.*, 1977; Stacher *et al.*, 1975). But for patients with chronic pain, the results were less convincing: true points were effective for 55%–85% of cases and sham points for 33%–85% of cases (Vincent and Richardson, 1986). In different animal studies, true points seem to be more effective than sham points in acute pain (Pomeranz and Chiu, 1976; Takashige, 1985; Toda and Ichioka, 1978). Mild stimulation should be used in order to avoid stress-induced analgesia since it has been well introduced (Pomeranz, 1985).

As for the anatomical structures, no special structure was found at acupuncture points. Since the local injection of anaesthetics before stimulation can block AA, many studies supported the close correlation of nerves with acupuncture points (Chiang *et al.*, 1973; Pomeranz and Paley, 1979). Neurophysiological studies showed the coincidence of acupuncture points with trigger points, and stimulation of muscle afferent is important for producing analgesia (Chiang *et al.*, 1973; Lu, 1983; Wang *et al.*, 1985). In 1952, Travell began to locate trigger points (Travell and Rinzler, 1952). In a manual, Travell stressed precisely needling of tender points and mild stimulation because the wrong location of tender points can aggravate the problem (Travell and Simmons, 1983).

How about physiological features of acupuncture points and meridians? Japanese and French researchers have made observations at skin and ear acupoints, respectively. Nakatani proposed that different parts of the body may have higher or lower impedance. Instead of the term "meridian", he used "Rydoraku channel" which means good conduction lines (Nakatani and Yamashita, 1977). Oleson *et al.* compared diagnosis with "point finder" machine on the ear and Western medical approach, and the results showed 72.5% correlation between the two methods (Oleson *et al.*, 1980). But the lower impedance was attributed to pressure artifacts from electrodes later. It has been known that stress from acupuncture can activate the sympathetic causing sweating, which has a profound influence on skin impedance. Vernjone injected a radioactive isotope subcutaneously into humans and found vertical lines resembling meridians in their distribution (Verneijoul *et al.*, 1985). Later, a doctor in North Korea published a monograph and claimed that he had discovered the nature of meridians and acupoints. However, the latter's findings contained technical errors, thus casting serious doubts. Despite all of the above findings, Melzack and Katz believed that there was no difference between acupoints and nearby control points in patients with chronic pain (Melzack and Katz, 1984).

Another interesting phenomenon related to meridians is that of propagated sensations along the meridians (PSM). It was estimated that about 10% of the population can feel a radiating sensation along the meridian in a direction inappropriate to that of the nerves. The PSM is from distal to proximal and its speed of transmission is about 10 cm/s, which is ten times slower than the slowest C-fibres (Bensoussan, 1994a and b).

Chiang *et al.* applied skin analgesia tests and found that acupoints in the arm produced equal analgesia in all parts of the body. In other words, the effect of acupuncture lacks of target specificity (Chiang *et al.*, 1973). Two more studies support Chiang's study, but they wrongly attributed the relief of pain to the placebo effect because they used the improper sham acupoints (Lim *et al.*, 1977; Lynn and Perl, 1977). Sham acupoints should refer to non-meridian acupoints, and not those located on the meridians separate from that of true acupoints. Maybe acupuncture has more or less the placebo effect that can never be the most important one. If not so, how can we explain the use of acupuncture in veterinary medicine for over 1000 years in China and for about 100 years in Europe (Stux and Hammerschalag, 2000).

7.8 Auricular Acupuncture — What is Its Mechanism?

Like foot reflexology and hand and scalp acupuncture, auricular acupuncture is one of the micro-acupuncture systems that is based on the theory of holographic homunculus pattern. Since Paul Nogier of Lyon, France described his inverted foetus map, auricular acupuncture has been redeveloped and widely applied in China.

Nogier thought that there are three different zones on the auricle that is related to different types of neural innervation and different categories of embryological tissue (Nogier, 1983). And there is a special somatotopic organisation of the acupoints on auricle. That is to say, the central concha of the auricle is innervated by the vagus nerve and serves as the region for autonomic regulation of pain and pathology produced from internal organs. The surrounding antihelix and antitragus ridges of the auricle represent somatic nerve processing of myofascial pain, back pain and headaches. The outer helix tail and earlobe represent the spinal cord and geminal neuralgia.

It has been known that there are both descending pain facilitation and descending pain inhibition systems in the central nervous system. Oleson proposed that the relief of pain by auricular acupuncture can be interpreted by the theory of stimulation-produced analgesia. The most potent area for obtaining stimulation-produced analgesia in rats is the midbrain periaqueductal gray, which is a region containing neurons specifically responsive to noxious stimuli. For higher species, deep brain stimulation in the subcortical thalamus is a more potent site for stimulation-produced analgesia. Similar results have been found in human patients (Hosobuchi *et al.*, 1979). Positron emission tomography (PET) scan activity in the periaqueductal gray, hypothalamus, somatosensory cortex and prefrontal cortex can be activated by nociceptive pain messages (Hsieh *et al.*, 1995).

In order to examine the bioelectric properties of auricular acupoints, Oleson conducted a double-blind assessment in which 40 patients with specific musculoskeletal pain were recruited (Oleson *et al.*, 1980). The medical diagnosis was previously established through Western medical technologies. Then a doctor with extensive auricular acupuncture knowledge will examine the patient's ear and he or she was not allowed to interact verbally with the patients. The results showed a positive correspondence between auricular acupoints (tender to palpation or exhibiting at least 50 μA of electrical conductivity) and the parts of the body where there was musculoskeletal pain. The overall correct rate was 75.2%. All these supported the fact that specific areas of the ear are related to specific parts of the body. Another assessment was conducted to examine the correspondence of heart diseases to the inferior concha and tragus (aurilular acupoint related to heart). Compared with the control group of healthy subjects (11%), the true group had correspondence of 84% in the inferior concha and 59% in the tragus.

In 1950s, Nakatani in Japan and Niboyet in France first reported their observations that auricular acupoints showed higher levels of skin conductance or lower levels of skin resistance than surrounding areas. The electrical resistance of skin ranged from 100 to 900 kOhm, while non-auricular acupoints from 1100 to 11,700 kOhm.

Clinically, auricular acupuncture is a popular selection by doctors and patients for certain conditions, including obesity and opiate drug dependence. A randomised controlled trial (RCT) study by Richards and Marley found women's weight loss was significantly greater in the auricular group than in the control group (Richards and Marley, 1998). It has been showed the appetite can be suppressed by stimulating the auricular branch of the vagus nerve and raising serotonin levels. Electrical stimulation was applied to the auricular acupoints of Stomach and Shen Men in the auricular acupuncture group, while in control group, transcutaneous electrical stimulation was given to the first joint of the thumb. Neuroanatomy recognised that two regions of the hypothalamus are responsible for weight control. The ventromedial hypothalamus (VMH) is referred to as the satiety centre, whereas the lateral hypothalamus (LH) as the feeding centre. Asamoto and Takeshige's study showed that electrical stimulation of auricular acupoints can selectively activate the neurons in VMH satiety centre but not in the lateral hypothalamic feeding centre (Asamoto and Takashige, 1992). The findings suggest that auricular acupuncture can selectively alter hypothalamic brain activity and is more likely to produce sensations of VMH than reduction of LH appetite.

Drug addiction is another condition in which auricular acupuncture was recommended. Wen discovered that auricular acupuncture can promote withdrawal from narcotic drugs (Wen and Cheung, 1973). Further studies showed that met-enkephalin levels have been raised in human heroin addicts and beta-endorphin levels raised in mice with morphine addiction. In another research, 14 patients with chronic pain taking oral methadone were studied (Kroening and Oleson, 1985). The auricular acupoints, "Lung" point and "Shen Men" point were needled bilaterally with electrical stimulation. All the patients were withdrawn from methadone within two to seven days, with only a few reported slight side effects of nausea and agitation.

7.9 Modern Technologies Involved in Acupuncture Research

With the rapid development of medical imaging technologies, Western medical doctors gained more powerful tools to make accurate diagnosis. Can these new instruments be used for explaining some possible mechanisms of acupuncture? A lot of work has been done in this field.

Computed tomography (CT), positron emission tomography (PET), magnetic resonance imaging (MRI), all these are more sensitive scanning techniques. It is confirmed that they are very useful in providing imaging diagnosis, especially for brain-related diseases. For example, a study has shown that the benefits of stroke patients from acupuncture can be objectively judged CT scanning through detecting the uptake of cerebral blood glucose or blood flow (Naeser *et al.*, 1992). The asymmetry of blood flow was found in the thalamus of those patients with chronic pain through PET technique. We have known that the thalamus is an important structure in pain transmission. But the asymmetry was greatly reduced after acupuncture treatment (Alavi *et al.*, 1996).

Many theories have been put forward to explain the anatomical bases of acupuncture and meridians. Peripheral nerves and blood vessels, surrounded by small nerve bundles, are considered to be the most relative structures (Chan, 1984; Chiang *et al.*, 1973). Chao *et al.* applied the MRI approach to test their hypothesis that sensory-related acupoints have brain cortical correspondence (Cho *et al.*, 1998). Visual cortex was observed following needling of acupoint UB. 67, which was commonly used to treat eye-related problems. Later, another two acupoints, GB 37 and GB 43, were used to study the MRI changes before and after needling in order to confirm whether or not they are specific points for eye-related and ear-related diseases, respectively. Furthermore, they compared the results with those of the initial study on UB 67. Needling of UB 67 was found to promote the blood flow, in other words, the MRI signals in several regions of the visual cortex. Also, UB 66 and UB 65 had the same effect of activation in the visual cortex. But no visual cortex activity was found following the needling of SP 1 on the large toe, which is irrelevant to the eye according to meridian theories. Interestingly, needling of GB 37 also showed strong activation in the visual cortex region. Another area, auditory cortex, was further explored after the needling of GB 43 and similar results were obtained. All of these findings express the idea that messages from certain acupoints are projected to specific region(s) of the brain via the spinal cord and brainstem, which explains part of the mechanism of acupuncture's effectiveness.

7.10 Some Issues in Acupuncture Clinical Trials

Acupuncture has spread worldwide during the last three decades. With the growing interest in the therapeutic applications of acupuncture, there is a strong desire to explain the mechanism of action in terms of modern scientific knowledge. Unfortunately, the quality of acupuncture clinical trials since the early 1970s is often poor. And there is a relative paucity of good clinical trials of acupuncture. The papers published in English are still few and of variable methodological quality. Whilst the outcomes of some trials support the efficacy of acupuncture, they are compromised by methodological flaws. To date, the use of acupuncture is still based mainly on traditional and personal experience. So appropriate scientific studies would be useful for the rational use and further development of acupuncture. WHO made an emphasis on investigating the mechanism of acupuncture effect, which is directly concerned with the promotion and delivery of acupuncture in health care services.

7.10.1 *The BRITS method*

The quality or adequacy of acupuncture in most clinical trials may be problematic (Cheng, 1987; Prance *et al.*, 1988; Stux, 1990). Considering this, some have discussed guidelines on what constitutes adequate treatment (Berman *et al.*, 2000; Stux, 1995). Birch developed a set of criteria for evaluating the adequacy of treatment in acupuncture studies. The following aspects are included: randomisation, adequate description of the acupuncture treatment, adequate acupuncture treatment, the training of the acupuncturist, adequate description of control treatment, appropriate control treatment, sample size calculation, blinded evaluators, follow-up

Table 7.1. The results of Birch's review from 33 studies.

Criteria	Number of studies	
	Yes	No
Adequate description of treatment	31	2
Adequate treatment	17	16
Mention of the qualifications of the acupuncturist	8	25
Appropriate control treatment if needed	17	11
Randomisation	25	5
Blinded evaluators	19	9
Follow-up of three months or more	13	12
Mention of side-effects	16	17

after three or more months and side-effects record. According to the above criteria, Birch reviewed 33 studies. The results are shown in Table 7.1.

A method, named "Birch Relevant and Irrelevant Treatment Selection" (BRITS), was developed by Birch in early 1993. It aims to establish treatment validity and improve generalisability of results through extensive literature reviews. In the United States, major clinical trials adopted this method (Birch *et al.*, 1999; Margolin *et al.*, 1995 and 1997). As an easily applied standardisable approach, it helps to ensure appropriateness and adequacy of the test treatment, to select and validate irrelevant acupoints for the control treatment, to allow a broad generalisation of the results, and to formulate assessment criteria to evaluate the quality of the test. Birch also offers specific guidelines on how to obtain the above objectives. For instance, the following three methods are advisable on selecting and validating the test treatment acupoints. First, the relevant texts or papers concerned with the method or tradition of practice being tested should be reviewed carefully. This is to confirm that all acupoints to be used are recommended in a minimum number of sources for some special condition, e.g. at least six. Second, in order to enhance the generalisability of the results, more treatment texts should be reviewed to make sure the acupoints recommended in first step are also indicated in this step. Third, although it is not considered to be necessary, to conduct a pilot study before going to a full-scale study would be very useful to adjust the original design and determine the size of the larger follow-up studies.

7.10.2 *The adapted FDA approach*

According to the FDA regulations, it generally demands three phases for a clinical trial. Each phase has its specific features. Berman *et al.* adapted these three phases and applied them to the clinical trials of acupuncture. The following would introduce the development of each phase in detail.

The aims of phase I trials are to establish preliminary information of dose and safety of acupuncture on the condition under investigation. These trials are generally of small sample sizes with no control groups. Several decisions should be made during this phase. The first question is whether formulated or individualised acupuncture will be suitable for the study. The answer depends on the conditions being tested. If the patients share the same Western medicinal and TCM diagnoses, in other words, the patients are homogeneous populations, a design of formulated acupuncture is a better choice. On the contrary, individualised acupuncture will be more suitable for heterogeneous populations wherein many symptoms are being treated. Therefore, the demand of the experience of the acupuncturist is much higher for individualised acupuncture than for formulated acupuncture. Since different textbooks always give the different selection of points for a specific condition, it is recommended to review a wide range of literature and also consider the personal clinical observations of effectiveness. As for the total number and frequency of treatments, it is not easy to find the answer from the literature. Frequent measurements to observe the change of improvement, if present, are necessary in order to determine these two parameters.

Compared with phase I, the control group should be applied in phase II. In this stage, the dose and safety are further confirmed and the preliminary information on efficacy is initially studied. It is commonly recognised that designing a suitable control group for a certain study is a really difficult task for investigators. Currently, there are several control designs being used in clinical trials, including no treatment control, sham acupuncture, placebo acupuncture, standard medical care, etc. All of them have advantages and disadvantages. Placebo acupuncture, for example, can explain whether or not the effect of true acupuncture is due to the placebo effect. But in nature, placebo design cannot resemble the true acupuncture completely, therefore the patients cannot be blinded.

Table 7.2. Different levels of evidence.

Level	Description of evidence
I	Strong evidence from at least one systematic review of well-designed RCTs
II	Strong evidence from at least one RCT
III	Well-designed trials without randomisation
IV	Non-experimental evidence
V	Expert opinion

The main objective of the large-scale phase III and multi-centred trials is to test the efficacy of the treatment. At this stage, proper inclusion and exclusion criteria based on the knowledge of the disease and acupuncture should be determined first. To set an appropriate statistical power is also a critical item since it directly relates to the results. Nowadays, the RCT is regarded as the golden standard for clinical trial. Adequate randomisation is responsible for avoiding the selection bias. Although it seems impossible to blind the acupuncturist, the patients and outcome evaluators must be completely blinded to the treatment being given.

The recent push to apply the principles of evidence-based medicine (EBM) to Chinese medicine is an important step for scientific research. EBM is defined as "the conscientious, explicit and judicious use of current best evidence in making decisions about the care of individual patients" (Sackett *et al.*, 1996). According to the principles of EBM, doctors should make decisions based on good quality evidence, and not simply on personal experiences or so-called "expert" opinions (Moynihan, 1993). The quality of studies can be divided into different levels by systematic review or meta-analyses of EBM approach. The details are shown in Table 7.2.

7.11 Some Indications for Acupuncture Treatment in Clinic

In early November 1997, the National Institutes of Health (NIH) held a consensus development conference on acupuncture in order to provide clinicians, patients and the general public with a responsible assessment of the use and effectiveness of acupuncture to treat a variety of conditions (NIH Consensus Conference, 1998). The results of this conference showed that some conditions can be effectively treated by acupuncture, including stroke rehabilitation, low back pain, nausea and vomiting associated with pregnancy and chemotherapy, etc. Many systematic reviews relating to the efficacy of acupuncture for various conditions appeared. The following are some examples.

Low back pain: In 1989, Patel and his colleagues made a meta-analysis of acupuncture for chronic back pain. Although they found acupuncture to be effective, some designing flaws existed as well (Patel *et al.*, 1989). A few years ago, using a three-arm parallel group design, Molsberger and his team workers recruited 186 low back pain patients to study the efficacy of acupuncture on this specific problem. The three arms were real açupuncture plus baseline treatment, sham acupuncture plus baseline treatment, and baseline treatment. They determined that the primary outcome was a pain reduction of 50% or more via VAS measurement at the end of treatment. After an intention to treat analysis was done, they found that the achievement of the primary outcome was 76.6% (real acupuncture), 29.3% (sham acupuncture) and 13.9% (conservative treatment). Thus, they concluded that acupuncture is an important supplement in the management of chronic back pain (Molsberger, 1998).

Nausea and vomiting: The consistently supportive evidence of acupuncture is for the treatment of nausea and vomiting (Vickers, 1996). In this systematic review, 27 of the 29 trials showed positive results. Among 12 trials with highest methodological quality, 11 trials supported acupuncture. In its consensus statement, NIH consensus panel said "there is clear evidence that needle acupuncture is efficacious for adult post-operative and chemotherapy nausea and vomiting and probably for the nausea of pregnancy" (Chan, 1984).

Headache: Headache (including migraine) is a big problem in clinic. Acupuncture has long been used to solve this problem, as its level of efficacy is very high. A systematic review was conducted to assess the efficacy of acupuncture on headaches and migraines (Melchart *et al.*, 1999). The results showed a trend in favour of acupuncture. But the reviewers also found that the trials included were of small sample size with methodological limitations. Furthermore, the types of acupuncture procedure used in these trials varied extremely, making it difficult for the reviewers to draw a clear conclusion.

Stroke rehabilitation: This is another condition covered by the NIH Consensus Development Conference. In China, acupuncture serves as a necessary rehabilitation approach for stroke patients. Some reviews showed the additional benefit of acupuncture to standard care regimen, although the subjects experienced different stroke histories (Ernst and White, 1996; Hopwood, 1996; Naeser, 1996).

7.12 Conclusion

The integration and incorporation of a new clinical intervention, like acupuncture, into the accepted mainstream of health care delivery system faces a lot of difficulties. Acupuncture should explore and establish its value in such areas as chronic pain, post-operative rehabilitation, immune-related diseases, allergic diseases, etc., for which Western medicine cannot provide good solutions. Basic research and clinical trials are both important to identify the possible mechanisms and the efficacies of acupuncture. Evidence-based medicine and RCTs should be more naturally applied into the studies of acupuncture in order to improve the credibility and validity of acupuncture research.

It has been more than a decade since I embarked on the study and research of acupuncture. For the love of Chinese traditional culture, I have chosen this ancient art of healing as my career. Though I have had moments of doubt and uncertainly, I have now come to accept and trust my choice. The following sums up my understanding of acupuncture over the years.

Acupuncture Education

Currently, the Chinese medicine education system in China places importance on both Chinese and Western medicine, the ratio being seven to three. Under the influence of two very different types of ▶

medical knowledge, it is normal for students to have contrasted answers to the same questions. And they began to doubt the choice of their profession. In my opinion, the confusion arose because we have become too accustomed to the Western medicine mode of linear thinking, the influence of which we were under from primary to secondary schools. However, Chinese medicine thinks in a totally fuzzy manner — correlative thinking — aptly represented by its theories of *Yin-Yang*, Five Elements and *Zang-Fu* (the viscera).

Acupuncture Research

Acupuncture, after undergoing a few thousand years of ups and downs, has accumulated a wealth of clinical experience. To a certain extent, it is a form of empirical medicine, and this practical knowledge is preserved as it passes down the generations. However, this does not imply that acupuncture is a product of empiricism. I believe that there exists concrete evidence of its effectiveness, which just have not been discovered yet. To prove my point, and also to look into the possibility of "the modernisation of Chinese medicine", I chose to attempt further studies in Chinese medicine. There are strengths and weaknesses in each type of medicine; the areas in which Chinese medicine is beneficial are chronic illnesses, viral diseases, immunological diseases and some intractable illnesses. Therefore, I chose to study asthma and senescence for my Masters and Ph.D. degrees, respectively. Asthma is a chronic illness for which there is no radical cure. It does not only cause damage to the patient's body, it also exerts a great burden on society and the economy. Based on my understanding that traditional Chinese medicine (TCM) is capable of increasing the body's immunity, my study focused on the efficacy of TCM prescription in controlling the symptoms of asthma and reducing its recurrence rate. Our results showed that the symptoms as well as data on the interleukins and the immunoglobulin have improved by different extents.

China is an ageing society and the medical expenses of the elderly account for a sizable portion. Most people develop chronic illnesses during the process of ageing. Therefore it would be a significant ▶

contribution if we can reduce the occurrence of these chronic illnesses for the elderly to ease into senescence in a relatively healthier state. In my research, I applied the traditional moxibustion therapy on the "Senescence-Accelerated Mouse" (SAM, developed by Kyoto University) to observe their ageing process. The results showed that although moxibustion could not completely reverse the path of ageing, it could actually delay its development. However, as the number of elderly people was insufficient for the clinical trials, the clinical effect of moxibustion therapy on old-age illnesses is inconclusive as yet.

The modernisation of Chinese medicine, including the modernisation of acupuncture, is an inevitable trend. In acupuncture, there are many areas worth researching into, such as the specificity of acupoints, the essence of channels and collaterals, clinical treatment of illnesses, etc. Nevertheless, before we discuss the modernisation of acupuncture, we need to know the correct way to modernise. China once invested a great amount of financial and human resources to study the essence of channels and collaterals, and it was a collaborative effort on a national scale no less. But in the end, scientists from different fields presented their studies from their own viewpoint. There was one similarity though: their vision became increasingly microscopic. In my opinion, the research would be more valuable if they could employ a macroscopic view for something that is macroscopic in nature, and it would be more helpful in clinical practice too. The study obtained some positive results too. For instance, in the use of electro-acupuncture to relieve pain, it is now widely recognised that electrical stimulation at a low frequency and a high intensity is a better choice. The purpose of basic research and clinical trials is to improve clinical efficacy, hence we should focus our attention on complex clinical problems. Only then would our research be useful.

Acupuncture Clinical Practice

I observed, in my clinical practice, that acupuncture works better for peripheral nerve and muscles, and displays better results in vascular diseases, central nervous system (CNS) and post-operative ▶

rehabilitation. As for facial paralysis, headache, trigeminal neuralgia, chronic low back pain, stroke rehabilitation, and some specialty diseases like myopia in children, bed-wetting, nausea and vomiting associated with pregnancy, menstruation disorders, etc. it has been shown that acupuncture can help to regulate the nerve-endocrine immunity circuit, after ruling out organic pathology.

Every patient is unique, requiring us to address each problem specifically. The dialectical approach in Chinese medicine has its necessity. On the other hand, some academics proposed to combine the dialectical approach with the concept of differentiation of diseases. In cases where the patient's pathology and diagnosis are clear and unambiguous, taking these two factors into consideration could certainly improve the efficacy of TCM. However, if the symptoms are constantly changing within a period of time, we should then refer to the dialectical approach. Moreover, I think it is futile to search for a specific acupoint for a certain kind of illness. The function of an acupoint is neither singular nor fixed, and it could affect the focus of infection in an indirect manner. I believe that this indirect path is the nerve-endocrine immunity circuit, which deals with illnesses by building up the patient's resistance to them. It should be the main mechanism in the use of acupuncture for treatment of illnesses.

References

Acupuncture-NIH Consensus Conference (1998) *J. Am. Med. Assoc.* **17**, 1518–1524.

Alavi, A., LaRiccia, P., Sadek, H., Lattannd, C., Lee, L., Reich, H. and Mozley, P.D. (1996) Objective assessment of the effects of pain and acupuncture on regional brain function with Tc99mm HMPAO SPECT imaging. *J. Nucl. Med.* **37**(Suppl. 5), 278.

Asamoto, S. and Takeshige, C. (1992) Activation of the satiety center by auricular acupuncture point stimulation. *Brain. Res. Bull.* **29**, 157–164.

Bensoussan, A. (1994a) Acupuncture meridians — myth or reality? Part 1. *Comp. Ther. Med.* **2**, 21–26.

Bensoussan, A. (1994b) Acupuncture meridians — myth or reality? Part 2. *Comp. Ther. Med.* **2**, 80–85.

Berman, B.M., Ezzo, J., Hadhazy, V., Jadad, A., Lao, L. and Singh, B.B. (2000) Penetrating the methodological issues in randomised controlled trials of acupuncture and chronic pain: a systematic review. *Pain* **89**, 217–227.

Bian, J.T., Sun, M.Z., Xu, M.Y. and Han, J.S. (1993) Antagonism by CCK-8 of the antinociceptive effect of electro acupuncture on pain-related neurons in nucleus parafascicularis of the rat. *Asia Pac. J. Pharmacol.* **8**, 90–97.

Birch, S.J. and Felt, R. and Robert, L. (1999) *Understanding Acupuncture.* Churchill Livingstone, Edinburgh.

Brockhaus, A. and Elger, C.E. (1990) Hypalgesic efficacy of acupuncture on experimental pain in men. Comparison of laser acupuncture and needle acupuncture. *Pain* **43**, 181–185.

Cao, X. (1999) Scientific basis of acupuncture. In: *Consultation Meeting on Traditional and Modern Medicine: Harmonising the Two Approaches.* WHO, Beijing, pp. 67–79.

Chan, S.H. (1984) What is being stimulated in acupuncture: evaluation of the existence of a specific substrate. *Neurosci. Behav. Rev.* **8**, 25–33.

Chapman, C.R., Chen, A.C. and Bonica, J.J. (1977) Effects of intrasegmental electrical acupuncture on dental pain: evaluation by threshold estimation and sensory decision theory. *Pain* **3**, 213–227.

Cheng, X.N. (1987) *Chinese Acupuncture and Moxibustion.* Foreign Languages Press, Beijing.

Chiang, C.Y., Chang, C.T., Chu, H.L. and Yang, I.L. (1973) Peripheral afferent pathway for acupuncture analgesia. *Sci. Sin.* **16**, 210–217.

Cho, Z.H., Chung, S.C., Jones, J.P., Park, H.J., Lee, H.J., Wong, E.K. and Min, B.I. (1998) New findings of the correlation between acupoints and corresponding brain cortices using functional MRI. *Proc. Natl. Acad. Sci. USA* **95**, 2670–2673.

Cox, B.A., Goldstein, A. and Li, C.H. (1976) Opiate activity of a peptide, β-lipotropin (61-91) derived from β-lipotropin. *Proc. Natl. Acad. Sci. USA* **73**, 1821–1823.

Dickenson, A.H., Sullivan, A.F. and Magnuson, D.S. (1992) CCK and opioid interaction in the spinal cord. In: *Multiple CCK Receptors in the CNS.* (eds.) Dourish, C.T., Cooper, S.J., Iverson, S.D., *et al.* Oxford University Press, Oxford, pp. 503–510.

Ernst, E. and White, A.R. (1996) Acupuncture as an adjuvant therapy in stroke rehabilitation? *Wien. Med. Wochenschr.* **146**, 556–558.

Fei, H., Xie, G.X. and Han, J.S. (1987) Low and high frequency electroacupuncture stimulation releases met-enkephalin and dynorphin A in rat spinal cord. *Chin. Sci. Bull.* **34**, 703–705.

Gellman, H. (2002) *Acupuncture Treatment for Musculoskeletal Pain.* Taylor & Francis Press.

Goldstein, A., Tachibana, S., Lowrey, L.I., *et al.* (1979) Dynorphin (1-13): an extraordinary potent opiate peptide. *Proc. Natl. Acad. Sci. USA* **76**, 6666–6670.

Han, J.S. (1992) The role of CCK in the electro acupuncture analgesia and electro acupuncture tolerance. In: *Multiple Cholecystokinin Receptors in the CNS.* (eds.) Dourish, C.T., Cooper, S.J., Iversen, S.D. and Iversen, L.L. Oxford University Press, Oxford, pp. 480–502.

Han, J.S. (1995a) Cholecystokinin octapeptide (CCK-8): a negative feedback control mechanism for opioid analgesia. *Prog. Brain. Res.* **105**, 263–271.

Han, J.S. (1995b) Molecular events underlying the antiopioid effect of CCK-8 in the central nervous system. In: *Pharmacological Sciences: Perspectives for Research and Therapy in the Late 1990s.* (eds.) Cuello, A.C. and Collier, B. Birkhauser Verlag, Basel, pp. 199–207.

Han, J.S., Chen, X.H., Sun, S.L., *et al.* (1991) Effect of low and high frequency TENS on met-enkephlin-Arg-Phe and dynorphin-A immunoreactivity in human lumbar CSF. *Pain* **47**, 295–298.

Han, J.S., Ding, X.Z. and Fan, S.G. (1985) Is CCK-8 a candidate for endogenous antiopioid peptide substrate? *Neuropeptides* **5**, 399–402.

He, C.M. and Han, J.S. (1990) Attenuation of low rather than high frequency electro acupuncture analgesia by micro injection of β-endorphin anti serum into the periaqueductal gray in rats. Acupuncture. *Sci. Int. J.* **1**, 94–99.

Hopwood, V. (1996) Acupuncture in the stroke recovery: a literature review. *Complem. Ther. Med.* **4**, 258–263.

Hosobuchi, Y., Rossier, J., Bloom, F.E. and Guillemin, R. (1979) Stimulation of human periaqueductal gray for pain relief increases immunoreactive beta-endorphin in ventricular fluid. *Science* **203**, 279–281.

Hsieh, J., Stahle-Backdahl, M., Hagermark, O. and Stone-Elander, S. (1995) Traumatic nociceptive pain activates the hypothalamus and the periaqueductal gray: a positron emission tomography study. *Pain* **64**, 303–314.

Huang, K.C. (1996) *Acupuncture, the Past and the Present.* Vantage Press, New York.

Hughes, J., Smith, T.W., Kosteritz, H.W., *et al.* (1975) Identification of two related pentapeptides from the brain with potent opiate agonist activity. *Nature* **258**, 577–579.

Hyman, S.E. and Cassem, N.H. (1989) In: *Pain.* (eds.) Rubinstein, E. and Federmann, D.D. Scientific American, New York.

Klide, A.M. and Kung, S.H. (1977) *Veterinary Acupuncture*. University of Pennsylvania Press, Philadelphia.

Kroening, R. and Oleson, T. (1985) Rapid narcotic dotoxification in chronic pain patients treated with auricular electroacupuncture and naloxone. *Int. J. Additions* **20**(9), 1347–1360.

Latshaw, W.K. (1975) Current theories of pain perception related to acupuncture. *J. Am. Anim. Hosp. Assoc.* **11**, 449–450.

Li, Y. and Han, J.S. (1989) Cholecystokinin octapeptide antagonizes morphine analgesia in periaqueductal gray of the rat. *Brain. Res.* **480**, 105–110.

Lim, T.W., Loh, T. and Kranz, H.S. (1977) Acupuncture effect on normal subjects. *Med. J. Aust.* **26**, 440–442.

Lu, G.W. (1983) Characteristics of afferent fiber innervation on acupuncture point Zu san li. *Am. J. Physiol.* **245**, R606–R612.

Lynn, B. and Perl, E.R. (1977) Failure of acupuncture to produce localised analgesia. *Pain* **3**, 339–351.

Margolin, A., Avants, S.K., Birch, S., Falk, C.X. and Kleber, H.D. (1997) Methodological investigations for a multisite trial of auricular acupuncture for cocaine addiction. A study of active and control auricular zones. *J. Subst. Abuse Treat.* **13**, 471–481.

Margolin, A., Avants, S.K., Chang, P. and Birch, S. (1995) A single blind investigation of four needle puncture conditions. *Am. J. Chin. Med.* **23**, 105–114.

Mayer, D.J., Price, D.D. and Raffia, A. (1977) Antagonism of acupuncture analgesia in man by the narcotic antagonist naloxone. *Brain. Res.* **121**, 368–372

Melchart, K., Linde, K., Fischer, P., Berman, B., White, A., Vickers, A. and Allais, G. (1999) Acupuncture for recurrent headaches (Cochrane review). In: *The Cochrane Library, Issue 3.* Update Software, Oxford.

Melzack, R. and Katz, J. (1984) Auriculotherapy fails to relieve chronic pain. *J. Am. Med. Assoc.* **251**, 1041–1043.

Melzack, R. and Wall, P.P. (1965) *Science* **150**, 971.

Molsberger, A. (1998) *Acupuncture in Chronic Low Back Pain.* Paper presented at the International Society for the Study of the Lumbar Spine, Brussels.

Moynihan, R. (1993) *Too Much Medicine?* ABC Books, Sydney.

Murai, M., Takeshige, C., *et al.* (1986) Correlation between individual variations in effectiveness of acupuncture analgesia and those in contents of brain endogenous morphine-like factors. In: *Studies on the Mechanism of Acupuncture Analgesia Based on Animal Experiments.* Showa University Press, Tokyo, p. 542.

Naeser, M.A. (1996) Acupuncture in the treatment of paralysis due to central nervous system damage. *J. Alt. Complem. Med.* **2**, 211–248.

Naeser, M.A., Alexander, M.P., Stiassny-Eder, D., Galler, V., Hobbs, J. and Bachman, D. (1992) Real versus sham acupuncture in the treatment of paralysis in acute stroke patients: a CT scan lesion site study. *J. Neurol. Rehab.* **6**, 163–173.

Nakatani, Y. and Yamashita, K. (1977) *Ryodoraku Acupuncture.* Ryodoraku Research Institute, Osaka.

NIH Consensus Conference (1998) Acupuncture. *J. Am. Med. Assoc.* **280**, 1518–1524.

Nogier, P. (1983) *From Auriculotherapy to Auriculomedicine.* Mainsonneuve, Moulins-les-Metz.

Oleson, T.D., Kroening, R.J. and Bresler, D.E. (1980) An experimental evaluation of auricular diagnosis: the somatotopic mapping of musculoskeletal pain at acupucture points. *Pain* **8**, 217–229.

Patel, M., Gutzwiller, F., Paccaud, F. and Marazzi, A. (1989) A meta-analysis of acupuncture for chronic pain. *Int. J. Epidemiol.* **18**, 900–906.

Peets, J. and Pomeranz, B. (1978) CXBX mice deficient in opiate receptors show poor electro acupuncture analgesia. *Nature* **273**, 675–676

Pomeranz, B. (1985) Relation of stress-induced analgesia to acupuncture analgesia. In: *Stress-induced Analgesia.* (ed.) Kelly, J. *Ann. NY Acad. Sci.*, pp. 444–447.

Pomeranz, B. and Chiu, D. (1976) Naloxone blocks acupuncture analgesia and causes hyperalgesia: endorphin is implicated. *Life Sci.* **19**, 1757–1762.

Pomeranz, B. and Paley, D. (1979) Electroacupuncture hypoalgesia is mediatedby afferent nerve impulses: an electrophysiological study in mice. *Exp. Neurol.* **66**, 398–402.

Prance, S.E., Dresser, A., Wood, C., Fleming, J., Aldridge, D. and Pietroni, P.C. (1988) Research on traditional Chinese acupuncture — science or myth: a review. *J. R. Soc. Med.* **81**, 588–590.

Richards, D. and Marley, J. (1998) Stimulation of auricular acupuncture points in weight loss. *Aust. Fam. Physician* **27**(Suppl. 2), S73–S77.

Sackett, D.L., Rosenberg, W.M.C., Gray, J.A.M., Haynes, R.B. and Richardson, W.S. (1996) Evidence based medicine: what is and what it isn't. *Br. Med. J.* **312**, 71–72.

Stacher, G., Wancura, I., *et al.* (1975) Effect of acupuncture on pain threshold and pain tolerance determined by electrical stimulation of the skin: a controlled study. *Am. J. Chin. Med.* **3**, 143–146.

Stux, G. (1990) Migraine treatment with acupuncture and moxibustion. *Acupunct. Sci. Int. J.* **1**, 16–18.

Stux, G. (1995) Qualitataskriterien fur die akupunktur bei linischen studien. In: *Einfuhrung in die Akupunktur*, 4th Ed. (ed.) Stux, G. Springer-Verlag, Berlin.

Stux, G. and Hammerschlag, R. (2000) *Clinical Acupuncture — Scientific Basis.* Springer-Verlag, Berlin.

Takeshige, C. (1985) Differentiation between acupuncture and nonacupuncture points by association with an analgesia inhibitory system. *Acupunct. Electrother. Res.* **10**, 195–203.

Toda, K. and Ichioka, M. (1978) Electroacupuncture relations between forelimb afferent impulses and suppression of jaw opening reflex in the rat. *Exp. Neurol.* **61**, 465–470.

Travell, J. and Rinzler, S.H. (1952) Myofascial genesis of pain. *Postgrad. Med. J.* **11**, 425–434.

Travell, J. and Simmons, D. (1983) *Myofascial Pain and Dysfunction. The Trigger Point Manual.* William and Wilkins, Baltimore.

Verneijoul, P. de, Parras, J.C., *et al.* (1985) Etude des meridians d' acupuncture par les traccurs radioactifs. *Bull. Acad. Natl. Med. (Paris)* **169**, 1071–1075.

Vickers, A.J. (1996) Can acupuncture have specific effects on health? A systematic review of acupuncture antiemesis trials. *J. R. Soc. Med.* **89**, 303–311.

Vincent, C.A. and Richardson, P.H. (1986) The evaluation of therapeutic acupuncture: concepts and methods. *Pain* **24**, 1–13.

Wang, K., Yao, S., Xian, Y. and Hou, Z. (1985) A study on the receptive field of acupoints and the relationship between characteristics of needle sensation and groups of afferent febers. *Sci. Sin.* **28**, 963–971.

Wang, Q., Mao, L.M. and Han, J.S. (1990a) Analgesic electrical stimulation of the hypothalamic arcuate nucleus: tolerance and its cross-tolerance to 2 Hz or 100 Hz electro acupuncture. *Brain. Res.* **518**, 40–46.

Wang, Q., Mao, L.M. and Han, J.S. (1990b) The arcuate nucleus of hypothalamus mediates low but not high frequency electro acupuncture analgesia in rats. *Brain. Res.* **513**, 60–66.

Wang, Q., Mao, L.M. and Han, J.S. (1990c) The role of PAG in mediation of analgesia produced different frequencies electro acupuncture stimulation in rats. *Int. J. Neurosci.* **53**, 167–172

Wang, Q., Mao, L.M. and Han, J.S. (1991) The role of parabrachial nucleus in high frequency electro acupuncture analgesia in rats. *Chin. J. Physiol. Sci.* **7**, 363–367.

Wang, X.J., Wang, X.M. and Han, J.S. (1990d) CCK-8 antagonize opioid analgesia mediated by μ- and η but not δ receptors in the spinal cord of the rat. *Brain. Res.* **523**, 5–10.

Wen, H. and Cheung, S. (1973) Treatment of drug addiction by acupuncture and electrical stimulation. *Am. J. Acupunct.* **1**, 71–75.

WHO (1995) *Guidelines for Clinical Research on Acupuncture.*

Zhou, Z.F., Du, M.Y., Jian, Y., *et al.* (1981) Effect of intracerebral microinjection of naloxone on acupuncture- and morphin-analgesia in the rabbit. *Sci. Sinica* **24**, 1166–1178.

Zhou, Z.F., Xuan, Y.T. and Han, J.S. (1984) Analgesic effect of morphine injected into habenula, nucleus accubens, or amygdala of rabbits. *Acta Pharmacol. Sin.* **5**, 150–153.

Chapter 8

The State of Chinese Medicine in China Today

Ping-Chung Leung

8.1 Introduction

Chinese medicine refers to an ancient art of healing that has developed and has continued to be popular in China. It originated from central China as a folk-art of healing, eventually spreading throughout the vast country. If *Huangdi Naijing* ("Internal Medicine") is considered the classical core knowledge from which other related text and information are derived, the geographic origin of Huangdi will thus be the centre of development of Chinese medicine. All archaeological excavations and historical deduction will tend to identify this centre to be at the historical Zhongyuan, i.e. Shenzi — Shanzi region of today (Hoizey and Hoizey, 1988).

Since China is a huge country largely influenced by once-dominating neighbouring powers like the Mongols and Jiangs (now Xinjiang), Chinese medicine of central China has mixed with medicine from the North-West, West and South-West. The Arabic influence has been brought in from the West. The Silk Route will have further introduced European concepts and methodology, whereas the South-West boundaries will be exposed to Ayurveda medicine from India (Hoizey and Hoizey, 1988; Farquhar, 1994; Cant and Sharma, 1966; Kleinman, 1975).

The imperial courts and scholars of China are well known for integrating knowledge and information from different sources. Presumably, the wide exposure, the centralisation and subsequent integration of the different streams of ancient medicine, created a most comprehensive and sophisticated system of medicine, called the Chinese medicine. The system is mastered by a unique system of philosophy which has clear links with the ancient philosophers. It is in command of huge volumes of material medica and instruction manures and documents passed down from generation to generation. The system is not only rich in diagnostics and herbal therapeutics, but also uniquely possesses an important section on acupuncture, which is later further developed into a comprehensive system of manual therapy (Huang Di).

The Chinese people used this a system of healing to serve its people for over 3000 years, since the beginning of human civilisation. It was only when the missionaries arrived at the scene, in the later part of the 19th century, that European medicine was brought into China (Wardwell, 1962).

To gain more insight into Chinese medicine today, we must first start from its place of origin (Ernst and Resch, 1995). When European medicine was introduced into China in the late 19th century, the state of art was still fragmented and did not possess the scientific appeal of subsequent years. Literal writers and scholars of this era used to make fun of these healers in their writings and ridiculed them as being incapable of maintaining life (Hoizey and Hoizey, 1988). Other writers laughed at their herbal counterparts and regarded them as circus clowns and quacks (Farquhar, 1994).

The most respected healers before the establishment of the People's Republic of China, must have been experienced herbalists who inherited the art of healing from a father or teacher of equivalent repute, or an odd chief missionary European physician serving in one of the few missionary hospitals in the provincial capitals.

8.2 Chinese Medicine in the People's Republic During the Early Days

The Communist Party earned support through mass participation and peoples' movements. One of the earliest mass movements that won peoples' enthusiastic support after the People's Liberation Army took over a city or district was mass activities aimed at public health promotion, such as street cleansing, hygiene promotion and pest control. This was the modern public health concept (Leung, 1971).

Due to the lack of scientific medicine professionals, Chinese medicine practitioners were highly regarded in the Peoples' Republic. One saw a real integration of modern and traditional medicine brought about by political administration. Ever since then, integration of modern and traditional medicine was very much advocated and had been adopted as a national policy on medical care. The Administration even put down in the revised version of the constitution of the People's Republic that Chinese medicine should be developed at the same time as modern medicine (Leung, 2001). This national policy enjoyed various intensities of support during different eras of the Republic's history and under special circumstances. During the Cultural Revolution, for instance, some hospital workers were forced to spend 50% on Chinese medicine and 50% on modern medicine. The result of such unwise administrative directions only induced distrust and misunderstanding among the two streams of practitioners. The political intension could have been integration, but the result turned out to be mutual suspicion and loss of goodwill and respect.

8.3 Chinese Medicine in China Today

Integration of modern and Chinese medicine has been a national policy for decades. Is there genuine integration since its advocation?

Integration should mean one mixed form of management for different diseases, modern practitioners using traditional practices and traditional practitioners going modern (Eisenberg, 2001). One sees more of the latter. Modern practitioners, on the whole, are satisfied with their scientific practice, whereas well-trained Chinese medicine graduates are keen on using modern means of diagnostics and treatment.

8.3.1 *Education in Chinese medicine*

There are three streams: university level, vocational school level and apprenticeship. For obvious reasons, apprenticeship is no longer acceptable in modern societies. It is therefore being phased out. There are around 20 high quality Chinese medicine universities in China providing a five-year training programme and a curriculum which includes 30%–60% of modern medicine. The vocational schools accept lower ranking students for a shorter period of training of three years and the contents of modern medicine in the curriculum varies from limited general knowledge to about 30% (Xu, 2001).

Some figures will show the actual governmental attitude towards the provision of education for Chinese medicine. For instance, the number of Chinese medicine universities is less than 20% of universities of modern medicine. The number of university level graduates in Chinese medicine is about equal to that of vocational school graduates (Korn, 2001).

In 1999, when a new ordinance on the national standard of medical practitioners was put into practice, a national examination on medical qualification was being organised that same year. The examination not only gives the chance of unification of standard, but also allows the lower ranking graduates (vocational) to apply for quality evaluation after some years of experience and with respectable recommendations (Legislation PRC, 1998).

The policy in education has been one that endorses the value of Chinese medicine because Chinese medicine is included in the curriculum of both the modern medicine schools and Chinese medicine Schools. Moreover, the graduates are given identical employment positions, and Chinese medicine graduates are allowed to take up specialty training (e.g. in surgery or obstetrics) provided the training is offered.

However, the policy of forcing the Chinese medicine stream into modern medicine is also obvious from the curriculum arrangement. However, modern medicine is also considered more important since only less than 20% of teaching venues are dedicated to Chinese medicine.

8.3.2 *Chinese medicine services*

China undoubtedly offers the best services in Chinese medicine. Three levels of services are offered: in modern hospitals, in Chinese medicine hospitals and in hospitals of integrated medicine.

In every modern hospital, there is a Chinese medicine unit ready to provide services on request.

On the other hand, specially named Chinese medicine hospitals provide more sophisticated services. Although named "Chinese medicine hospital", such hospitals also provide diagnostic and treatment services in modern medicine. In fact, most of the Chinese medicine hospitals run an annual budget spending of 50%–70% on modern medicine, which truly indicates the dependence on Western medicine in areas such as diagnostics, emergencies and resuscitations. After all, the number of Chinese medicine hospitals in any city is small compared to that of modern medicine hospitals. The ratio will not be more than one in ten (Korn, 2001).

Hospitals of integrated practice, specialising in areas such as dermatitis, vascular diseases and rheumatology, are rare in big cities. These rare entities do have a major emphasis on the use of Chinese medicine in problem areas of modern medicine (Hospital of Integrated Therapy, 1999).

Some still think that Chinese medicine Hospitals offer only Chinese medicine services. In actual fact, a hospital is strictly a modern setup built to facilitate different forms of investigations and modern treatment. Chinese medicine services, in the traditional sense, do not require hospital services.

In a consumer-driven community, where people enjoy the fruits of science and technology, patients will demand modern investigations as means of diagnosis and modern technology as means of treatment. Today, no hospital can survive or function without modern equipment and technology.

Therefore, "Chinese medicine hospital" is just a misnomer describing a modern setting which also offers Chinese medicine as additional forms of treatment.

8.3.3 *Research in Chinese medicine*

If the national policy of integration of Chinese medicine and modern medicine were genuine and practical, the equivalent research should have enjoyed a good record.

The research on Chinese medicine has followed a main line of herbal analysis: explorations of their bio-activities and identification of the active components. These were conducted in chemistry, biology and biochemistry laboratories. There have only been a few successful examples: crude preparations like Sennakot for constipation and extract formulae like Qinghao for malaria.

On the clinical side, there were numerous reports on the successes of the use of various well-known herbal treatments. But these reports may not reflect a genuine integration of the scientific and traditional streams. Some extreme examples were found during the Cultural Revolution when Party Administration wanted to replace acupuncture anaesthesia with other forms of anaesthesia, and herbal treatment to replace some standard emergency surgery like appendicectomy and laparotomy. Clinical studies and reports seldom applied the evidence-based concepts. The randomised sampling technique and double-blinding principle were seldom followed. Most reports, if not anecdotal, were just cohort studies. Tang in 1999 reviewed clinical papers published in Chinese journals and found that only a small proportion (15%) attempted to apply the modern biostatistics principles which follow evidence-based approaches (Tang *et al.*, 1999).

Looking at the scientific periodicals on Chinese medical research, the total number of journals today is 147, with 116 devoted to clinical sciences, 16 to integrated medicine, five to acupuncture, four to Qikong, and ten to herbal drugs. From 1950 to 1959, only ten journals were published. In the next ten years (1960–1969), no new journals appeared. What followed after the years of turmoil was a thriving development, so that in the 1970s, 12 new journals were added. The number continued to increase: 53 new journals in the 1980s and 34 in the 1990s (Xu, 2001).

8.3.4 *Overall situation*

The general trend of the education, service and research on Chinese medicine indicates that Chinese medicine is under going modernisation, whereas modern medicine has been following its own way of development.

In 2000, a special investigating team of academics from Hong Kong and the United Kingdom embarked on a fact-finding trip to China, to visit the most important academic and service institutions in Chinese medicine. A report of the trip included the following facts: "around 170 registered research institutions in Chinese medicine exist in China. They focus mainly on three types of research, namely basic, clinical and applied research. Further scientific development of Chinese medicine hinged very much on the successful establishment of the therapeutic properties of the individual elements contained in Chinese herbs. However, this was very difficult because their patients, having paid for their treatment, were often unwilling to take part in trials in which one arm might be a placebo. They had also found an inherent suspicion of clinical trials amongst Chinese patients. A further problem was that many herbal products had a distinctive smell, which made the creation of an appropriate placebo difficult (Tang *et al.*, 1999)."

Actually, Chinese medicine emphasises on individual cases and individualisation of treatment. This approach greatly hinders the objectivity and generalisation that is inseparable from scientific research. Traditional healers will naturally object to the scientific approach and will have no interest in the Western way of trials and research. It is up to the scientists and modern healers to try to persuade the traditional healers before any proper research in the modern scientific sense can be started. Thus, it is not surprising that reports of scientific research on Chinese medicine were so rare in the period of time before the 1970s.

The Hong Kong Institute for Promotion of Chinese Culture launched a scientific contest — "The First Li Shi Zhen Award for Scientific Manuscripts on Traditional Chinese Medicine" in 1991–1992. The participants came from China, Taiwan, Hong Kong and the United States. A total of over 10,000 articles were collected, screened and studied separately in China and Hong Kong, using standard objective methods of assessment for scientific papers. The following conclusions were made:

(1) There were a lot of active scientists and clinicians involved in Chinese medicinal studies.
(2) Most manuscripts were clinical in nature.
(3) Basic science research was limited.
(4) Manuscripts of the best quality belonged to the category of traditional classical writings.
(5) Using Western method of assessment, the quality of manuscripts and the methodology of research were of low standard (Leung and Wong, 2002).

8.3.5 *The changing trend*

With the modernisation of economy, China is showing immense changes in all areas, including Chinese medicine. As convergence of the two streams, i.e. scientific and Chinese medicine, is actively taking place, diligent workers of Chinese medicine have to demonstrate their ability and expertise by engaging more actively in research. The appearance of more journals on Chinese medicine, and notably those specially created to serve the "integrated approach", is a timely event which will significantly contribute towards the need.

One expects this group of medical scientists who is in command of both modern methodology and traditional knowledge, to bring Chinese medicine research to a new level. Although biostatisticians will want to see more randomised, double-blind trials, reports are not forthcoming. Nevertheless, reports on the use of Chinese medicine alternatives aimed at supplementing modern medicine, are becoming more common.

8.3.6 *Effects of modern economic development on Chinese medicine*

Chinese medicine has enjoyed special attention and protection from the Chinese government and yet it is being carried along in a process of "convergence" towards modern practice. Now that hospitals and medical services are being divorced from state subvention, Chinese medicine hospitals may be facing a tougher time than modern hospitals. There is a high demand from lay-people to use more modern technology in both diagnosis and treatment. Chinese medicine hospitals, therefore, will be facing heavy pressure to go modern, i.e. acquiring modern diagnostic equipments, giving up some traditional practices, sending their staff for training on surgical and other interventional manoevres and reinforcing their ability on emergencies and resuscitations. There will be more "convergence" to modern practice. The pressure of "going modern" is growing as Chinese medicine hospitals spend their budget on more and more modern equipment and modern pharmaceuticals to please their patients. On the other hand, Chinese medicine remains the cheaper form of treatment which less well-off people can afford. The decline in Chinese medicine can therefore be balanced out by a more popular demand from the less well-off citizens.

8.3.7 *Drug development*

Chinese medicine started as a discipline relying very much on herbal concoctions. In the modern society, the inconvenience of steaming has always been felt, especially among the working class who may not possess proper cooking facilities. Chinese medicine practitioners have thus developed a tradition of providing supplementary medicine in the form of pills or drinks in an effort to replace herbal brews, or to supplement the effects of the conventional form of administration. This practice has led to an industry of proprietor drugs of herbal origin.

Proprietor drugs in market target at commonly occurring symptoms like cough, diarrhea and pain, or common ailments like the common cold and fever. A lot of varieties claim superiority because of some traditional "secret formula".

One should not ignore the commercial value of proprietor products because the production cost is very low while the number of users can be vast.

With the rapid expansion of China's economy and the establishment of private enterprises, production of proprietor Chinese medicine is expected to escalate. The increased productivity in this area might have little to do with health promotion, but rather, it reflects the enthusiasm for short-term investments with quick returns. In the eagerness to create popularity and to boost the market, there is a surge in advertising activities which try to impress people with dramatic results of treatment. One just needs to watch television programmes in China to witness the vibrant but chaotic scenes of market competition for the sale of proprietor herbal preparations.

This is particularly worrying in a country where medical practitioners are still given plenty of freedom to differentiate between advertising and legitimate promotion, and the code of practice is either deficient or considered unimportant.

However, although the Central Administration is mainly concerned with productivity gain, it still sees the need for a national policy on herbal drug production, and is in the process of formulating such a policy.

China has over 6000 drug makers. They are capable of producing over 1000 chemical drugs and more than 8000 traditional Chinese drugs.

According to the *Journal of Chinese Medicine in China* (1999), there are over 1000 Chinese medicine factories of which 178 are medium to large sizes. The total output from the drug industry in 1999 was RMB194.6 billion (US$23.5 billion), showing an increase of 14.4% from 1998. The top five provinces in term of sales revenues were Guangdong, Zhejiang, Jiangsu, Shandong and Hunan.

Traditionally, the development of the Chinese medicine industry was stronger in the coastal region compared with the central and western regions. However, the rich natural resources of the central and western regions are beginning to turn into new economic strengths. This is why Sichuan was selected as the first national industrial base for the modernisation of Chinese medicine (Fung, 2000a and b).

The Ministry of Science and Technology has worked out an "Action Plan for the Modernisation and Development of Chinese Medicine" to improve product quality and to elevate its ability to compete on world markets. Sichuan was selected as the first national industrial base for the modernisation of Chinese medicine. The action plan includes the construction of a research and development system. The system includes screening centres for Chinese medicine, a safety evaluation centre, a centre for the standardisation of Chinese medicinal products and a centre for clinical research. Other goals include the establishment of several competitive enterprises by the year 2010 — to build a research centre for Chinese medical engineering technologies, to form transnational alliances with foreign businesses, research organisations and investors. The ultimate aim is to increase China's market share in the international market of Chinese and herbal medicine to 15%. (In 1997, the share was only 4%, i.e. US$660 million.) Research and development will focus on disease areas where modern medicine is either ineffective or deficient. These include chronic diseases, difficult and complicated illnesses and geriatric ailments. In addition, national and provincial level innovation centres are to be established to build information databases and websites on Chinese medicine, and to develop special technology and research on promising traditional formulae.

Requirements for drug manufacturing like certification and business licensing are tightened.

According to the new "Regulations on the Approval of New Medicines", new medicines are divided into three major categories, viz. chemical medicine, biological medicine and Chinese medicine. Each category is further classified into five groups. The five groups for Chinese medicine are as follows:

Group 1

- Synthetic materials from Chinese medicinal raw materials.
- Newly discovered Chinese medicinal raw materials and their semi-finished compounds.
- The active ingredients and their semi-finished components derived from Chinese medicinal raw materials.
- The active ingredients derived from a complex prescription.

Group 2

- Injections manufactured from Chinese medicinal raw materials.
- New medicinal applications and their semi-finished components from anatomical components of existing Chinese medicinal raw materials.
- The active components and its semi-finished components derived from existing Chinese medicinal raw materials and their derivatives.
- Medicinal products extracted from animals, and its semi-finished components obtained from artificial means.
- The active components cluster derived from complex prescription.

Group 3

- New semi-finished components from complex prescription.
- Semi-finished components from Chinese medicine and synthetic drugs based on theory of Chinese medicine prepared from a complex prescription.
- Common imported medicinal raw materials and their semi-finished components introduced from overseas.

Group 4

- Alteration of preparation and form of intake.
- Domesticated animal and herbal medicine introduced from overseas.

Group 5

- Newly discovered Chinese medicinal material demonstrating effects of existing drugs.

These clear guidelines indicate China's intention to effectively boost the Chinese medicine industry.

We look forward to the consolidation of professionalism by which clinical trials can be conducted strictly according to good clinical practice along an evidence-based direction (The Ministry of Health PRC), so that drug production and marketing can enjoy a solid base of efficacy.

8.3.8 *Will Chinese medicine continue to play an important role in modern medical practice in China?*

We have earlier discussed the observation that convergence of the old and modern systems of medicine is occurring in China. Convergence means the old system is applying more and more scientific means of diagnosis and treatment, whilst the modern system, is in fact gradually accepting Chinese medicine on a systemic scale. The subordinate role of Chinese medicine may not be preferred by the herbalists and bone setters, but it has already taken place, while integration of the two streams remains a politically correct concept.

The almighty modern medicine is not solving all the problems. On the other hand, a subordinate, supporting alternative, which is only traditionally accepted and observed to be effective, is starting to gain recognition. Chinese medicine will therefore survive well, while scientific medicine assumes its own way of development.

In fact, there is increasing disappointment and dissatisfaction with modern medicine. Technically, modern medicine does not solve all problems. When the pathology is simple, clearly located and well defined, treatment is equally simple and effective. However, when the pathology is more complicated, treatment becomes ineffective and defective. Disappointed people look for alternatives.

Other reasons for disappointment include the over-priced specialisation fees and over-specialisation: segmented care, indifference, poor teamwork and unaffordable costs. This disappointment is not confined to public hospital dwellers but to all levels of people looking for medical service in all parts of the world today. This is reflected in the rising popularity of and the increasing expenditure on alternative medicine (Eisenberg, 1998).

The United States National Institutes of Health (NIH) had the most realistic proactive arrangements. After forming a working group to look at alternative medicine to see whether it deserves more analysis, a special committee was founded to establish an office which was, in 1999, endorsed. There are, by now, nine national alternative medicine centres receiving special assignments from NIH (NIH, 2000), and the number is increasing. Acupuncture was already recognised as a means of removing pain in 1998 (NIH, 1998). The World Health Organization (WHO) has also taken an accommodating stand on alternative medicine. Developing countries are encouraged to keep and promote useful alternative medicine including folk medicine (WHO, 2000).

NIH and WHO have taken an admirable open stand on alternative medicine. At the same time, they formulated a new line of approach to the research. Past experiences on herbal research were very narrow. Research work was mainly confined to the laboratory where active ingredients were being extracted from herbs. Only a few successful examples, like Qinghao for malaria, can be quoted (Jonas, 1998). The laboratory-orientated approach had been slow, expensive and unreliable. A new approach was then proposed: the efficacy-driven approach. The new direction starts with clinical trials using appropriate herbal formulae in evidence-based, randomised trial protocols. When efficacy is proven, the formula used is further authenticated and considered for drug development. Before the trial, ingredients of the herbal formulae need to be checked for toxicity both from available literature and directly through laboratory screening. With a few exceptions of toxic herbs, the overwhelming majority of herbal preparations are harmless and safe. The long history of consumption of simple herbs in China also adds to the accountability of the practical utilisation.

This new approach focuses on special problem areas in modern medicine that need support and has limited the laboratory investment to clinically efficacious areas. Clinical trials start at phase 2. China can seriously look towards this direction of commitment.

The national policy of China on Chinese medicine for the past 50 years has been emphasising on "integration". The reality, as observed by outsiders, is one of Chinese medicine converging towards modern medicine. In fact, a group of well-respected herbalists presented repeated petitions to the People's Congress, expressing their concern about Chinese medicine not receiving the due respect and recognition it deserved. They considered "integration" a process by which Chinese medicine would lose its identity (Chinese Medicine Practitioners Group, 2000).

Users, on the other hand, are adopting a practical attitude. They use a service that they can afford. The expensive investigations of modern medicine are technology dependent. Those who can afford will hardly rely on traditional Chinese medicine alone. In fact, hardly anyone today will claim that Chinese medicine can replace modern medicine. Chinese medicine is at best a specialty that takes care of the deficiencies in modern medicine.

Now that research opportunities have improved in China and Chinese medicinal research often leads to drug production, Chinese medicine workers in China can follow a practical direction where specific items are used to enhance treatment programmes in which modern medicine is used, i.e. to supplement modern treatment and improve the overall results. Once the results are proven efficacious, the value-adding procedures, i.e. the efforts spent on upgrading the drugs, will become worthwhile.

There are so many herbs and formulae that offer good potential for the supplementary treatment of difficult problems. These can be collected and subjected to scientific trials using the principles of good clinical practice. Once their efficacy is proven, practical promotion of their proper role as a supplement can follow. This way of "integration" will be a solid means of enriching medical treatment, promoting drug production and marketing.

8.4 Conclusion

Chinese medicine in China is not just a folk-lore or a belief, it is a practical way of treating ailments and diseases and has enjoyed centuries of cultural identification. Although nowadays, most sick people in China rely mainly on modern medicine, they still turn towards Chinese medicine when they need an alternative.

The day-to-day behaviour of the average Chinese reminds us of the anthropological influences: local herbal compresses and ointments are folk-related and are still widely used in today's Chinese communities. The caring mother almost invariably prepares food and dishes believed to be good for various physiological needs at different circumstances for her beloved offspring. Likewise, different ethnic groups are keeping their traditional practice of supplying different varieties of food and herbal formulae for different stages of life, e.g. puberty, marriage, pregnancy and post-partum periods.

While such traditional practices are slowly fading in China, surprisingly, affluent societies in America and Europe are beginning to embrace Chinese medicine's traditional approach. The boostering effects on the attitude and production of Chinese medicine in China from these outside influences are obvious.

For the past 50 years, China is modernising on all fronts. Modernisation means bringing the research activities closer to what is considered world level of science and technology. Actually both Western and Chinese medicine in China require modernisation, i.e. scientific and technological enhancement. The national policy for Chinese medicine has been "integration", i.e. integrating with modern medicine. If integration carries no substance of science and technology, the two different streams of medicine will not integrate. Therefore, after 40 years of "practice", integration today means subjecting Chinese medicine to scientific tests (Wong *et al.*, 1993).

Judging from the popularity of the efficacy-driven approach in the U.S., perhaps a realistic way of modernising Chinese medicine in China is to use a similar approach. How far should the modernisation go? If convergence towards modern medicine is happening in the two streams of medicine in China, should one facilitate the convergence, which in a way dissuades people from using Chinese medicine?

China should value its tradition and make the best out of Chinese medicine while at the same time continue its scientific pursuit. With the vast territory and divergent economic abilities of the people, Chinese medicine offers an inexpensive means of treatment, while carers and patients alike should be made aware of the need for scientific investigation whenever serious pathology is suspected. Large-scale studies can start on the preventive value of herbal treatment for common illnesses such as osteoporosis, dementia and other aspects of ageing. Drug production should not be based on market demand alone. Evidence-based trials aimed at the proof for efficacy followed by drug manufacture should be made a standard practice.

References

A Group of Senior Chinese Medicine Practitioners (2000) *Petition to the Standing Committee of the People's Congress.* Internal Publication, People's Congress Bureau.

Cant, S. and Sharma, U. (1966) *Complementary and Alternative Medicines: Knowledge in Practice.* Free Association Press, London.

Eisenberg, D. (2001) Complementary, alternative and integrative medicine in the United States: overview and opportunities for collaboration. In: *Proceedings on Health Care, East and West, Moving Into the 21st Century.* Harvard.

Eisenberg, D.M. (1998) Trends in alternative medicine use in the United States, 1990–1997: results of a follow-up national survey. *JAMA* **280**(18), 1569–1575.

Ernst, E. and Resch, K.L. (1995) Complementary medicine — a definition. *Br. J. Gen. Pract.* **45**, 506.

Farquhar, J. (1994) *Knowing Practice — The Clinical Encounter of Chinese Medicine.* Westview Press, San Francisco, Oxford.

Fung, S.K.W. (2000a) *Investing in Biotech and Chinese Medicine in China and Hong Kong.* Technology Assessment, Rotary Club, September 1st.

Fung, S.K.W. (2000b) *Biotechnology Development in China and Hong Kong.* British Chamber of Commerce in Hong Kong, July 6th. http://www.most.gov.cn

Hoizey, D. and Hoizey, M.J. (1988) *A History of Chinese Medicine.* Edinburgh University Press.

Hospital of Integrated Therapy Hospital Brochure (1999) Rainbow Mouth Integrated Hospital, Shanghai.

Huang Di. *Internal Medicine (Nai-jing).* Chinese Classic.

Huang Di. Dialogue, *Questions and Answers (Zu-run).* Chinese Classic.

Jonas, W.B. (1998) Alternative medicine: learning from the past, examining the present, advancing to the future. *JAMA* **280**, 1616–1618.

Kleinman, A. (1975) *Medicine in Chinese Cultures: Comparative Studies of Health Care in China and Other Societies.* U.S. Department of Health, Education and Welfare, Washington D.C.

Korn, D. (2001) *Report After a Special Visit to China to Understand the Situation of Chinese Medicine in China.* Internal Publication, Medical Panel, University Grant Council.

Legislation on the Registration of Medical Practitioners, Peoples' Republic of China (1998) Paper of Standing Committee, People's Congress.

Leong, C.H. (2001) The role of traditional and complementary alternative medicine. In: *Proceedings on Health Care, East and West, Moving Into the 21st Century*. Harvard.

Leung, P.C. (1971) Medical and health care in China since 1949. In: *Communist China.* World Christian Federation.

Leung, P.C. and Wong, M.W.N. (2002) A critical analysis of professional and academic publications on traditional Chinese medicine in China. *Am. J. Chin. Med.* **30**(1), 177–181.

National Institutes of Health (2000) *Report on Complementary and Alternative Medicine.* NIH publication.

National Institutes of Health (1998) Report on special seminar on acupuncture. *JAMA* **280**, 1518–1524.

Tang, J.L., Zhau, S.Y. and Ernst, E. (1999) Review of randomized controlled trials of traditional Chinese medicine. *Br. Med. J.* **819**, 160–161.

The Ministry of Health of the People's Republic of China. http://www.moh.gov.cn

Wardwell, W. (1962) Limited, marginal and quasi practitioners. In: *Handbook of Medical Sociology* (ed.) Freeman, H. Englewood Cliffs.

Wong, T.W., Wong, S.L. and Donnan, S. (1993) Traditional Chinese medicine and Western medicine in Hong Kong. *J. Hong Kong Med. Assoc.* **45**, 278–284.

World Health Organisation (2000) *Strategic Plan on the Promotion of Folk Medicine.* WHO publication.

Xu, M. (2001) *A Review of Chinese Journals on Chinese Medicine in the Past 20 Years.* Report of Institute of Chinese Medicine, Chinese University.

Xu, Q.Y. (2001) Medical education in China. In: *Proceedings on Health Care, East and West, Moving Into the 21st Century.* Harvard.

Chapter 9

Globalisation of Chinese Medicine*

Yung-Chi Cheng†

Abstract

During the past century, Western medicine has made major advances in treating and controlling many human diseases. In recent years, the development of new technologies, including genomics, proteomics, combinatorial chemistry, high throughput chemistry, computational chemistry, bioinformatics and a more profound understanding of human biology has accelerated the discovery and development of new medicines. The scope of medicine is also rapidly changing. Today, the emphasis includes the treatment, prevention of chronic and age-associated disease, e.g. metabolic disorders, neurodegenerative disease and cancer, as well as improvement of quality of life. The paradigm of mainstream pharmaceutical discovery is to identify single compounds that can regulate a given target associated with a disease. Such compounds are expected to have potency and selectivity for the treatment of the disease targeted. This reductionist approach is good if the targeted diseases are the result of one aetiological factor. However, it may not be the ideal approach in trying to find drugs for the treatment and prevention of chronic and age-associated diseases since the aetiology of those diseases may be multifactorial and hence more complex. This is recognised, an integrated and systematic approach should be taken.

Chinese medicine and Chinese medicine theories have evolved over the past 4000 years. The approach taken is an integrated and systematic approach. Although there is a scientific basic, due to the limitation

*This is a modified version of the manuscript which was originally published in *2001 Traditional Chinese Medicine and Natural Products, China*, pp. 27–35 by Era Resources Publisher, Hong Kong, and subsequently reproduced in the proceedings of several meetings.

†A "Western medicine"-trained pharmacologist with no claim to be an expert in Chinese medicine.

of technologies and scientific knowledge in the past to verify its claim, Chinese medicine has not made major advances during the past 400 years. As a result, Chinese medicine has had only a relatively minor impact on mainstream medicine, and while in current use around the world, is not globally accepted.

One claimed usage of Chinese medicine is for the treatment and prevention of chronic and age-associated diseases. Some of the botanical formulas used for this purpose were discovered thousands of years ago and continue to be used today in China, Korea, Japan and Chinese predominant areas. There are indications that these formulas may indeed be helpful in the treatment or prevention of chronic diseases. It could be very useful today in meeting clinical needs for which there are inadequate mainstream medicine approaches. The potential usefulness of Chinese medicine embodies the belief of maintaining healthy homeostasis of the body through the balance of a mixture of chemicals at different organs or tissues. This integrative concept is different from Western medicine and inplies that multiple compounds may act on multiple mechanisms of action to maintain the balance of the complex web of biology. This is very important in view of our current direction to integrate fragmented information to develop future medicines. If the effectiveness of the botanical formulas proves to be true, the scientific basis of the mechanism of action of these formulas could be very powerful in advancing the basic knowledge of medical science and developing more effective treatments.

While there is a different emphasis on how to treat human disease, the science behind mainstream medicine and Chinese medicine could in fact be very complementary. To integrate these two apparent different approaches in medicine could be the most efficient way to develop new medicines for the treatment and prevention of diseases in this new century. In order to achieve this, modern science and technology has to be utilised to address the efficiency and to study the action of Chinese medicine and botanicals. The following is suggested

- Botanicals should be cultivated under defined conditions, authenticated and certified including sources, chemical composition, and conditions of their cultivation.
- The manufacturing and preparation process of Chinese medicine or individual botanicals should be carefully monitored and standardised employing modern methodologies for quality assurance.
- Methodologies for quality control should be further improved for a given botanical of formula employing modern technologies.
- Rigorous clinical trials of quality assured Chinese medicines should be used to verify the claims of Chinese medicine.

- Methodologies used for individualisation of botanical prescriptions used by Chinese medicine practitioners should be examined and the scientific basis of those methodologies should be studied.
- Pharmacological interactions of Western single-compound medicines and Chinese medicines should be carefully studied.
- The mechanism of action of Chinese medicine needs to be addressed and an explanation of the principles of Chinese medicine using modern scientific terminology should be attempted.
- The philosophy, principles and practices of Chinese medicine should be introduced to the medical establishment using concepts and language of modern science.
- A comprehensive, accessible-related database should be established to include chemical composition and biological activity of herbs, chemical and biological properties of the chemicals in herbs and the growth conditions and storage of each herb. The composition, preparation and potential indication and toxicity of different formula, etc.
- The number of herbs used for preparing Chinese medicine formula could be decreased to avoid redundancy of their biological activity.
- A simplified, more efficacious and friendly version of formula based on scientific investigation should be developed.

This will be a major undertaking requiring international collaboration and participation. For areas of the world that do have a strong focus on using Chinese medicines or botanicals, it is the moral obligation of the government and private enterprise to take steps to ensure the health of their population by improving Chinese medicine. In those areas that are not familiar with Chinese medicine, they should take advantage of the knowledge accumulated, through many centuries, by the Chinese in order to fulfill the clinical needs that remain poorly treated. There are a growing number of patients using Chinese medicine or botanicals for various reasons in Western societies. A joint effort among different governments and enterprises across the international borders should be strongly encouraged to insure the safety and efficacy of botanical pharmaceuticals. It is believed that a convergence of Western and Chinese traditional medicines, may evolve into a greatly improved method of human health care in the coming century.

9.1 Introduction

Chinese medicine has not been globally accepted for the treatment of diseases. For Chinese medicine to be considered as a credible form of medicine, there is a minimum of two-and-a-half requirements. Preparations should be prepared with consistent and reproducible pharmacological properties. Clinical efficacy and potential side effects of medicine should be documented through vigorous clinical trials. Possible placebo effects should be ruled out. Some understanding of its mechanism of action and the active compounds responsible for the action and its interaction with other drugs used by patients should be provided. In this article, my personal perspective of globalisation of Chinese medicine and its impact on the development of future medicine is discussed.

9.2 Current Status of Chinese Medicine and Its Bottleneck in Its Advancement

Chinese medicine theories and practice have evolved over the past 4000 years. Although the evolution is empirical, it has its own scientific basis. This includes the means to perform herbal identification and cultivation, methodologies of preservation and preparation, subjective selection of the quality of herbs for use, principles of formulation, methodologies for diagnosis and functional interaction among organs and tissues, and finally the individualisation of treatment based on diagnosis and physiological status. A brief summary based on a textbook and its content and the number of herbs used as described through history is shown in Fig. 9.1. The principle of formulation and interaction of different herbs is shown in Tables 9.1 and 9.2. While Chinese medicine has made contributions to serve human health, particularly the Chinese and other people in Asia,

Table 9.1. Four considerations in establishing Chinese medicine formulas.

• Imperial herb	君	Key herb
• Ministerial herb	臣	To promote the action of key herb
• Assistant herb	佐	To decrease the side effect of herb
• Servant herb	使	To help the formulation

Note: Different formulas are used depending on the symptoms. Variation in the amounts of each component in a formula will depend on the physiology of each patient.

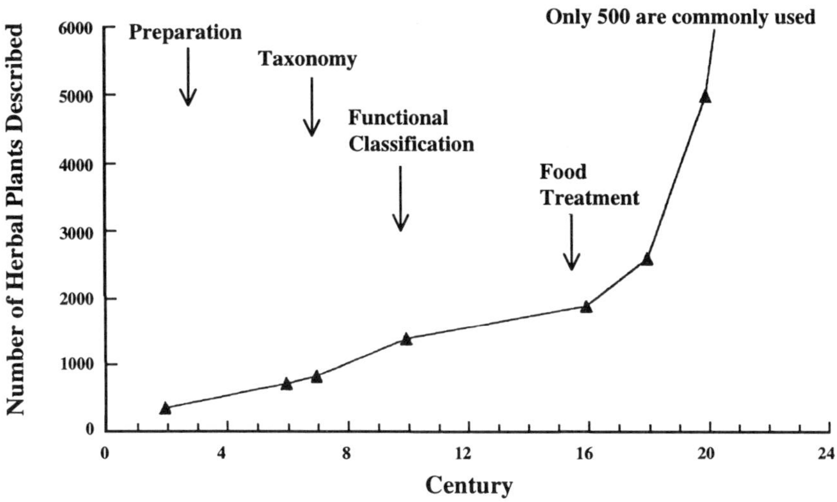

Figure 9.1. Chinese medicine discovered.

Table 9.2. Interaction of different ingredients of Chinese formula (described by Tao Hongjing, 451–526).

Chinese	English translation	Explanation
1. 相助	Help or reinforce each other	Additive or synergistic enhancement of pharmacologic action by two or more substances with similar properties
2. 相需	Need each other	Potentiation or synergism; enhancement of therapeutic action by substances with different properties
3. 相畏	Mutual respect or restraint	Inhibition or reduction of pharmacologic effects by two or more substances with properties in common
4. 相惡	Mutual dislike	Inhibition or reduction of an effect of one drug by another with an opposing action
5. 相殺	Kill each other	The specific nullification of the effect of one compound by another agent through competitive antagonism, such as between agonist and antagonist compounds
6. 相反	Oppose each other	Incompatibility, not suitable for combination due to severe adverse effects

the scientific basis of Chinese medicine has not made much progress during the past 400 years, except for the identification of new herbs, the isolation of biologically active natural products from herbs, and the preparation of injectable formula as well as more user friendly formula. As a result, traditional Chinese medicine has had only a relatively minor impact on today's global mainstream medicine. The lack of progress could be due to many reasons including:

(1) Clinical efficacy of Chinese medicine has not been tested vigorously using today's clinical methodology, which has only evolved during the past 40 years. The practice of the individualised treatment based on the methodology of diagnosis practiced by Chinese medicine practitioners has certainly complicated clinical trial design.
(2) The validity of the approaches of using mixtures of herbs versus a single active compound for the treatment of diseases was not well established. This has raised the question as to whether Chinese medicine approaches would eventually be replaced by a single active compound approach, which is popular in mainstream medicine.
(3) The quality control of Chinese medicine is difficult to maintain given the fact that herbs are grown or collected from the wild and that the composition of herbs may vary with time of harvest, conditions of growth, location of plantation and methodologies used in herbal preparation. Furthermore, it is not even clear which of the same herb harvested under different conditions or locations could be better for a given indication given the complexity of chemicals of different strain of herb.
(4) The methodologies to be used for quality control of medicine could be complicated given the active compounds could be many, which could target on multiple targets, in different origins.
(5) The mechanism of the action of Chinese medicine is difficult to study since the active compounds may have more than one target and the targets of action are likely involved in multiple cellular pathways and tissues.
(6) The concept that Chinese medicine is safe since it is "natural" and has been used for thousands of years has mistakenly

neglected the issue of toxicity and the need for regulatory mechanisms.

(7) Methodologies and technologies of reductionism science which are mainstream approaches in current medicine may not be sufficient to study the complexities inherent in phytochemical compositions and multiple modes of action of botanical medicines.

(8) The methodologies used by Chinese medicine in diagnosis are very subjective and the significance of the methodologies has not been verified using today's technologies. In addition, the terminology used in Chinese medicine is quite different from that used in mainstream medicine, contributing to difficulties in the practices of Chinese medicine and the research or Chinese medicine utilising modern scientific approaches.

(9) Lack of knowledge of potential interaction of Chinese medicine and current mainstream medicine can result in undesirable clinical consequences.

(10) Governments in specific areas where Chinese medicine is practiced do not have a cohesive programme or feel the need in promoting the advancement of the science of Chinese medicine.

(11) Industry in the area of Chinese medicine does not have sufficient commitments or resources to perform in-depth research required to upgrade the products.

9.3 Advancement of Western Medicine

During the past century, Western medicine has made major advances in treatments for many human diseases. This rapid rise of Western medicine has been driven by many factors, including:

- The evolution of the dedicated scientific spirit that defines the essence of the inquisitive, inquiring need to know about the universe around us.
- Hypothesis-driven, experimental investigations that define the rigorous and reproducible construction of facts, knowledge on which to build understanding.

- Open-minded approaches in making scientific conclusions and peer review to assure quality and reproducibility.
- Powerful advances in scientific technologies and methodologies that provided more precise tools with which to probe and understand nature.
- The enthusiastic support given by society and government to further our understanding of human biology.
- The emergence of private enterprise to rapidly capitalise on developing laboratory results into high-valued commercial products.
- A global vision of the overall role and importance of medicine in advancing the human condition.

In recent years the advancement of medicine has only accelerated and is now being driven by increasingly powerful technologies. These technologies now include:

- Gene cloning and sequencing that has fueled the mapping of complete species genomes.
- Functional and structural genomics and proteomics.
- Analytical technology such as c-DNA array, proteomics, mass spectrometry, macromolecular sequence, and high performance liquid chromatography completed with different detection system.
- Chemical synthesis and combinatorial chemistry.
- Laboratory automation and high-throughput bioassay and pharmacology surrogates.
- Micro- and nano-scale engineering.
- Computation and data processing.
- Data management, data mining and information technology.

These technological revolutions have allowed scientists around the world to develop a more profound knowledge of human biology. Today, this is leading to a more detailed genetic and molecular understanding of the epidemiology of diseases, more efficient methods to identify relevant targets for drug design and discovery, produce predicative *in vitro* and *in vivo* models, and new approaches in molecular and genetic diagnosis. Tommorrow, we will see this knowledge utilised in consideration of individualised patient treatment using pharmacogenomic and pharmacophenomic information.

9.4 Current Mainstream Medicine and Chinese Medicine are Complementary

In recent years, with the advancement of mainstream medicine, the following were recognised.

9.4.1 *The combination of chemicals with different modes of action or different target specificities, could achieve better therapeutic effects than a single compound, targeted on single biochemical sites for certain diseases*

However, in these cocktails of chemical therapeutics, it is not always easy to optimise the combination. One unique characteristic of Chinese medicine is the use of a combination of herbs, prepared in a formula for treatment. The principle of the combination is to combine herbs that could enhance the therapeutic action, decrease the toxicity, improve the pharmacokinetic and pharmacodynamic features, and increase the absorption or modification of the metabolism of the active components of key herb(s) that are essential for the treatment. Thus, it is conceivable that the principles of herbal combination and the choice of selecting certain herbs for any given purpose, in a formula of Chinese medicine, could provide new leads in the development of combination therapy, which could include both mainstream medicine and Chinese medicine, and discovery of more effective drugs.

9.4.2 *The multiple symptoms associated with the side effects of cancer or viral chemotherapy are often severe and limiting depending on the drugs that are used*

The therapeutic index in many cases is very narrow, the mechanism of toxicity may or may not be the same and different organs or tissues may react differently to the same drugs. In order to overcome the side effects, the use of additional drugs, which are known to treat these symptoms, are a common practice. While this may relieve one symptom, it rarely addresses multiple symptoms and may in fact exacerbate other side effects. Chinese medicine often has multiple claims in terms of its therapeutic effects, which is not surprising given the multiple chemicals and mechanisms of action of these chemicals. It is conceivable that some Chinese medicines may be useful in relieving multiple side effects without compromising the therapeutic effects of a given chemotherapy through alterations of physiology or enhancement of the recovery of organ responsible for side effects directly or indirectly.

9.4.3 *Chronic disease and age-associated illness are major challenges in today's medicine*

The pathogenesis of these diseases and symptoms may not only be multifactorial, they could vary from one individual to another. Current mainstream medicine approaches in developing drugs are to identify a single target, responsible for the initial pathogenesis, and to discover drugs to regulate that target. The approach is based on the assumption that the biochemical step responsible for the pathogenesis is responsible for the eventual symptoms expressed in all patients and that the initial cause of the pathogenesis does not change with the progression of the disease. While this assumption may be true for some diseases, the assumption may not be true in chronic and age-associated diseases, including cancer, neurodegeneration and metabolic disorders, since the aetiology of those diseases may multifactorial and hence more complex. The complex, difficult and changing nature of these chronic diseases has certainly slowed Western science's approach to finding treatments or prevention, leaving today a large medical need that has not yet been met. It is known that the human body is in homeostasis, involving cellular processes, cell-cell interactions and inter-organ interactions mediated through chemicals such as hormones, chemokines or cytokines and neuralelectrical impulses. Currently, not all the cytokines, chemokines, inter-organs or intracellular regulators are known. The progression of chronic disease or age-associated symptoms could be due to the off balance of the complex biochemical web that maintains the feedback loops that regulate the state of homeostasis in the body. Disease, then, would result in changing some key element(s) that will take the state of homeostasis out of the "buffering zone". Once this happens, it may not be reversible, but it could be possible to establish a new state of homeostasis to prevent further progression or relieve some of the symptoms. Despite the advances of medical science and technology, our knowledge to understand the process involved in the homeostasis of the body is still not at all clear. A key and unique approach of Chinese medicine practices are to treat patients in a holistic way. The potential usefulness of Chinese medicine embodies the belief that maintaining healthy homeostasis of the body involves the balance of a mixture of chemicals at different organs or tissues. It takes the interaction of "organ systems" (functional rather than anatomic term) into consideration, to re-establish the homeostasis of the body in patients with the hopes to treat disease. Many Chinese medicine treatments claim to be useful for chronic disease and age-associated symptoms. If some of these treatments are clinically proven, it will be useful not only for treating patients, but will provide us with new leads to understand the regulation of homeostasis and the further advancement of human medicine.

9.4.4 *Prevention of disease is preferable to treatment of a disease both from the quality of life, health care and economic perspectives*

To initiate a prevention clinical trial, however, is often time-consuming, costly and not always in the financial interest of the health care industry. Often, the scientific basis of these clinical trials is based on laboratory studies, which may not be applicable in human or epidemiology studies. Given that the causes of some of those diseases could be multifactorial, the mainstream approach in developing drugs is unlikely to be useful in preventing the majority of the population from multifactorial diseases. The role of preventative treatments is going to be more important in the future. Preventative medicine is always an important area of Chinese medicine. Many herbs or formulas have been used for centuries with claims of preventing diseases, improving the quality of life, or prolonging life. Most of these remedies are taken on a daily basis and therefore the safety of the dosage used is well documented. Recent studies indicate that some of the herbs could modulate immunofunctions or serve as antioxidants, which is the scientific basis of some current approaches in prevention medicine. Most important of all, chemicals of those herbs could have multiple functions which could prevent different aetiological causes of a given disease. Thus, the past experiences of using those herbs in Chinese medicine for preventative purposes could serve as a major and valuable source of information in developing preventative medicine in the future.

9.4.5 *The response to a given drug during therapy for different individuals could be quite different*

This was attributed to the differences in genetic makeup of individuals in terms of drug metabolism of tissue or targets. It could be also due to the differences of drug metabolism as the result of environmental factors and food (including health food) habits. An important area of current medical research and biotechnology development is pharmacogenomics and pharmacophenomics. It is anticipated that prescribed drugs to individuals could be optimised based on certain diagnostic tests for each individual in the future. For centuries, Chinese medicine practices not only diagnoses but also prescribes medicine based on the individual conditions using a unique system that includes the spectrum of the variation of pulse, colour of the eyes, tongue, and skin, smell, etc. It is conceivable that some of these methodologies may reflect the functional state of organs or tissues as defined by the genetic makeup and environmental exposure of the individual. If this is indeed the case, these methodologies once standardised should be very useful for the clinical practices of the future and may provide a bridge to the ongoing research in pharmacogenomics and pharmacoghenomics.

9.5 Step to be Taken to Advance Chinese Medicine

While there is a different emphasis on how to treat human diseases, the mainstream medicine and Chinese medicine could in fact be very complementary. Chinese medicine may well find value not only for the treatment of illness and management of human health or as the source for the isolation of drugs or lead compounds for Western drug discovery, but also as the scientific basis for the evolution of future medicine. It is worthwhile to make a major effort to advance Chinese medicine through our understanding of the theories of Chinese medicine as well as the therapeutic value of Chinese medicinal formulas or herbs for the treatment and prevention of human diseases. These efforts may eventually provide medicines that will overcome significant unment clinical needs of current medicine. In order to bring Chinesse medicine into mainstream and global medicine, certain steps should and could be taken.

9.5.1 *Herbs should be authenticated and their source as well as conditions of cultivation should be well defined and documented*

The problem arises in that some herbs have similar Chinese names but belong to different genesis of the plants. Thus, their composition and biological activity could be very different. Han fang ji (*S. tetrandra*) and Guang-fang ji (*A. fongchi*) are totally different in terms of their chemical composition and biological indication. Guang-fang ji has aristodochic acid, which can cause renal toxicity and have carcinogenic properties (Marcus and Grollman, 2002; Arlt *et al.*, 2002; Nortier *et al.*, 2000; Luyckx *et al.*, 2002), whereas Han fang ji does not. In a weight control formula sold in Europe, labelled as having Han fang ji, Guang fang ji was probably mistakenly used by the manufacturer. A tragedy occurred in those patients using this prepared formula. Many of them developed renal failure and urothelial carcinoma (Marcus and Grollman, 2002; Arlt *et al.*, 2002; Nortier *et al.*, 2000; Luyckx *et al.*, 2002). Thus, botanicals used in preparation should be authenticated.

In addition to the descriptive classic methodologies described previously, some modern technologies, which are more precise and quantitative in terms of chermical and biochemical composition, should also be used. These methodologies include FT-IR, DNA fingerprints, LC-MS and LC-contour, etc. It was described that the chemical composition and biological activity of a given part of the plant could vary with climate, soil conditions, and the season of harvesting and age of the plant. As the first step for quality control of Chinese medicine, the herbs used in formula preparation should be carefully monitored and conditions well defined in terms of their growth, levels of inorganic contamination, herbicide, fungicide, pesticide and fertilisers and harvest conditions to insure the highest level of consistency in the raw botanical product. Modern agriculture technology can be employed to solve many of these cultivation problems as long as it does not change the pharmacological properties of the herbs intended for use in TCM preparation.

Good Agriculture Practice (GAP) for botanical cultivation, which has been initiated recently in China, is one of the most important steps forward. While this is not a small undertaking, it should be strongly encouraged and enforced in order to have high quality Chinese medicine preparation for human health. There are several issues that need to be addressed. This includes which strain of herb to use, where is the best place to cultivate, when will be the right time to cultivate and harvest, whether the herb should be grown without other plants, how to present insect by growing the herb in conditions without insecticide, which part of the herb should be used, what are the best conditions to store, and should a given herb be grown in only one area, which could be dangerous in the case of natural disaster. Research in those areas is badly needed. It should be pointed out that a lot of this knowledge was described in traditional Chinese medicine literature, which can be used as reference.

The choice of herb for preparation of desirable Chinese medicine was in use based on the appearance, colour, taste stiffness, etc. by Chinese pharmacists. Attempts should be made to translate those experiences into objective measurements. As a matter of fact, some commonly used herb, selected by experienced Chinese pharmacists may not be varied that much (less than one fold) in terms of chemical amount from one source to another. As an example, the content of baicalin, baicalein and wogonin in ten scut Radix samples collected from herb stores was measured, less than one fold variation in all except for one sample (Lai *et al.*, 2001) was found. If the dose response curve is not steep, this variant of the content may not change efficiency that much. To identify the herb which does not vary much from one source to another requires systemic study. Since different commercial sources for the same formula may involve different manufacture methodology and source of herb, the chemical composition or biological activity may vary quite a bit from one source to another. For instance, by comparing the ginseng products of 25 preparations, there is a big variation of the chemical content (Harkey *et al.*, 2001). It should not be assumed that the same formula prepared by different commercial sources has the same pharmacological claims (Straus, 2002).

9.5.2 *The manufacturing and preparation process of Chinese medicine or individual botanicals should be carefully monitored and standardised employing modern methodologies for quality assurance*

The traditional methodologies used in preparing different formulas of herbs include hot water extraction, ethanol, extraction, acetic treatment for hydrolysis and esterfication as well as the condensation process. For a manufacturer with the aim to prepare Chinese medicine based on historical claims, the methodologies for preparation should be kept as authentic as possible. Once the original procedure for preparation, such as the extraction procedure is modified, the historical claims may no longer be valid since the composition of an extract may no longer be the same.

Recently, several groups are making an attempt to extract chemicals from herbs using several modern technologies such as critical temperature CO_2 extractions. If the purpose is to extract natural product from a given herb more thoroughly, this is a reasonable approach. If the purpose is to use the extract for preparing Chinese medicine to be used based on historical claims, this should not be allowed since the chemical compositions of the extract will be very different from those using traditional methodologies. Studies should be done to address these issues.

Good Manufacture Practice (GMP) should be enforced to ensure the consistency and quality of the manufacturing process of both herbal mixtures as well as single herbs that may be used in individualised herbal formulations. CMC practices should be implemented. In addition to GMP for the production of new herbal drugs, increased attention must also be directed to address the chemical and biological activity of the *stability* of a formulation. Without making those attempts, the proper and standard methods, which would be eventually needed to bring Chinese medicine into the mainstream of medicine, will never be able to be developed.

9.5.3 *Methodologies for quality control should be further improved for a given botanical or formula employing modern technologies*

Currently, the content of marker compounds or compounds proposed to be the active ingredients are typically examined using one or more chemical analysis methods. In most cases, it is not clear whether the marker compounds(s) are even responsible for the biological activity of the herb or formula. For example, *berberine* is the major active constituent in both *Cortex phellodendri* and *Rhizoma coptidis* and used as a marker compound for both herbals. Usage of both herbals in Chinese medicine by Chinese medical practitioners is very different, which is attributed to the presence of other chemicals in those herbals. Thus, the value for the determination of the content of those marker compounds(s) for quality control of herbs or formulas is questionable.

With the advancement of analytical and separation technologies, it is now possible to measure the content of several compounds in herbs and formulas without difficulty. Chemical fingerprints can be established for each herb and formula that can then be compared using sophisticated computer algorithms. The question is whether there is an analytical methodology that is suitable for most herbs or its preparations.

Each methodology has its own limitation. The use of HPLC coupled with MS, light scattering or UV-visible wavelength spectrum should be the minimum requirement. The chemical fingerprint of different preparations of formula should be as similar as possible. No chemical should be considered inactive or insignficant unless it is proven. The significance of the content of each measurable chemical can be eventually deduced though bioassays using bioinformatics strategies. While it is not possible at this time to define a simple bioassy that will reflect all the activity of a given Chinese medicine, the use of *in vivo* assays, relevant animal models and a panel of surrogate pharmacological assays are a possible approach. This approach clearly has the same caveats as animal models in conventional drug discovery: namely the possibility of different chemical metabolism, the relevance of the animal model to human diseases, and the inherent labour and expense of animal studies.

The use of cell culture in looking for a particular response or of *in vivo* assay such as the interaction with specific receptors while useful, are only able to measure a limited number of biological parameters of possible herbs or formula action. Since the bioactivity of the collections of phytochemicals can be multiple targets, multiple pathways, multiple cell types and perhaps even interact with each other at the different sites of action, a system that can monitor more global changes in cells upon the action of the herb or formula can be useful.

Several newly developed technologies such as c-DNA array and proteomics that can monitor thousands of parameters simultaneously, provides a powerful signature to measure the influence of chemicals from herbs or formulas on living cells or cellular systems. As in animal model work, it should also be noted that these *in vitro* or cell culture studies may not reflect the potential chemical metabolism as found in humans. Thus the information obtained while useful for quality control may not reflect the mechanism of action of a given formula or herb in humans. At the present time, the best approach for quality control of herbs or formulas is to employ multiple parameter measurement approach, termed "phytomics", which include chemical and biological fingerprints. Eventually, the approaches can be simplified once we learn what the active compounds are and what parameters are most relevant to clinical outcomes. Bioinformatics support is a must element in this venture.

9.5.4 *Rigorous clinical trials of quality assured and consistent Chinese medicine should be used to verify the claims of Chinese medicine*

Although Chinese medicine practitioners prescribe medicine by sometimes individualising a prescription by adding or subtracting herbs in a given formula based on their diagnosis, it is not clear whether this practice is necessarily required for a majority of patients. In view of the fact that some formulas were used without much variation for hundreds of years and continue to report to be useful for certain intended indication, it is logical to test the effectiveness of those formulas first before engaging in the more challenging clinical trials that will assess the value of individualisation of prescriptions. The priority of clinical studies should target on the current unmet clinical needs with Chinese medicine formulas that claim to be useful.

The quality of medicine used for clinical trials should be prepared with GMP criteria and characterised using the "phytomics" chemical and biological fingerprints. This will give greater confidence to the reproducibility of clinical results. Double-blind and random clinical trials with placebos should be entertained whenever possible. Placebo treatment was shown to have an impact on the course of diseases. A critical review of herbal remedies was recently published (De Smet, 2002). Chinese medicine practitioners should be encouranged to participate in the diagnosis of patients using their traditional methodology of diagnosis so that they can be carefully recorded and later correlated with the final outcome of the clinical trial. This will be helpful in assessing the value of traditional diagnosis since some of the patients may respond better than others. The clinical end-point should be well defined without ambiguity. Good Clinical Practice (GCP) should be employed so that the final clinical outcome will be generally acceptable to the worldwide medical community.

So far, almost all the clinical trials of Chinese medicine or herbs no matter how well they are designed can only be considered as pilot studies if the quality of medicine used cannot be consistently prepared and is not well characterised.

To establish the validity of the methodology used for individualisation of prescriptions used by Chinese medical practitioners, these practitioners should participate in the diagnosis of the patients under clinical trials. If the outcomes of clinical trials are correlated with the diagnosis of Chinese medicine practitioners, it would suggest the value of individualised prescriptions by Chinese medicine practitioners. Then, clinical studies should be designed to assess the value of standard formula(s) treatment and individualised prescription treatment. Double-blind clinical trials could still be designed to ensure the quality of the clinical trial. The herbs used in the clinical trial preferably from sources with GAP should be well characterised with respect to its chemical and biological fingerprints.

9.5.5 *Methodologies used for individualisation of botanical prescripts used by Chinese medicine practitioners should be examined and the underlying scientific basis of those methodologies should be studied*

One approach to mainstream medicine is to develop a methodology for the individualisation of chemotherapy treatment for individual patients based on individual pharmacogenomic and pharmacophenomin characteristics. This raises the possibility that some of the methods of diagnosis used by Chinese medicine practitioners could in fact be a reflection of some of those characteristics. For a given "Western medicine" treatment for a disease, not all the patients respond equally. Clinical studies should be designed to assess whether the means of diagnosis used by Chinese medicine practitioners could be useful in predicting the outcome of a "Western medicine" treatment or in adjusting the dosage of "Western medicine". The information obtained will be useful in establishing the value of the methodologies used by Chinese medicine practitioners as well as giving a possible scientific basis of those methodologies or directions for scientific investigation.

Since most of these methodologies for diagnosis used by Chinese medicine practitioners are still quite subjective, instruments or a quantitative measure should be developed to make those diagnoses more objective. Such instruments could be a valuable asset to clinicians or researchers who wish to use the verified methodology used by the methodologies evolved from Chinese medicine practitioners and have no training in Chinese medicine. The validity of such an instrument should also be established using a double-blind approach. For a given patient, several Chinese medicine practitioners should participate in diagnosis without knowing the diagnoses of others, so as to ensure the consistency of diagnosis.

9.5.6 *Pharmacological interaction of "Western drug(s)" and Chinese medicine should be studied and the information should be centralised into accessible databases*

"Western drugs" are today the mainstream drugs for the treatment of disease. The effectiveness and the therapeutic index of many of these compounds are dependent on how the body metabolises those drugs. It is well known that the metabolism of each drug can vary from one individual to another and that liver metabolic enzymes, such as the primary oxidative enzymes (e.g. the cytochrome P450 isozymes) or the secondary metabolising enzymes (e.g. gluthathione transferase), often play important roles. In addition, different chemicals can stimulate or inhibit as well as induce or suppress metabolising enzymes. Phytochemicals in botanicals and Chinese medicine are no different. The increase or decrease of metabolism of the drug can have a positive or negative impact on its effectiveness. In order to use either "Western drugs" or Chinese medicine effectively, the information whether there is a pharmacological interaction between "Western drugs" and Chinese medicine including herbs, dietary supplements and many foods, is needed. For instance, many people use St. John's wort as an OTC antidepressant. It is now known that this herb, upon long term usage, can alter pharmacokinetics of several "Western drugs", including anti-HIV protease inhibitors or cyclosporine (Fugh-Berman, 2000; Moore *et al.*, 2000). Wine and MAO inhibitors and aspirin and anticoagulants are other well known examples.

Understanding the full spectrum of drugs being taken, and understanding the drug-drug interactions and effects on metabolism is critical for physicians to prescribe the proper doses and determine the level of drug level monitoring. Pharmacogenetic approach is taken by assessing the genotype of drug metabolising enzymes. Drug metabolising enzyme activities are not only determined by gene but also by environmental factors as mentioned before. This approach does have its limitations. The activities of these enzymes controlling drug metabolism (termed "pharmacophenomics") ultimately determine how a drug is metabolised. It is conceivable that traditional diagnosis by Chinese medicine practitioners may actually measure metabolic function of individuals since they prescribe herbs based on their diagnosis.

With over 50% of the general population of Western countries now ingesting unregulated or well documented neutriceuticals, dietary supplements or health foods, and the increasing popularity of botanicals or Chinese medicine by the general population, this issue of drug interaction is becoming even more important (Vickers and Zollman, 1999). The treatment failure or poorly optimised treatments by "Western drugs" can be the result of insufficient information concerning the impact of using herbal medicine by their patients. However, physicians who practice mainstream medicine often advise their patients not to take botanical medicines to avoid the potential complication or leave it up to patients to make the decision. Since some Chinese medicines may have value in relieving certain symptoms or preventing certain diseases, both patients and physicians have difficult decisions to make. Clearly more information regarding the interaction of Western medicines and herbal medicines will be beneficial to both the patient and the healthcare professional.

9.5.7 *Mechanism of actions of Chinese medicine needs to be addressed and an explanation of the principles of Chinese medicine using modern scientific terminology should be attempted*

In order to use Chinese medicine more effectively and advance Chinese medicine to the level of global medicine, it is important to understand issues of mechanism(s) of action and to identify the active compounds that may be acting at the different sites. For many years, attempts were made in this area by trying to identify a single active compound for a defined biological system. The result of these studies while useful can only serve as a reference in our understanding the mechanism of action. Attempts were also made using *in vivo* systems in studying the effects of Chinese medicine at different sites of action. However, again, the choice of animal models is an important issue, which should be verified since the metabolism of animals, are different from humans and the diseases in the animal models may have different aetiological reasons from humans. Furthermore, the quality of Chinese medicine used for *in vivo* studies in most cases is not well defined and the results obtained may be difficult to reproduce. In many instances, the route of administration of the medicine did not consider how those particular Chinese medicines were even used. Given that the composition of active compounds can be quite different depending upon the route of administration (oral, I.V. or I.P.), the significance of the study in understanding the mechanism of drug actions is questionable.

The mechanism of action of nearly all Chinese medicines is still a black box. In the past, one of the major reasons for the lack of progress could be due to the availability of technologies. Recent advances in technology including bioinformatics and high throughput, information rich bioassays should be useful to address the issue in a more systematic fashion. It is conceivable that many of these herbals share some common properties, cluster analysis could be employed to identify those herbs. Based on the chemical composition of these herbs, certain chemicals can be identified to be responsible for certain pharmacological responses. The molecular targets associated with different pharmacological responses are known in many cases. Those chemicals identified can be tested against their targets. Data mining bioinformatics technology based on the chemical fingerprint and their target activity of different preparations could be an efficient way of identifying active compound candidates instead of using traditional natural product bioassay directed isolation technology. The information obtained will be useful for our understanding of the mechanism of action of these herbs. An understanding of the mechanism of actions of Chinese medicine, the role of each botanical in the formula and identification of active compounds within each botanical will facilitate future drug development including discovering new therapy uses of known formulas, optimisation of more potent botanical medicines and a more global acceptance of the value of Chinese medicine.

9.5.8 *A comprehensive, accessible and related database should be established to include chemical composition and biological activity of herbs, chemical and biological properties of the chemicals in herbs, the growth conditions storage of each herb and the composition, preparation, potential indication and toxicity of different formulas, etc.*

Currently, several databases of Chinese medicine and herbs have been established, each of them have unique features but none of them are comprehensive enough. Most of the databases are not easily accessible and the quality of these databases is questionable. Furthermore, traditional Chinese medicine terminology was often used and is not easily understood with today's medical terminology. Some of the databases are in Chinese and this will limit their usage. Also, the translation of traditional Chinese medicine terminology into English is sometimes incorrect. Toxicity information is also very limited. A comprehensive database which encompasses the chemical composition, physical as well as biological activities of herbs, the perferred source of herbs to be grown, the methodology to be cultivated and the type of insects causing cultivation problem, part of herbs that should be chosen for the preparation of medicine, chemical and biological variation of herbs grown or stored under different conditions or sessions, the medical use of those herbs, the bases of using those herbs in Chinese medicine formulation, medical use of these formulas in classic traditional way (even though we may not understand them yet), and its potential use in diseases defined with today's medical terminology, the literature to support the claims if it is available, the dosage and scheduled to be used, the interaction with other chemicals in pharmacological terms, the toxicity of some of the Chinese medicine if available, etc. This database should be available to the general public who may be interested in using or studying Chinese medicine. For instance, the potential toxicity of herbs on Liver was recently summarised (Stedman, 2002). Development of Chinese Herbal Toxicity database was also initiated (Bensoussan *et al.*, 2002). The establishment of such a comprehensive database will require continuous updating. The availability of such a database will be critically important in facilitating the advancement of Chinese medicine as an industry. It will also help the regulatory agency with should establish guidelines in regulating Chinese or herbal medicine. A collaboration effort of different institutions is required and should be encouraged to make this important venture possible.

9.5.9 *The number of herbs used for preparing Chinese medicine formula can be minimised due to the redundancy of their biological activity*

Through the years, there are more than 5000 different herbs being identified and used in the preparation of Chinese medicine. Among them, less than 500 herbs are commonly used. Some of those herbs were claimed to have similar pharmacological properties. Given that the same biological or active chemicals are found in different herbs or different chemicals can act on the same target, it is highly likely that many of these herbs can be redundant in terms of their biological activity. Then there will be no need to have that many herbs available. This will be helpful in establishing the priority of cultivating herbs with GAP, preparation or prescription of Chinese medicine. In order to achieve this, it will require not only research in multidisciplinary areas but also a good database with many of the required information for mining. Modern bioinformatics technology will be required.

9.5.10 *A simplified, more efficacious and friendly version of formula based on scientific investigations should be developed*

Traditional Chinese medicine was used for many years for different claims. Any new change in the source of herbs or the methodology for preparation of Chinese medicine should be considered as a new drug and its historical claims will become invalid. Regulations should be put in place to protect the population from using those preparations which deviate from those used in the past. One major drawback of some of these Chinese medicines is their unfriendly user nature such as taste, smell, colour and size of preparation. Another difficulty is the methodologies of making consistent preparations with so many variables. With the advancement of our understanding of how Chinese medicine works through research, it is possible that a simplified, more efficient and friendly version of Chinese medicine formula could be developed. The products with modification of content or preparation of formula without solid scientitic information of their claims, which are commonly practiced in many Chinese medicine companies, should be carefully monitored. The industry of Chinese medicine will have no bright future without research on their new products. A heavy investment of these companies together with other organisations such as government, foundation, etc. in research is strongly encouraged. Most Chinese medicine companies are trying to develop their businesses as a grocery store with many products — constantly changing packaging and using advertisements with often non-substantiated claims, they should instead focus more on a few products with research in-house or in collaboration with academia.

9.5.11 *The philosophy, principles and practices of Chinese medicine should be introduced to the medical establishment using the language and concepts of modern science*

In order for Chinese medicine to benefit humankind worldwide, it is important that all the principles are understood and accepted by the global scientific community. Today the scientific basis of Chinese medicine is not in keeping with the path of modern scientific development. In many instances, the languages used may be the same, but the meaning can be very different. In other cases, the science and technology developed over the past 50 years is still not sophisticated enough to understand the complexities and principles of Chinese medicine. Using the technologies of genomics, cell manipulation and biochemical informatics and knowledge of neural, endocrine, immune and other biological sciences that have been developed over the past ten years, it may now be possible to explore the scientific foundation that lies beneath the philosophy and principles of Chinese medicine. For instance, it is suspected that the diagnosis used by Chinese medicine practitioners is not only for diagnosis of the disease associated with different organs in their functional sense, it may even stratify the same disease patients based on the stage of disease, the aetiology of disease and the individual response to a given treatment. Furthermore, it may also indicate the activity of drug metabolic enzymes, which can be one of the rationales for the prescription of drugs based on their diagnosis. Those possibilities can be systematically proven using today's technologies. Once it is proven, the information will not only substantiate the validity of their diagnosis to be accepted globally but also provide the scientific basis for the diagnosis used by traditional Chinese medical practitioners. As a result, their vast experience, accumulated through thousands of years of practice can now be very useful for the development of future medicine in combination with current mainstream medicine.

One immediate approach to open the black box behind the diagnosis used by Chinese medicine practitioners is its possible association with the profiles of serum or urine proteins including cytokine and chemokines. Recently, it was recognised that the unique profiles of chemokine, cytokines and clusters of serum proteins can associate with different diseases (Vlahou *et al.*, 2001; Petricoin *et al.*, 2002; Li *et al.*, 2002; Qu *et al.*, 2002; Cazares *et al.*, 2002; Adam *et al.*, 2002; Kingsmore and Patel, 2003; Schweitzer *et al.*, 2002). Although it is not proven, the serum protein profiles including cytokine and chemokine may also reflect the activity of different drug metabolic enzymes such as CYP450 isozymes. If the association of the unique profile of the protein serum profiles with the stratification of patients based on the diagnosis of the Chinese medicine practitioner, such as hot versus cold, weak versus strong, functional organ state, etc. can be established, this can help us understand the significance of their unique way of diagnosis. It can also provide an alternative objective way of diagnosis evolved from their subjective methodologies.

Multiplex assays for cytokines and chemokines as well as high throughput technology of proteomics serum proteins together with bioinformatics methodology to do cluster analysis are all available. A well-designed clinical study, which has more than one experienced TCM practitioner involved in the diagnosis of the same individual in order to avoid subjective errors being made by different TCM practitioners, and blind analysis of serum protein profiles or urine samples from individuals once the bioinformatics algorithm for each diagnosis is established, should be designed to test the hypothesis. The participation of mainstream medical doctors in their independent diagnosis based on modern medical technology is also important. This should be very helpful in advancing the science of Chinese medicine and in facilitating the development of future medicines.

9.6 Summary

In summary, the development of Chinese medicine is based upon the accumulation of experience and knowledge gathered over the centuries. The approaches taken are holistic and empirical. There is a need to understand their actions at molecular levels with more rational, objective and scientific studies. The development of mainstream medicine is based upon our current understanding of biological systems at the molecular level. Integration of the actions of drugs that are targeted at the molecular level on the whole body is needed. Today, with the emphasis and need for effective therapies shifting towards the treatment and prevention of chronic and age-related diseases, e.g. metabolic disorders, neurodegenerative diseases and cancer, the paradigm of mainstream pharmaceutical discovery of identifying single compounds to regulate a single associated target may not be sufficient. Today, it appears that chronic and age-associated diseases may be multifactorial and hence more complex. A different approach may be required.

One claimed usage of Chinese medicine is for the treatment and prevention of chronic and age-associated illnesses. Some of the botanical formulas used for this purpose were discovered thousands of years ago and continue to be used today. There are indications that these formulas may indeed be helpful in the treatment or prevention of chronic diseases. This multi-component medicine should not only be useful in meeting clinical needs, it must also define a more synergistic therapy that supports and maintains the boby's natural curative abilities. The potential usefulness of Chinese medicine embodies the belief of maintaining healthy homeostasis of the body through the proper balance of a mixture of chemicals at different organs or tissues. This concept is different from Western medicine and implies that multiple compounds may act on multiple mechanisms of action to maintain the balance of the complex web of biology. This is very important in view of sciences current direction to integrate fragmented information to develop future medicines. If the effectiveness of the botanical formulas proves to be true in rigorous clinical trials, the scientific basis of the mechanism of action of these formulas will provide an important step forward in advancing the basic knowledge of medical science and developing more effective treatments. The Western and Eastern approaches to human health and disease are complementary to each other. The best approach in developing future medicines is to integrate both approaches.

To integrate current mainstream medicine and Chinese medicine will be a major undertaking requiring international collaboration. For areas of the world that do have a strong focus on using Chinese medicines or botanicals, it is the (moral) obligation of governments and private enterprises to take the necessary steps to ensure the health of their population by improving the quality and verifying the effectiveness of Chinese medicine. In those areas that are not familiar with Chinese medicine, serious attempts should be made to take advantage of the knowledge accumulated, through many centuries, by the Chinese people in order to fulfill the clinical needs that remain poorly treated. There are a gowing number of patients using Chinese medicine or botanicals for various reason in Western societies. A joint effort among different governments and enterprises across the international borders should be strongly encouraged to insure the safety and efficacy of these botanical pharmaceuticals. It is believed that a convergence of Western and Chinese traditional medicines may evolve into a greatly improved method of humam health care in the coming century.

It is anticipated that the evolution of Chinese medicine in this century will be:

Traditional Chinese Medicine (TCM)
↓
Modern Chinese Medicine (MCM)
↓
Globally accepted Chinese Medicine (GCM)
↓
Future New Medicine (NM) ← Other Folk Medicine (FM)
↑
Current Mainstream Medicine (CMM)
↑
Western Medicine (WM)

Demonstrating the clinical efficiency of a well-characterised Chinese medicine formula, which can be made in a consistent matter with respect to its pharmacological properties with modern clinical study approach, should be the first priority in advancing Chinese medicine. This will establish the credibility of Chinese medicine. To do research in understanding the principle of formulation, its active compounds and mechanism of their actions of Chinese medicine will also be essential in introducing Chinese medicine to the world for the advancement of future medicine. Today, we sit at the juncture of transitional TCM through MCM to GCM. Eventually, there should be only one medicine.

Acknowledgements

Yung-Chi Cheng is a Fellow of the National Foundation for Cancer Research. I would like to thank Dr. Robert Tilton, Vice-President, PhytoCeutica, Inc. (A Yale University-sponsored company with a focus on Chinese medicine) for his reading and correcting this manuscript and Ms. Jennifer Visaggio for her assistance in the preparation of this manuscript.

References

Adam, B.-L., Qu, Y., Davis, J.W., Ward, M.D., Clements, M.A., Cazares, L.H., Semmes, O.J., Schellhammer, P.F., Yasui, Y., Feng, Z. and Wright, G.L. Jr. (2002) Serum protein fingerprinting coupled with a pattern-matching algorithm distinguishes prostate cancer from benign prostate hyperplasia and healthy men. *Cancer Res.* **62**, 3609–3614.

Arlt, V.M., Stiborova, M. and Schmeiser, H.H. (2002) Aristolochic acid as a probable human cancer hazard in herbal remedies: a review. *Mutagenesis* **17**, 265–277.

Bensoussan, A., Myers, S.P., Drew, A.K., Whyte, I.M. and Dawson, A.H. (2002) Development of a Chinese herbal medicine toxicity database. *Clin. Toxicol.* **40**(2), 159–167.

Cazares, L.H., Adam, B.-L., Ward, M.D., Nasim, S., Schellhammer, P.F., Semmes, O.J. and Wright, G.L. Jr. (2002) Normal, benign, preneoplastic and malignant prostate cells have distinct protein expression profiles resolved by surface enhanced laser desorption/ionization mass spectrometry. *Clin. Cancer Res.* **8**, 2541–2552.

De Smet, P.A.G.M. (2002) Drug therapy. *N. Engl. J. Med.* **347**(25), 2046–2056.

Fugh-Berman, A. (2000) Herb-drug interactions. *Lancet* **355**, 134–138 [Erratum, *Lancet* **355**, 1020 (2000)].

Harkey, M.R., Henderson, G.L., Gershwin, M.E., Stern, J.S. and Hackman, R.M. (2001) Variability in commercial ginseng products: an analysis of 25 preparations. *Am. J. Clin. Nutr.* **73**, 1101–1106.

Kingsmore, S.F. and Patel, D.D. (2003) Multiplexed protein profiling on antibody-based microarrays by rolling circle amplification. *Curr. Opin. Biotechnol.* **14**(1), 74–81.

Lai, M.-Y., Chen, C.-C., Hsiu, S.-L. and Chao, P.-D.L. (2001) Analysis and comparison of Biacalin, Baicalein and Wogonin contents in traditional decoctions and commercial extracts of Scuttellariae Radix. *J. Food Drug Anal.* **9**(3), 145–149.

Li, J., Zhang, Z., Rosenweig, J., Wang, Y.Y. and Chan, D.W. (2002) Proteomics and bioinformatics approaches for identification of serum biomarkers to detect breast cancer. *Clin. Chem.* **48**(8), 1296–1304.

Luyckx, V.A., Ballantine, R., Claeys, M., *et al.* (2002) Herbal remedy-associated acute renal failure secondary to Cape aloes. *Am. J. Kidney Dis.* **39**, E13.

Marcus, D.M. and Grollman, A.P. (2002) Botanical medicines — the need for new regulations. *N. Engl. J. Med.* **347**(25), 2073–2076.

Moore, L.B., Goodwin, B., Jones, S.A., *et al.* (2000) St. John's wort induces hepatic drug metabolism through activation of the pregnane X receptor. *Proc. Natl. Acad. Sci. USA* **97**, 7500–7502.

Nortier, J.L., Martinez, M.-C.M., Scheiser, H.H., *et al.* (2000) Urothelial carcinoma associated with the use of a Chinese herb (*Aristolochia fangchi*). *N. Engl. J. Med.* **342**, 1686–1692.

Petricoin, E.F. III, Ardekani, A.M., Hitt, B.A., Levine, P.J., Fusaro, V.A., Steinberg, S.M., Mills, G.B., Simone, C., Fishman, D.A., Kohn, E.C. and Liotta, L.A. (2002) Use of proteomic patterns in serum to identify ovarian cancer. *Lancet* **359**, 572–575.

Qu, Y., Adam, B.-L., Yasui, Y., Ward, M.D., Cazares, L.H., Schellhammer, P.F., Feng, Z., Semmes, O.J. and Wright, G.L. Jr. (2002) Boosted decision tree analysis of surface-enhanced laser desorption/ionization mass spectral serum profiles discriminates prostate cancer from non-cancer patients. *Clin. Chem.* **48**(10), 1835–1843.

Schweitzer, B., Roberts, S., Grimwade, B., Shao, W., Wang, M., Fu, Q., Shu, Q., Laroche, I., Zhou, Z., Tchernev, V.T., Christiansen, J., Velleca, M. and Kingsmore, S.F. (2002) Multiplexed protein profiling on microarrays by rolling-circle amplification. *Nat. Biotechnol.* **20**(4), 359–365.

Stedman, C. (2002) Herbal hepatotoxicity. *Semin. Liver Dis.* **22**, 195–206.

Straus, S.E. (2002) Herbal medicines — what's in the bottle? *N. Engl. J. Med.* **347**(25), 1997–1998.

Vickers, A. and Zollman, C. (1999) ABC of complementary medicine herbal medicine. *Br. Med. J.* **319**, 1050–1053.

Vlahou, A., Schellhammer, P.F., Mendrinos, S., Patel, K., Kondylis, F.I., Gong, L., Nasim, S. and Wright, G.L. Jr. (2001) Development of a novel proteomic approach for the detection of transitional cell carcinoma of the bladder in urine. *Am. J. Pathol.* **158**(4), 1491–1502.

Chapter 10

Practice and Research on Chinese Medicine Outside of China

Qunhao Zhang

10.1 Introduction

During the past 30 years, Chinese medicine is increasingly used by a significant percentage of the world population. In the 1970s, under programmes sponsored by the World Health Organization, physicians from many countries came to China to study in one- to three-month acupuncture programmes. Since the early 1980s, many two- to three-month programmes have been established for both physician and non-physician acupuncturists from around the world. Today, Chinese medicine is widely used and has become a rapidly growing health system of increasing importance to the world economy. In China, it accounts for approximately 40% of all healthcare delivery, while in Hong Kong, 60% of the population has consulted Chinese medicine practitioners. The WHO estimates that Chinese medicine is being used for healthcare in over 100 countries. The use of Chinese medicine remains widespread in developing countries such as China, Vietnam and Africa; it is also rapidly increasing in developed countries, such as the United States, Germany, Singapore, Japan, Australia, Canada, and the United Kingdom. In many developed countries, complementary/alternative medicine (CAM, including mainly Chinese medicine) is becoming more and more popular. The percentage of the population which has used CAM at least once is 48.5% in Australia, 70% percentage in Canada, 42% in the U.S., 75% in France, and 38% in Belgium. In many parts of the world, expenditure on CAM is significant, and rapidly expanding. In Malaysia, an estimated US$500 million is spent annually on Chinese medicine, compared to about US$300 million on conventional medicine (WHO Traditional Medicine Strategy for 2002–2005, 2002). In the U.S. in 1997, the estimated total number of visits to CAM practitioners exceeded the estimated total number of visits to all primary care physicians. In addition, the total number of out-of-pocket expenditures relating to CAM therapies during 1997 is US$27, which was comparable to the projected out-of-pocket expenditures for all U.S. physician-rendered services in that year (Eisenberg *et al.*, 1993). In Australia, Canada and the U.K., the annual CAM expenditure is estimated at US$80 million, US$2400 million and US$2300 million, respectively. In Japan, 72% of conventional doctors prescribe Kampo medicine for their patients and according to an October 2000 survey, the herbal medicine market was worth US$2.4 billion. A survey of 610 Swiss doctors showed that 46% had used some forms of CAM, mainly acupuncture and homeopathy. In the U.K., almost 40% of all general conventional medicine doctors offer some form of CAM referral or access. The world market for herbal medicines based on traditional knowledge is now estimated at US$6 billion. The WHO Complementary/Alternative Medicine Facts and Figures (2002) says that, up to 80% of people in the southern hemisphere use traditional medicine (mainly Chinese medicine) as part of primary health care. In Africa, up to 80% of the population use traditional medicine to help meet their healthcare needs, and in France, 75% of the population has used traditional medicine at least once (WHO Complementary/Alternative Medicine Facts, 2002). Traditional medicine has been fully integrated into the health systems of China, North and South Korea and Vietnam. The global market for traditional therapies stands at US$60 billion a year and is steadily growing.

As one of the most important parts of Chinese medicine, acupuncture is especially popular. Originating in China, it is now used in at least 100 countries and practiced not only by acupuncturists, but also by conventional doctors. According to the World Federation of Acupuncture-Moxibustion Societies, there are at least 50,000 acupuncturists in Asia. In Europe, there are an estimated 15,000 acupuncturists including conventional doctors who also practice acupuncture. In Belgium, 74% of acupuncture treatment is administered by conventional medicine doctors. In Germany, 77% of pain clinics provide acupuncture. In the U.K., 46%

of conventional medicine doctors either recommend patients for acupuncture treatment or treat their patients with acupuncture themselves. The U.S. has about 20,000 licensed acupuncturists; the practice of acupuncture is legal in 41 states and the District of Columbia, and the other states are developing acupuncture practice policies.

A World Health Organization Inter-regional Seminar on Acupuncture, Moxibustion and Acupuncture Anaesthesia was held in Beijing in June 1979. The seminar drew up the following provisional list of diseases that lend themselves to acupuncture treatment. The list is based on clinical experience, and not necessarily on controlled clinical research. Furthermore, the inclusion of specific diseases are not meant to indicate the extent of acupuncture's efficacy in treating them.

The following is a list of conditions which the World Health Organization determined may respond to acupuncture:

Upper Respiratory Tract

- Acute sinusitis
- Acute rhinitis
- Common cold
- Acute tonsillitis

Respiratory System

- Acute bronchitis
- Bronchial asthma (most effective in children and in patients without complicating diseases)

Disorders of the Eye

- Acute conjunctivitis
- Central retinitis
- Myopia (in children)
- Cataract (without complications)

Disorders of the Mouth

- Toothache, post-extraction pain
- Gingivitis
- Acute and chronic pharyngitis

Gastro-intestinal Disorders

- Spasms of esophagus and cardia
- Hiccough
- Gastroptosis
- Acute and chronic gastritis
- Gastric hyperacidity
- Chronic duodenal ulcer (pain relief)
- Acute duodenal ulcer (without complications)
- Acute and chronic colitis
- Acute bacillary dysentery
- Constipation
- Diarrhoea
- Paralytic ileus

Neurological and Musculo-skeletal Disorders

- Headache and migraine
- Trigeminal neuralgia
- Facial palsy (early stage, i.e. within three to six months)
- Paralysis following a stroke
- Peripheral neuropathies
- Sequelae of poliomyelitis (early stage, i.e. within six months)
- Meniere's disease
- Neurogenic bladder dysfunction
- Nocturnal enuresis
- Intercostal neuralgia
- Cervicobrachial syndrome
- "Frozen shoulder", "tennis elbow"
- Sciatica
- Low back pain
- Osteoarthritis

The most common conditions treated effectively by acupuncture include:

Chronic Pain

- Neck and back pain
- Migraine headaches

Acute Injury-related Pain

- Sprains
- Strains

Gastrointestinal Problems

- Indigestion
- Ulcers
- Constipation
- Diarrhoea

Cardiovascular Conditions

- High and low blood pressure

Genitourinary Problems

- Menstrual irregularity
- Infertility
- Impotence

Muscle and Nerve Conditions

- Paralysis
- Deafness

Addictive Behaviours

- Substance abuse
- Over-eating
- Drug dependence
- Smoking

Surgery

- Anaesthesia

10.2 The United States

The transmission of Chinese medicine into the U.S. can be traced back to the 18th century. At that time, Chinese herbal medicine and tea were imported directly from China to the U.S. or through Europe.

In the early 19th century, acupuncture was used in patients in Europe, and was later transmitted to the U.S. through Europe. The papers and books about Chinese medicine research and practice were translated into English and published in the U.S. In the 1840s, the discovery of gold in California attracted hundreds of thousands of Chinese to the U.S., most of them were Cantonese. Together with them, they brought Chinese medicine and used it in Chinese communities as the main source of healthcare. During this period, Chinese medicine was practiced mostly among Chinese and very few Americans. Most Americans had not heard of Chinese medicine at the time.

The true transmission of Chinese medicine into the U.S. was in the 1970s. On 26 July 1971, James Reston published a report in the *New York Times* introducing how Chinese physicians in Beijing (Chaoyang Hospital) eased his post-surgery abdominal pain and discomfort with needles. For most Americans, this was their first glimpse of Chinese medicine and its potential uses (Reston, 1971). The following year, on 21 February 1972, President Nixon visited China, thus opening the gates of China to the West.

Since then, Chinese medicine has caused great interest in the U.S. As more Chinese medicine practitioners immigrated to the U.S., an increasing number of Americans began to use Chinese medicine for their medical condition. In 1973, Oregon and Nevada approved the acupuncture practice and issued acupuncture licenses, which officially announced the acceptance of acupuncture by the U.S. government. In 1974, Hawaii and Montana approved acupuncture; 1975, Louisiana, 1976, California, etc. Today, 40 out of 50 U.S. states including the District of Columbia approved acupuncture. In 1979, the first acupuncture school in the U.S., the New England School of Acupuncture, was established in Boston, Massachusetts. Today, there are over 50 acupuncture or Chinese medicine schools in the U.S. (Zhang, 2001). In 1992, the National Institutes of Health (NIH) established Office of Alternative Medicine (OAM). In 1993, the first survey of the prevalence of CAM in the U.S. was published, showing that one-third of Americans were CAM users (Eisenberg *et al.*, 1993). In 1996, FDA classified acupuncture needle as a class II medical instrument. In November 1997, a consensus development conference on acupuncture was convened at the National Institutes of Health. In November 1998, based on OAM, Congress established the National Center for Complementary and Alternative Medicine (NCCAM). At the same time, a special issue of the *Journal of the American Medical Association* devoted to Complementary medicine was published (Eisenberg *et al.*, 1998). Twelve National Centers for CAM were established in 12 famous universities and institutions (Zhang, 2000). In 2000, a growing number of Americans are using alternative approaches to health promotion and medical treatment. As a result of public interest and the use of unconventional health care, President Clinton established the White House Commission on Complementary and Alternative Medicine Policy (WCCAMP). Executive Order 13147 (http://govinfo.library.unt.edu/whccamp/eo.html) authorizing the Commission was issued on 7 March 2000. The Commission, which is composed of individuals knowledgeable in both conventional and CAM, has been charged with addressing:

(1) Research on CAM practices and products.
(2) Dissemination of reliable information on CAM to health care providers and the general public.
(3) Delivery of and public access to CAM services.
(4) Appropriate licensing, education and training of CAM health care practitioners.

The Final Report of the White House Commission on Complementary and Alternative Medicine Policy in accordance with Executive Order 13147 was submitted to the White House in March 2002. It is also available on the Internet at http://govinfo.library.unt.edu/whccamp/finalreport.html

10.2.1 *What is the prevalence of CAM in the U.S.?*

Due to the dramatic increase in the prevalence of chronic conditions for which conventional therapies have provided only modest gains, the past decade has witnessed an acceleration both in consumer interest in and use of CAM practices. Those with the most serious and debilitating medical conditions, such as cancer, chronic pain, asthma, depression, infertility, hypertension, hepatitis and HIV, tend to be the most frequent users of CAM practices (Richardson *et al.*, 2000; Morris *et al.*, 2000; Sparber *et al.*, 2000; Astin, 1998; Krauss *et al.*, 1998; Lerner and Kennedy, 1992).

A 1997 national survey estimated that in the previous year, 42% of the adult population in the U.S. has used at least one of the complementary therapies (including acupuncture, massage and herbal medicine) included in the survey. This is an increase from 33.8% in 1990. The probability of patients visiting a complementary medical practitioner increased from 36.3% to 46.3% between 1990 and 1997. The total number of visits to complementary medicine practitioners increased from 427 million in 1990 to 629 million in 1997, exceeding total visits to all primary care physicians. Estimated expenditure for professional complementary medical services increased 45.2% between 1990 and 1997. In 1997, the expenditures were conservatively estimated at US$21.2 billion with at least US$12.2 billion of this paid out-of-packet. Total out-of-packet expenditures relating to complementary medicine therapies were conservatively estimated at US$27 billion, which is comparable to the projected out-of-pocket expenditures for all U.S. physician services (Eisenberg *et al.*, 1998).

There are about 20,000 acupuncture practitioners in the U.S., among them, 5000 are physicians who practice acupuncture. There are approximately 50,000 qualified massage therapists in the U.S., providing 45 million one-hour massage sessions per year. Most of the CAM practitioners have their own clinics, which are distributed widely all over the countries. During the past five years, more and more hospital and clinical centres in the U.S. offer acupuncture services, such as Massachusetts General Hospital of Harvard University, UCLA Hospital, University of Maryland, Memorial Sloan-Kettering Cancer Center, etc.

Under the U.S. Constitution, the Federal government has no jurisdiction over the licensing of professionals. Therefore, each of the 50 states regulate the professionals independently, setting licensing standards, scopes of practice, and education and examination requirements. Forty-one of the 50 states, and the District of Columbia, regulate the practice of acupuncture and Oriental medicine as a licensed or registered health care profession. Most states have their own professional organisation to represent the members of Chinese medicine profession.

10.2.2 *What can CAM treat?*

The nature of CAM allows it to treat a wide variety of conditions, including pain, headaches, digestive problems, menstrual cramps, sports and work-related injuries, and many others. However, it generally can be used as the treatment of choice for sprains and strains, allergies, poor digestion, menstrual problems, menopause, headaches, neck and back pain, fatigue, stress, and other minor and self-limiting illnesses. CAM is also a wonderful adjunct for speeding recovery from major trauma, surgery and strokes, treating the side effects of cancer chemotherapy, and enhancing the effectiveness of alcohol and substance abuse recovery programmes.

California Occupational Survey

In 1996, an occupational survey was conducted under contract by the California State Acupuncture Committee in order to update the content of the California Acupuncture Licensing Exam. This survey identified well over one 100 conditions or categories of conditions treated. The following is a top 25 conditions the Licensed Acupuncturists treated.

25 Commonly Treated Conditions

- Anxiety and Depression
- Arthritis, Tendonitis and Joint Pain
- Asthma and Allergies
- Auto Injuries
- Bladder and Kidney Infections
- Cardiac Palpitations (Irregular Heartbeat)
- Chronic Fatigue Syndrome
- Common Cold and Influenza
- Degenerative Disk Disorders
- Diet, Nutrition and Weight Control
- Fibromyalgia
- Headaches and Migraines
- Hypertension (High Blood Pressure)
- Indigestion, Gas, Bloating, Constipation

- Insomnia
- Menopause Symptoms
- Musculoskeletal Pain
- Nausea
- Orthopaedic Conditions
- Pain — Other Kinds
- Pre-mentrual Syndrome (PMS) and Menstrual Irregularity
- Sports Injuries
- Tension/Stress Syndromes
- Tinnitus
- Work Injuries

Maryland Patient Survey

The Maryland Acupuncture Society contracted for a patient survey to be conducted in 1999, with the results being published in January 2000. The Patient Satisfaction Survey — Final Report lists the following 13 most common conditions for which patients sought treatment from an acupuncturist. Over 80% of the respondents also found these treatments to be very effective or moderately effective.

Thirteen Commonly and Effectively Treated Conditions

- Stress/Tension
- Depression/Mood
- Fatique/Energy
- Back Pain
- Other Musculoskeletal Pain
- Arthritis
- Migraine
- Other Headaches
- Female Concerns
- Gastrointestinal
- Allergies
- Asthma
- Health/Wholeness

Soon after the California and Maryland Survey in 1997, acupuncture received its highest confirmation of credibility to date in the U.S. (NIH, 1997). In November 1997, a Consensus Development Conference sponsored by the National Institutes of Health and several other agencies concluded: "there is sufficient evidence... of acupuncture's value to expand its use into conventional medicine and to encourage further studies of its physiology and clinical value". The panelists recommended that the Federal government and insurance companies expand coverage of acupuncture so more people can have access to it. These conclusions were based on the review of numerous studies, of which few were done in English and up to rigorous scientific standards. In spite of this, they found ample evidence to support its continued practice and to recommend further research.

Specifically, the NIH Consensus Statement on Acupuncture states: "Acupuncture as a therapeutic intervention is widely practiced in the United States. While there have been many studies of its potential usefulness, many of these studies provide equivocal results because of design, sample size and other factors. The issue is further complicated by inherent difficulties in the use of appropriate controls, such as placebos and sham acupuncture groups. However, promising results have emerged, for example, showing efficacy of acupuncture in adult post-operative and chemotherapy nausea and vomiting and in post-operative dental pain. There are other situations such as addiction, stroke rehabilitation, headache, menstrual cramps, tennis elbow, fibromyalgia, myofascial pain, osteoarthritis, low back pain, carpal tunnel syndrome and asthma, in which acupuncture may be useful as an adjunct treatment or an acceptable alternative or be included in a comprehensive management programme. Further research is likely to uncover additional areas where acupuncture interventions will be useful...".

"There is clear evidence that needle acupuncture is efficacious for adult post-operative and chemotherapy nausea and vomiting and probably for the nausea of pregnancy. Much of the research is on various pain problems. There is evidence of efficacy for post-operative dental pain. There are reasonable studies (although sometimes only single studies) showing relief of pain with acupuncture on diverse pain conditions such as menstrual cramps, tennis elbow and fibromyalgia...".

"Although many other conditions have received some attention in the literature and, in fact, the research suggests some exciting potential areas for the use of acupuncture, the quality or quantity of the research evidence is not sufficient to provide firm evidence of efficacy at this time". (See the NIH Consensus Statement on Acupuncture.)

10.2.3 *What CAM research is being done in the U.S.?*

As a result of the rapid rise of interest in and use of CAM in the U.S., the research to take a serious look at both safety and efficacy of CAM is growing dramatically fast. In 1992, the NIH established the Office of Alternative Medicine (OAM). Based on this, Congress established the National Center for Complementary and Alternative Medicine (NCCAM) in 1998. Its mission is "to prevent and alleviate human suffering through research on the safety and effectiveness of CAM modalities and through research training and information dissemination for healthcare providers and consumers".

NCCAM has received progressive budget increases since its establishment. The budget was US$2 million in 1992, US$2 million in 1993, US$3.5 million in 1994, US$5.5 million in 1995, US$7.8 million in 1996, US$12 million in 1997, US$20 million in 1998, US$50 million in 1999, US$68 million in 2000, and risen to US$93 million in 2001 (NIH, 2003b). Currently, NIH supports over 200 studies involving CAM therapies, the diseases being treated include coronary heart disease, hypertension, diabetes, arthritis and allergies (Eisenberg, 2003). Examples are: acupuncture for nausea and dental pain, acupuncture for fibromyalgia, acupuncture for post-operative nausea, acupuncture for headache, acupuncture for low back pain, massage for low back pain, moxibustion for breech presentation, Chinese herb for irritable bowel syndrome, Gingko for Alzheimer's Dementia, Garlic for hypercholesterolemia, PC-SPES for prostate cancer, herbal remedies for asthma, acupuncture for tinnitus, acupuncture for peripheral neurophy, acupuncture for stroke, functional MRI studies of acupuncture in normal subjects, Taichi for balance disorder, acupuncture for arthritis, etc. In 2000, Massachusetts General Hospital of Harvard University accepted a multi-million dollar grant from NIH to study acupuncture's effect on hypertension. The study, called SHARP

(Stop Hypertension with Acupuncture Research Program), is the biggest of its series in the U.S.

To date, NCCAM has funded the establishment of 17 national research centres to explore the safety and efficacy of a wide range of CAM therapies for a host of conditions (NIH, 2003a). A list of centers follows:

Center for Addiction and Alternative Medicine Research

Specialty: Addictions
Principal Investigator: Thomas J. Kiresuk, Ph.D.

Address:
Center for Addiction and Alternative Medicine Research (CAAMR)
Minneapolis Medical Research Foundation
914 South Eighth Street, Suite D917
Minneapolis, MN 55404
URL: www.mmrfweb.org/research/addicton&alt_med/index.html

Center for CAM Research in Aging and Women's Health

Specialty: Aging and Women's Health
Principal Investigator: Fredi Kronenberg, Ph.D.

Address:
Center for CAM Research in Aging and Women's Health
Columbia University
College of Physicians and Surgeons
630 West 168th Street
New York, NY 10032
URL: cpmcnet.columbia.edu/dept/rosenthal/

Center for Alternative Medicine Research on Arthritis

Specialty: Arthritis
Principal Investigator: Brian M. Berman, M.D.

Address:
Center for Alternative Medicine Research on Arthritis
University of Maryland School of Medicine
Division of Complementary Medicine
2200 Kernan Drive
Baltimore, MD 21207-6693
URL: www.compmed.ummc.umaryland.edu/

Center for Frontier Medicine in Biofield Science

Specialty: Biofield
Principal Investigator: Gary E. Schwartz, Ph.D.

Address:
Department of Psychology
University of Arizona
PO Box 210068
Tucson, AZ 85721-0068

Botanical Center for Age-Related Diseases

Specialty: Botanicals
Principal Investigator: Connie M. Weaver, Ph.D.

Address:
Botanical Center for Age-Related Diseases
Purdue University West Lafayette
Division of Sponsored Programs
West Lafayette, IN 47907-1021

Botanical Dietary Supplements for Women's Health

Specialty: Botanicals
Principal Investigator: Norman R. Farnsworth, Ph.D.

Address:
Botanical Dietary Supplements for Women's Health
University of Illinois at Chicago
809 S. Marshfield Avenue
Chicago, IL 60612-7205

Center for Dietary Supplements Research: Botanicals

Specialty: Botanicals
Principal Investigator: David Heber, M.D., Ph.D.

Address:
UCLA Center for Dietary Supplements Research: Botanicals
University of California at Los Angeles
10945 Le Conte Avenue, Suite 1401
Box 951406
Los Angeles, CA 90095-1406

Center for Phytomedicine Research

Specialty: Botanicals
Principal Investigator: Barbara N. Timmermann, Ph.D.

Address:
Arizona Center for Phytomedicine Research
University of Arizona College of Pharmacy
1703 E. Mabel
P.O. Box 210207
Tucson, AZ 85721-0207

The Center for Cancer Complementary Medicine

Specialty: Cancer
Principal Investigator: Adrian S. Dobs, M.D.

Address:
Johns Hopkins Center for Cancer Complementary Medicine
Johns Hopkins University
720 Rutland Avenue
Baltimore, MD 21205
URL: www.hopkins-cam.org

The Specialized Center of Research in Hyperbaric Oxygen Therapy

Specialty: Cancer
Principal Investigator: Stephen R. Thom, M.D., Ph.D.

Address:
Specialized Center of Research in Hyperbaric Oxygen Therapy
University of Pennsylvania
133 South 36th Street (6463801)
Research Services, Mezzanine
Philadelphia, PA 19104-3246

CAM Research Center for Cardiovascular Diseases

Specialty: Cardiovascular Diseases
Principal Investigator: Steven F. Bolling, M.D.

Address:
Center for Complementary and Alternative Medicine Research in CVD
Adult Cardiac Surgery/Thoracic Transplantation
The University of Michigan Taubman Health Care Center
2120, Box 0344
Ann Arbor, MI 48109
URL: www.med.umich.edu/camrc/index.html

Center for Natural Medicine and Prevention

Specialty: Cardiovascular Disease in Aging African Americans
Principal Investigator: Robert H. Schneider, M.D.

Address:
Center for Natural Medicine and Prevention
Maharishi University of Management
504 North 4th Street, Suite 207
Fairfield, IA 52557
URL: www.mum.edu/CNMP

Consortial Center for Chiropractic Research

Specialty: Chiropractic
Principal Investigator: William C. Meeker, D.C., M.P.H.

Address:
Consortial Center for Chiropractic Research
Palmer Center for Chiropractic Research
741 Brady Street
Davenport, IA 52803
URL: www.palmer.edu

Oregon Center for Complementary and Alternative Medicine Research in Craniofacial Disorders

Specialty: Craniofacial Disorders
Principal Investigator: B. Alexander White, D.D.S.

Address:
Center for Health Research
Kaiser Foundation Hospitals
3800 N. Interstate Avenue
Portland, OR 97227-1110

Oregon Center for Complementary and Alternative Medicine in Neurological Disorders

Specialty: Neurological Disorders
Principal Investigator: Barry S. Oken, M.D.

Address:
Oregon Center for Complementary and Alternative Medicine in Neurological Disorders
Oregon Health Sciences University
3181 SW Sam Jackson Park Road
Portland, OR 97201

Center for CAM in Neurodegenerative Diseases

Specialty: Neurodegenerative Diseases
Principal Investigator: Mahlon R. Delong, M.D.

Address:
Center for CAM in Neurodegenerative Diseases
Department of Neurology
Emory University School of Medicine
1639 Pierce Drive
Atlanta, GA 30322
URL: www.emory.edu/WHSC/MED/NEUROLOGY/CAM/index.html

Pediatric Center for Complementary and Alternative Medicine

Specialty: Pediatrics
Principal Investigator: Fayez K. Ghishan, M.D., D.C.H.

Address:
University of Arizona Health Sciences Center
Department of Pediatrics
1501 N. Campbell Avenue
P.O. Box 245073
Tucson, AZ 85724-5073

10.3 Australia

The first recorded material on Chinese medicine is traced back to the 3rd century B.C. It has existed in Australia since the intake of Chinese immigrants into the Australian gold fields in the 19th century. By 1911, Chinese herbal medicines were available in Australia with English labels and directions.

In 1996–1997, the Australian Commonwealth Health Insurance Commission paid over US$17.7 million in Medicare rebates for 960,000 acupuncture treatments by registered medical practitioners. There has been a similar increase in the practice of other aspects of Chinese medicine, including herbal medicine, therapeutic massage, manipulation, dietary therapy and exercise therapy. Approximately A$1 billion are spent on CAM (Chinese medicine) each year (WHO, 1997; Bensoussan, 2000), and a 1996 study claims that 48.5% of the population has used at least one non-medically prescribed alternative medicine (Chinese medicine) (MacLennan, 1996). A study on the practice of Chinese medicine done by the Victorian Department of Human Services in 1995 found that Chinese medicine accounts for an increasing percentage of total health care services. There are at least 2.8 million consultations on Chinese medicine each year, representing an annual turnover of over A$84 million. In 1995, over 1500 primary practitioners reported their principal health occupation as Chinese medicine. There are 23 professional associations of Chinese medicine with a total of 2029 members, most of these associations were established after 1985.

In Australia, Chinese medicine treatment is provided to patients of all ages, including infants. Approximately 70% of patients are aged between 23 and 57 years old. Two out of three patients seeking treatment with Chinese medicine are female, 50% have a tertiary education, and over 80% have English as their first language. Approximately 40% are employed full-time and 39% are employed in the managerial or professional sectors. A wide range of illnesses are treated, with the profile of disorders varying significantly between medical practitioners and Chinese medicine practitioners. Fifty-eight per cent of all cases treated by medical practitioners are rheumatological or neurological in origin, in contrast to 40% of all cases for non-medical practitioners. Over 75% of patients are being treated for a recurrent complaint from at least the past three months. The regular fee for each acupuncture treatment in Australia is A$30. The average weekly cost of Chinese medicine treatment to the patient including any herbal medicine is A$98, with the full course of treatment amounting to approximately A$670. Private health insurance coverage for Chinese medicine treatment is used by one in three patients seeking Chinese medicine treatment. Substantial differences exist in the use of private health insurance between states. About 65% of Chinese medicine patients are first-time users of Chinese medicine. The majority (83%) are self-referred, i.e. by other patients, word of mouth, or in response to advertising; while 14% are referred by medical or other health practitioners. Seven out of ten patients have consulted another healthcare practitioner before starting Chinese medicine treatment, and in six of the seven, this is a medical practitioner. Thirty-five per cent of patients taking Chinese herbal medicines are taking them concurrently with one or more of a broad range of pharmaceutical drugs. There are 1500 Chinese medicine doctors and 3000 physicians who practice Chinese medicine. Fifty-five per cent used acupuncture only, 3% use herbs only, and 28% use both acupuncture and herbal medicine. There is currently no direct regulation by governments of Chinese medicine practitioners in Australia. Regulation of Chinese medicine practitioners is handed by the State governments, not the Federal government (MacLennan, 1996).

In 1995, the University of Western Sydney (Macarthur) and Southern Cross University won the tender to conduct a research project. Departments of Health in New South Wales and Queensland agreed to fund the research jointly with Victoria, resulting in a total research grant of A$125,000 (A$80,000 from Victoria, A$40,000 from New South Wales and A$5000 from Queensland). The resulting research report, "Towards a Safer Choice: The Practice of Traditional Chinese Medicine in Australia", was launched by the Victorian Minister for Health in November 1996. It is also available on the Internet at: http://www.dhs.vic.gov.au/phd/hce/chinese/report/contents.html

Royal Melbourne Institute of Technology (RMIT) has tested the effect of Chinese medicine (acupuncture and Chinese herbal medicine) for management of seasonal allergic rhinitis (commonly known as hey fever). They were awarded several research grants totaling A$325,000 for studies into Chinese herbal medicine (https://www.rmit.edu.au). The first grant is a joint project with Hong Kong Baptist University funded by Xinghuo Herbal Pharmaceutical Company with a total of A$130,000 to conduct research into the pharmacological actions of herbs used in Chinese medicine for the treatment of dry eye syndrome. This research may lead to the development of new products for its management. Another NHMRC research grant has allotted A$260,000 to study the mechanisms involved in a new mode of neurotransmission, which plays an important role in the regulation of functions of various systems in the body, and the effect of Chinese medicine on this new mode of neurotransmission.

The number of Chinese medicine programmes offered by universities and private colleges is growing. These programmes, some of which lead to diplomas, range from 50 hours to over 300 hours of contact time. There are also Chinese medicine programmes available for qualified medical doctors. These range from 50 to 250 hours. The Royal Melbourne Institute of Technology, the University of Technology at Sydney, and the Victoria University of Technology have degree programmes in Chinese medicine. With growing acceptance of acupuncture by the public and by conventional doctors, graduates are able to play a larger part in the public health sector of the community, working in hospitals, community health centres, and in areas of specialised health services.

10.4 Singapore

Chinese medicine has been widely practiced in Singapore for centuries, where three-quarters of the 3.6 million population are ethnic Chinese. Although Western medicine is the main form of healthcare in Singapore, Chinese medicine continues to enjoy considerable popularity. Chinese medicine practice in Singapore is confined to outpatient care. About 12% of daily outpatient attendance is estimated to be seen by Chinese medicine practitioners, the majority of whom are trained locally by Chinese medicine schools (WHO, 1998). A report by the Committee on Traditional Chinese Medicine, Singapore Ministry of Health in October 1995 said about 45% of the population have consulted traditional medicine (mainly traditional Chinese medicine) providers (Singapore Ministry of Health, 1995). About 10,000 persons visit Chinese medicine clinics each day, compared to 74,000 persons who visit conventional medicine clinics. Chinese medicine is the most prominent traditional therapy in Singapore. A list published by the local Chinese medicine community in 1997 reported 1807 practitioners of Chinese medicine in Singapore. Half of them practiced Chinese medicine on a full-time basis, one-third practiced part-time, and the others were not practicing at the time of the listing (Chea, 1995; WHO, 2001). Chinese medicine is restricted to outpatient services in Singapore. The health authorities recognise the importance of traditional Chinese medicine in the provision of health care and have initiated efforts to promote and ensure the safe practice of traditional Chinese medicine. The Ministry of Health established a traditional Chinese medicine unit in November 1995. The Traditional Chinese Medicine Practitioners Act of 2000 was passed by Parliament on 14 November 2000. The Act requires Chinese medicine practitioners who practice the prescribed practice of Chinese medicine to be registered and issued with a license to practice. The Traditional Chinese Medicine Practitioner Board was established as the licensing body to approve or reject applications for registration and to accredit courses in the practice of Chinese medicine, among other things. This accreditation is intended to facilitate registration. The Register of Traditional Chinese Medicine Practitioners shall be kept by the Registrar appointed by the Board. A registered practitioner who desires to obtain a certificate to practice must apply to the Board. Unlawful engagement in prescribed practices of traditional Chinese medicine is punished by a fine, imprisonment, or both. Currently, there are 1388 registered acupuncturists available for search on the net by the Traditional Chinese Medicine Practitioner Board (http://web9.internet.gov.sg/moh/owa/chinese.main).

10.5 Japan

Chinese medicine in Japan is called Kampo medicine. Kampo medicine is widely practiced in Japan, and is fully integrated into the modern health care system. Kampo is based on traditional Chinese medicine but adapted to Japanese culture. Kampo literally means the Han Method, referring to the herbal system of China that developed during the Han Dynasty. Although Kampo encompasses acupuncture, moxibustion and other components of the Chinese medical system, it relies primarily on prescription of herb formulas.

A factor that has strongly influenced the practice of Kampo medicine was the formal recognition by the Japanese Ministry of Health of certain traditional Chinese herb formulas as suitable for coverage by national health insurance. These formulas are prepared in factories under strict conditions. In 1967, four Kampo remedies were approved for reimbursement under Japan's national health insurance. In 1976, the Japanese government gave official approval to 82 prescriptions of the Kampo system; these could be purchased under the National Health Insurance System and were available as over-the-counter remedies. In addition, the Department of Pharmaceutical Affairs of the Ministry of Health and Welfare approved 210 herbal formulas for use in medical facilities, where they were also available over-the-counter. These formulas were adopted as medicines without having to go through the lengthy registration process that was required for modern drugs. Today, 148 prescriptions are covered by the national health insurance and more than half of them are the focus of modern Kampo practice.

Kampo medicine spread rapidly during the period 1985–1995; after that, the number of practitioners stabilised at a nearly constant level. By 1985, it was reported that about 20–25% of the medical doctors in Japan were including some herb prescribing in their practice. The proportion of doctors that provide some Kampo medicines has risen to about 50% or more by some estimates, with a proportional increase in Kampo specialists. In addition, there are about 10,000 pharmacies in Japan that dispense herb formulas. About 2% of total drug expenditures in Japan are herbal medicines, the largest part of them provided by Tsumora Juntendo, with contributions from about 20 smaller manufacturers. Kampo medicine research is conducted at the Toyama Medical and Pharmaceutical University in Toyama, the Kitazato Institute in Tokyo, and the Kinki University Medical Teaching Hospital near Osaka, as well as at other sites. Surveys conducted in Japan have revealed that the main uses of Kampo medicines are treatment of hepatitis, menopausal syndrome, common cold and other upper respiratory tract infections, autonomic nervous dysfunctions, constipation, cough and asthma, skin diseases (mainly eczema and other categories of dermatitis), lumbago and neuralgia, and gastro-intestinal disturbances. The top list of Kampo medicine used in Japan are from Shanghanlun: Xiaocaihutang, Gegentang, Xiaoqinglongtang, Jiaweixiaoyaosan, Dangguishaoyaosan, Guizhihulingwan, Dacaihutang, Shenqiwan, Buzhongyuqitang, Caihuguizhitang and Maimendongtang.

In the early 1980s, there were about 6000 physicians practicing acupuncture. Current estimates are over 60,000 national licensed medical doctors using acupuncture, moxibustion, massage and herbal medicine. There are about 15,000 Chinese medicine practitioners, 30,000 researchers and ten Kampo medicine research institutes. Over 20 universities have established Kampo medicine research centres; 40,000 Kampo pharmacies sell 20,000 kinds of products. A survey in 1991 showed that over 65% of Japanese believe Kampo medicine to be effective for chronic conditions, and 65.6% believe it is effective for anti-ageing. In Tokyo, 29% of population has used acupuncture, 73% will consider Kampo medicine when they are diseased, and 69% of physicians used Kampo medicine in their practice.

10.6 Canada

The transmission of Chinese medicine into Canada started in the late 19th century, but it was not until the 1990s that Chinese medicine caused great interest and became popular in Canada. Between 15% and 70% of the Canadian population had used CAM (mainly Chinese medicine) in the proceeding six to 12 months. According to Health Canada 2001 report, 70% of Canadians had used one or more natural health products in the proceeding six months, but only 24% consulted one or more CAM practitioners (WHO, 1996; Millar, 1997). A significant proportion of Canadians reportedly spent Can$30 or more per month on CAM services or natural health products. From 1996 to 1997, a total of Can$3.8 billion was spent on CAM health care in Canada. The *Canadian Journal of Public Health* reported that the use of CAM health care in Canada is more frequent among the young age group, women, people with higher formal education and higher incomes, and in West Canada, users of CAM have better health habits and better overall health. Users of CAM make fewer visits than non-users to both conventional general practitioners and specialists (WHO, 1996). The most common reasons for which patients consult CAM practitioners are problems of the musculo-skeletal system and connective tissue. These complaints account for 56% of consultations. Other problems include respiratory diseases, injuries, poisonings, ill-defined conditions and special investigations.

Health Canada, through the Therapeutic Products Program, is actively pursuing the National Initiative on Traditional Chinese Medicine. British Columbia, Alberta and Quebec include acupuncture among their regulated health professions. The Ministry of Health in British Columbia has agreed that traditional Chinese medicine and acupuncture should be regulated. In April 1998, the British Columbia Health Professions Council recommended designating "the profession of traditional Chinese medicine as a health profession under the Health Profession Act". The Health Disciplines Act of 1980 set out a framework for the recognition and regulation of health disciplines in Alberta. Acupuncture is governed by the accompanying Acupuncture Regulation. In order to be registered as a member of the acupuncture health profession, an applicant, who need not be an physician, must complete both an approved programme of study and an examination. Under the Section 44 of the Medical Act of Quebec, no person can claim to be an acupuncturist unless he or she is a registered non-physician or physician who has undergone the required training in acupuncture (Blais *et al.*, 1997).

10.7 France

Chinese medicine was brought to France by businessmen and travellers in the 17th century. It is the main component of CAM in France, which is very popular in France. The most commonly used CAM in France are homeopathy, acupuncture and herbal medicine. A 1987 survey found that 36% of medical doctors, mostly general practitioners, used at least one form of CAM in their medical practices. Among the medical doctors using CAM, 5.4% used it exclusively, 20.7% used it often and 72.8% used it occasionally. An additional 50,000 non-MD practitioners provide complementary/alternative therapy in France (Maddalena, 1999). In 1993, there were 2600 Chinese medicine clinics in France, providing acupuncture and Chinese herbal medicine. The first Chinese medicine hospital in France was established in 1996 in Paris, supported by the Chinese and French governments, as well as the World Health Organization. One survey found 49% of the people questioned — 53% of the women surveyed and 44% of the men — had used CAM at least once during the previous year. CAM is most popular among people between the ages of 35 and 45. Fifty-nine per cent of persons in this age group have reported using CAM. Sixty-eight per cent of exclusives and academics had used CAM, compared to 60% of middle managers and intermediate professionals and 40% of farmers, the least likely group to use CAM for minor diseases (49%), chronic symptoms (54%), serious illness (3%), and the prevention of disease and promotion of a healthy lifestyle (17%).

Seventy per cent of patients of CAM consider it effective for minor diseases, 65% for chronic diseases, and 9% for serious illness. Only 11% of patients considered these therapies ineffective for minor diseases, 15% for chronic diseases, and 38% for serious illness. In France, social security and private insurance reimburse some forms of CAM as long as a medical doctor provides them (Maddalena, 1999).

10.8 Germany

CAM is very popular in Germany. In 1994, there were between 10,000 and 13,000 practitioners of CAM, 8000 of whom were members of professional associations. The increased use of CAM is also reflected in increased interest from medical doctors who integrate CAM into their daily practice. Three-fourths of medical physicians use CAM and 77% of pain clinics provide acupuncture treatments (Maddalena, 1999). In 1992, the Federal German Ministry of Research and Technology initiated an extensive research programme on complementary medicine coordinated by the University of Hedecke. There were 20 million patients who visited practitioners of CAM in 1992. The most frequently sought complementary/alternative therapies include homeopathy and Chinese medicine including acupuncture, herbal medicine and massage. Between 20% to 30% of the population had used CAM, with 5% to 12% having used it during the previous year. Complementary/alternative therapies are more popular with women than men. Most CAM users are between the ages of 18 and 65, and have a relatively high level of education. In most cases, patients have first sought treatment with conventional medicine (Maddalena, 1999).

In Germany, public and private insurance provides the same kind of coverage. Both currently reimburse some complementary/alternative treatments and are moving towards broadening this coverage, even though there is no constitutional right to obtain reimbursement. In the 27 clinics of the medical universities, 19 of them offer acupuncture therapy, which is reimbursed by the insurance company. There are over 40 CAM societies in Germany, the four main societies have over 8000 members totally. They all use acupuncture and herbal medicine in their daily practice. The most successful case of Chinese medicine development in Germany is Koetzting Chinese Medicine Hospital. It was established on 18 March 1993 by a private German founder and Dongzhimen Hospital of Beijing University of Traditional Chinese Medicine. It is the first and only Chinese medicine hospital in Germany. It has 80 beds and 18 Chinese medicine doctors who provide healthcare, education and research services. All the treatments are reimbursed by insurance companies. It provides Chinese herbal medicine, acupuncture, massage and Qigong therapies. According to its president, Dr. Jiazhen Liao, "Normally, a patient needs to wait at least six months to be hospitalise".

10.9 The United Kingdom

Chinese medicine began to emerge in the U.K. in the 1960s. At that time, a group of doctors went to Beijing, Shanghai and Guangzhou to learn basic techniques of acupuncture. They opened Chinese medicine clinics and schools in the early 1970s. British Acupuncture Association and Regulation (BaaAR) was established as a national organisation in the 1980s. British doctors went to Beijing, Shanghai, Nanjing and Guangzhou to learn Chinese medicine, including acupuncture and herbal medicine in the 1990s. Another council, British Acupuncture Council (Bacc) was established in 1990, with about 3000 members. During this time, more experienced and well-educated Chinese immigrated to the U.K. They practiced both Chinese herbal medicine and acupuncture, and extended the range of Chinese medicine usage. A good example is Dr. Dinghui Luo, who came from Guangdong Provincial Chinese Medicine Hospital of China. Dr. Luo set up her clinic near Chinatown in London and used Chinese herbal medicine to treat eczema. Eczema is a very common skin disease in London; Western medicine cannot do much other than to temporarily soothe the irritation with balms, or to resort to cortisone, a powerful but hazardous anti-inflammatory cream. Atopic eczema often affects young children and parents are naturally concerned about the treatments. Many of the patients Dr. Luo was seeing had tried and had been disappointed by many other therapies. These therapies included allergy treatments, prescriptions for balm and ointments, diets and various other alternative remedies. While all else was failing, Dr. Luo was getting remarkable results. Gradually, as many of her patients reported back to their dermatologists, Dr. Luo could not be ignored anymore. On 26 April 1993, British Broadcasting Corporation (BBC) reported the successful story of Dr. Luo, and his research papers were published in the *Lancet* and *Journal of Dermatosis*. Chinese medicine started to get a good reputation in London and all over the U.K.

Currently, no license is required for Chinese practitioners in the U.K., as its practice is allowed by common law. There is no clear estimate of the total number of Chinese medicine practitioners. Before 1980, only a small number of Chinese medicine doctors practiced in London's Chinatown. Most of them came from Hong Kong or Taiwan, and their patients are mainly Chinese. Since 1980 (especially 1990s), more and more Chinese doctors came to the U.K. from China. Most of them are trained in Chinese medicine colleges and have practiced in Chinese hospitals for years. This group of well-trained Chinese medicine doctors treated a large number of different conditions and showed the U.K. the numerous benefits of Chinese medicine, opening a new era of Chinese medicine in the U.K. In London alone, there are hundreds of Chinese medicine clinics, and it is estimated that there are 3000 Chinese medicine clinics in the U.K. The British government allows Chinese medicine clinics to hire Chinese medicine practitioners from China, which also promoted the development of Chinese medicine.

A new survey published in *Complementary Therapies in Medicine* has documented the use of CAM in the U.K. (Ernst and White, 2000). The survey, one of the first of its kind to track CAM use in the U.K., found that one-fifth of all adults had tried alternative care in the previous year, with herbal medicine and acupuncture ranking among the most popular therapies being used.

The survey was conducted by the BBC in conjunction with ICAM Research, a market research organisation based in London. A total of 1204 British adults aged 18 and older were contacted randomly by telephone and asked to answer the following five questions:

(1) Have you (or any members of your household) used any alternative or complementary medicines or therapies within the last year, at least once?
(2) What, specifically, do you or have you used or done?
(3) Would you say you are using alternative or complementary medicines and therapies more or less than five years ago?
(4) What is the main reason why you use alternative or complementary medicines or therapies?
(5) Can you estimate how much you spend a month on alternative or complementary medicines or therapies?

Responses to the questions were analysed according to gender, social class, working status, tenure of residence, number of children and geographic region. Percentages were then adjusted to give a more representative profile of the population in the U.K.

Of the 1204 interviewees, 254 (20%) reported using CAM within the preceding year. Herbal medicine was the most commonly used therapy (34%), followed by aromatherapy (21%) and homeopathy (17%). Acupuncture and acupressure ranked fourth, with 14% of adults having used it in the past year.

Overall use of complementary therapies was higher among females (24%) than males (17%), with the greatest percentage of CAM use occurring among people between the ages of 35–64 (26%).

A vast majority of participants (78%) believed that CAM use was increasing. Six per cent thought it had decreased over the last five years; eight per cent perceived no change.

When asked why they used complementary therapies, most respondents cited the perceived effectiveness of CAM, the user's liking it, and the therapy's "relaxing effects". Interestingly, 11% of the respondents said they used complementary therapies because their doctor had either recommended it or referred them to an alternative health practitioner.

Participants were also asked to estimate the amount of money they spent each month on complementary therapies. According to the survey, the average user spent £13.62 (approximately US$20.36) on CAM per month, with those between the ages of 18–24 spending the most (£18.61/US$27.81). Allowing for inaccuracies, those figures were extrapolated to an annual expenditure on CAM of £1.6 billion in the U.K., an amount deemed "considerable" by the reviewers of the survey.

References

Astin, J.A. (1998) Why patients use alternative medicine: results of a national study. *J. Am. Med. Assoc.* **279**, 1548–1553.

Bensoussan, A. (2000) Risks associated with the practice of traditional Chinese medicine. *Arch. Fam. Med.* **9**, 1071–1078.

Blais, R.B., Maiga, A. and Aboubacar, A. (1997) How different are users and non-users of alternative medicine? *Can. J. Public Health* **88**, 169–176.

Chea, C.H.A. (1995) *The Development of Policy on Traditional Medicine in Singapore.* Presented at the Workshop on Development of National Policy on Traditional Medicine, Beijing, China, 11–15 October.

Eisenberg, D.M., Kessler, R.C., Foster, C., *et al.* (1993) Unconventional medicine in the United States: prevalence, costs, and patterns of use. *New Engl. J. Med.* **328**, 246–252.

Eisenberg, D.M. (2003) *Complementary and Integrative Medicine — Current Status and Future.* CAM Continuing Education Course, Harvard Medical School.

Eisenberg, D.M., Davis, R.B., Ettner, S.L., Appel, S., *et al.* (1998) Trends in alternative medicine use in the United States. *J. Am. Med. Assoc.* **280**, 1569–1675.

Ernst, E. and White, A. (2000) The BBC survey of complementary medicine use in the U.K. *Complement. Ther. Med.* **8**, 32–36.

Krauss, H.H., Godfrey, C., Kirk, J. and Eisenberg, D.M. (1998) Alternative health care: its use by individuals with physical disabilities. *Arch. Phys. Med. Rehabil.* **79**(11), 1440–1447.

Lerner, I.J. and Kennedy, B.J. (1992) The prevalence of questionable methods of cancer treatment in the United States. *Cancer J. Clin.* **42**(3), 181–191.

MacLennan, A., Wilson, D. and Taylor, A. (1996) Prevalence and cost of alternative medicine in Australia. *Lancet* **347**, 569–572.

Maddalena, S. (1999) *The Legal Status of Complementary Medicine in Europe — A Comparative Analysis.* Bern, Stampfli.

Millar, W.J. (1997) Use of alternative health care practitioners by Canadians. *Can. J. Public Health* **88**, 154–158.

Morris, K.T., Johnson, N., Homer, L. and Walts, D. (2000) A comparison of complementary therapy use between breast cancer patients and patients with other primary tumor sites. *Am. J. Surg.* **179**(5), 407–411.

NIH (2003a) *National Center for Complementary/Alternative Medicine — Newsletter.*

NIH (2003b) *Research Centers Program*, National Center for Complementary/ Alternative Medicine.

NIH (1997) *NIH Consensus Statement: Acupuncture*, Vol. 15(5), 3–5 November. Office of the Director.

Reston, J. (1971) Now, let me tell you about my appendectomy in Peking. *NY Times*, 26 July.

Richardson, M.A., Sanders, T., Palmer, J.L., Greisinger, A., *et al.* (2000) Complementary/Alternative medicine use in a comprehensive cancer center and the implications for oncology. *J. Clin. Oncol.* **18**(13), 2501–2504.

Singapore Ministry of Health (1995) *Traditional Chinese Medicine: A Report by the Committee of Traditional Chinese Medicine.*

Sparber, A., Bauer, L., Curt, G., Eisenberg, D., *et al.* (2000) Use of complementary medicine by adult patients participating in cancer clinical trials. *Oncol. Nurs. Forum* **27**(4), 623–630.

University of Technology (1994) *Acupuncture College Handbook.* Sydney, Australia.

WHO (2001) *Legal Status of Traditional Chinese Medicine and Complementary/ Alternative Medicine: A World Review.*

WHO (1998) *Technical Briefing on Traditional Medicine.* Presented at the 49th Regional Committee Meeting, Manila, Philippines. WHO Regional Office for Western Pacific, 18 September.

WHO (1997) *Memorandum on the Draft Process Report by the Director-General to the 51st World Health Assembly on TRM.* Manila, Traditional Medicine, WHO Western Pacific Regional Office, 20 March 1997.

WHO (1996) The work of WHO in the Western Pacific Region. Proposed program budget 1995–1996. In: *Diagnostic, Therapeutic and Rehabilitative Technology.* WHO Western Pacific Regional Office, Manila.

WHO Complementary/Alternative Medicine Facts and Figures (2002) WHO, Geneva.

WHO Traditional Medicine Strategy for 2002–2005 (2002) WHO, Geneva.

Zhang, Q. (2001) The education of traditional Chinese medicine and license examination in USA. *Chin. J. Integ. Tradit. West. Med.* **21**, 862–864.

Zhang, Q. (2000) Twelve national centers for CAM in USA. *Chin. J. Integr. Tradit. West. Med.* **20**, 710–711.

Chapter 11

Clinical Trials Using Chinese Medicine

Ping-Chung Leung

11.1 Introduction

Chinese medicine relies on a philosophy that guides the practitioner to serve his patient according to the special need at a special time and circumstance. It is an extremely individualised, personal and flexible, person to person, expert to client relationship, so much so that the details would need to change, not only according to the symptom changes of the patient, but also in relation to the season, the climate, the time of the day and any other environmental factor possibly affecting the recipient of service.

Such practice is very much unfavourable to scientific research which, whether clinical or non-clinical, aims at revealing the general truth. If there were only individual cases and no generalization, there would not be general truth. Scientific research aims at the discovery of the laws of Nature. Chinese medicine individualises its treatment plan and practice and refukes any general law (Bensky and Gamble, 1993).

Chinese medicine practitioners therefore do not have the tradition of research. Experience of the respectable practitioners and the process of application of the experiences are considered most important. The patient trusts the practitioner and relies on his experience. He is not so much concerned whether some general law has been worked out through the same expert.

Given such tradition for Chinese medicine, there is really no need for clinical research.

The need comes only when scientists start asking: it is good to realise that Chinese medicine works for this condition, but does it work all the time? If it does, how does it achieve such uniformity? If it does not, when does it work and when does it not? Modern practitioners make use of Chinese medicine as an alternative to their conventional treatment or to supplement their routines. Naturally, they ask the same questions, and they demand clinical trials (Tang and Eisenberg, 1992).

11.2 Fundamental Considerations

Generally speaking, the successes of modern medicine is well known in most areas. It is therefore necessary to look to complementary medicine only in those areas that the scientific mainstream finds deficiencies.

11.2.1 *Where are the deficiencies?*

The deficient areas lie where modern medicine, in spite of the recent advances, have failed to obtain good solutions.

Modern medicine has developed from the logic of modern science which follows the empirical approach. The problem is first thoroughly understood by identifying the cause. The cause could then be removed by working out an effective means. In the situation of a disease when the cause is simple and straightforward, removing it would be easy. On the other hand, when the cause is either complicated, not well understood or multiple, removal becomes difficult or impossible. Simple disease-inducing causes include straightforward infections, and simple physiological deficiencies. The former is easily tackled with an efficient antibiotic while the latter could be treated with some replacement.

When the causative agent is not yet thoroughly known, e.g. viral infections, treatment becomes difficult. When the cause is complicated, e.g. in allergic conditions, treatment does not guarantee effective results.

When the cause is complicated, e.g. involving many factors like physiological, social and psychological, modern scientific medicine becomes obviously deficient or incapable (Leung, 2001).

Therefore, the deficient areas in modern medicine that deserve contributions from complementary medicine include:

- Allergic conditions
- Autoimmune diseases

- Cancers
- Chronic pain
- Chronic derangements
- Degenerative diseases
- Nerve damages
- Viral infections
- Other areas that modern conventional therapy fails.

11.2.2 *How does herbal medicine really work?*

Traditionally the system of herbal medicine was built on the rich experience of herb users or herbalists, accumulated for over more than 2000 years in China since the birth of Chinese culture. For some reason, even as basic medical science, viz. anatomy and physiology, gradually developed in European territories around the Renaissance period, Chinese healers never felt the need to explore the subject. Without sound knowledge of anatomy and physiology, i.e. biological structure and function of the human body, it would not be possible to investigate on abnormal structures and functions such as pathology. Without understanding the pathology, it would not be possible to apply a direct means of removing the pathology. Herbal practitioners therefore, try to heal, not by direct confrontation with the pathological problem, but by indirectly supporting the individual to overcome his own difficulties (Su, 1992; McGuire, 1988).

11.2.3 *How does the individual overcome its own pathological problems?*

Firstly, by surviving the harmful disturbances imposed by the pathological processes. Secondly, by supporting the unaffected organs and systems on their proper functions, and thirdly by preventing future pathological mishappenings while the current problem is being solved.

The herbal practitioner has means to suppress the symptoms which are manifestations of the pathology. Suppression of symptoms like cough, diarrhea or dyspnoea, helps the sick individual to survive.

While waiting for the pathological damages to heal naturally, the unaffected organs and systems need to be supported to maintain their efficient function which in turn will support the overall function and metabolic harmony of the living individual.

Prevention in the modern biological sense, frequently refers to an immunological mechanism through which the individual becomes more resistant to future attacks of similar pathological nature (Kaptchuk and Eisenberg, 1998).

The main focus of disease management for Chinese medicine is often the control of adverse symptoms. The ultimate goal is maintaining the well-being of the biological system. The aetiological consideration is therefore not directed towards the actual cause of the disease (which the herbal expert has no idea) but a general conceptual state of the biological balance of the human bodily functions. The ancient healers correlated this conceptual state with the Taoist philosophy and imagined that bodily function was kept at a balanced state between Yin and Yang (i.e. negative and positive). Any loss of balance led to ailment and disease.

The aim of treatment is therefore to maintain the balance. Yin and Yang includes other contrasting opposing forces like cool and heat, superficial and deep, emptiness and solid. The causes of imbalance could be traced to a lack of balance of any pair of opposing forces. In the actual treatment, therefore, all efforts are spent on the maintenance of balance, by a supplement of the deficient force, or a decrement of the excessive.

Since the pathological causes of the symptomatology is unclear to the herbal expert, he would need to observe the changes of symptoms and adjust his day to day protocol accordingly. This approach differs very much from the conventional modern medicine which successfully identifies a pathological cause of disease, choose a method of cure with good chance of success, then administers it with all efforts and persists on the commitment, until the total removal of the pathology is achieved.

While the aetiology, epidemiology and natural course of a disease affect the design of clinical trials for modern medicine, it is now clear that in Chinese medicine, there is little analogy of aetiological and epidemiological considerations. The course of events in a disease, for a herbal expert, is the appearance of the symptoms: the loss of biological well-being due to the lack of balance between the vital forces. The aim of treatment is the re-establishment of balance; once balance is re-established, either naturally or through herbal intervention, well-being will be re-established. Treatment consists of a dynamic application of symptomatic relief with the goal of re-establishing the balance (Ng, 1986).

Therefore, clinical trials for Chinese medicine or herbal medicine could follow the line of thought for scientific planning on data collection and subsequent data meta-analysis, however the pre-treatment data would be mainly confined to symptomatology. Other parameters would carry little weight for the herbal expert but could still be included for more scientific knowledge and for more proper assessment of the effects of treatment (Lai, 2001a).

11.3 General Considerations for Clinical Trials on Chinese Medicine

In the modern scientific world, only up-to-date methodology should be adopted. The set of common methodology for conducting clinical trials on modern medicine has been logical, useful and has made wonderful contributions on the clinical testing of new drugs and new methods of clinical treatment. The proper analysis of data and the use of statistics have shown the reliability of certain accumulated experience, while at the same time reveal the fallacies of some well accepted and widely practiced methods (Chalmers, 1993).

The common methodology of random selection, blinding and placebo control, followed by statistical analysis, should be adopted. In the design of the trial, good clinical practice should be the objective. However, because of the nature of the herbs, which come from different origins and carry different species, it is not uncommon that the basic principles could not be strictly kept adhered to (Lai, 2001b).

Good clinical practice insists that the prescribed drug for the clinical trial is thoroughly understood and uniform. However, using herbal preparations for clinical trials faces the difficulties of thorough technical knowledge and uniformity.

Pharmaceutical tests demand that details be known about the chemistry, the mode of action and metabolic pathways before clinical tests are conducted. How is the chemistry of herbs like? What are the pathways of action and metabolic degradation? Are there adverse effects in the process of metabolism? A lot of work has been done in the past 50 years on these basic concepts without much success. Each and every herb contains so much complicated chemistry that even extensive research might not provide the answers. At least 400 herbs are popular and possess records of action and impressive efficacy. Obtaining thorough knowledge on just this proportion of herbs is not practical, not to mention the less commonly used 1000–2000 varieties (Kong, 1998).

Uniformity is another difficult area. Strictly speaking, since herbs are agricultural products, uniformity should begin at the site of production. These sites have different weather, different soil content and different methods of plantation. At the moment, about 50% of popular Chinese herbs are produced in special farms in China. However, these farms are scattered over different provinces, which have widely different climatic and soil environments. Good agricultural practice demands that environmental and nurturing procedures are consistent. Procedures include soil care, watering, fertilizer use, pest prevention and harvesting. When such procedures are not uniform and no efforts are taken to ensure a common practice, good agricultural practice is not possible.

Not only is there lack of uniformity in the mode of herb production, but different species of the same herb are found or planted in different regions and provinces. These different species may have different chemical composition. Herbal experts have extensive experience and knowledge about some special correlations between the effectiveness of particular herbs and their sites of production. Some commonly used herbs are even labelled jointly with the best sites of production. With the development of molecular biology, coupled with modern means of assessment for active ingredients within a chemical product, species-specific criteria could be identified, using the "finger-printing" technique. Uniformity today should include screening using "finger-printing" techniques (Fair, 1999).

When we consider the other 50% of herbs that are only available in the wild, i.e. around mountains, highlands or swamps, and cannot be grown from agricultural farms, the insistence on product uniformity becomes even more difficult.

Based on what we have discussed, insistence on good clinical practice in clinical trials for herbal medicine is largely impossible. Thus, a compromise must be reached.

Indeed in the past 50 years, many attempts have been made on the proper analytical study of herbal preparations. The objectives were:

extract the herb, analyse its components, then try to work out the chemical formulae which could be responsible for its clinical effects.

Extraction helps to separate the useless components from the effective ones, which not only cuts down the volume of herbs used but also intensifies the biological actions. Knowing the actual effective ingredients and working out the chemical formulae would be ideal for modernisation of herbal preparations with the aim of converting the preparations into proper pharmaceuticals.

In spite of the time and effort put into herbal extractions and chemical analyses in the past 50 years, successful examples had not been impressive. The results certainly do not warrant the amount of resources needed (Leung, 2001).

The unsatisfactory outcome has initiated a new approach. Instead of following the scientific pathway previously taken by pharmaceuticals (which is lined with too many obstacles), a more practical line has been endorsed. Since most, if not all, herbs have been used for hundreds of years, they should be more or less reliable. The safety and efficacy of the herbs are already well documented, but their practical utilisation in specific clinical circumstances needs to be further established. The traditional use of the herbs had been focused on symptomatic control. Nowadays, the aim of clinical management is directed towards curing of a disease entity. We need to acquire an updated understanding on the effectiveness of the herbal preparations on disease entities. That is why we should not be satisfied with records on efficacy alone but should start a series of clinical trials to further prove the efficacy of the herbs (Eisenberg *et al.*, 1993).

The National Institutes of Health of the United States have openly endorsed the approach of accepting traditional methods of healing as safe measures and also conducting proper clinical trials (NIH, 2001). The recognition of acupuncture as a practical effective means of pain control started in 1998 (NIH, 1997). The subsequent formation of a special section devoted to research on complementary/alternative treatment followed. The National Centre for Complementary and Alternative Medicine (NCCAM) was properly formed and given a substantially large budget.

Today, new Chinese medicine-related drugs in China are divided into five categories:

Group 1

- Synthetic materials from Chinese medicinal raw materials.
- Newly discovered Chinese medicinal raw materials and their semi-finished compounds.
- The active ingredients and their semi-finished components derived from Chinese medicinal raw materials.
- The active ingredients derived from a complex prescription.

Group 2

- Injections manufactured from Chinese medicinal raw materials.
- New medicinal applications and their semi-finished components from anatomical components of existing Chinese medicinal raw materials.
- The active components and its semi-finished components derived from existing Chinese medicinal raw materials and their derivatives.
- Medicinal products extracted from animals, and its semi-finished components obtained from artificial means.
- The active components cluster derived from complex prescriptions.

Group 3

- New semi-finished components from complex prescriptions.
- Semi-finished components from Chinese medicine and synthetic drugs based on the theory of Chinese medicine prepared from complex prescriptions.
- Commonly imported medicinal raw materials and their semi-finished components introduced from overseas.

Group 4

- Alteration of preparation and form of intake.
- Transplanted from overseas or domesticated animal and herbal medicine.

Group 5

- Newly-discovered demonstrate applications of existing drugs (Wang, 1995).

In China, regular steps are recommended for the research on Chinese medicine drugs. Four stages are recommended:

Phase I

Studies on the general acceptance of the human being after consumption of the herbal preparation.

Normally phase I refers to toxicity studies. The code of practice given under "Code of Practice for the Scrutiny of New Drugs" in China recommend that the general well-being of the individual after consumption be observed (Lai, 2001). The logic of skipping toxicity tests is probably based on an assumption that Chinese herbal preparations have been used safely for centuries, therefore screening is not necessary. However, the author has strong reservations on this attitude and would recommend that toxicity clearance remains as the first phase of clinical trials.

Phase II

Studies on the safety and efficacy while working out the effective dosage.

Phase III

Expand on Phase II studies, collecting more reliable data on the safety and efficacy of the herbal preparation.

Phase IV

Further studies on the safety and efficacy after the new drug is put on the market. More observations on adverse effects are expected.

One realises that the four phases follow closely the staged trials currently recommended for any pharmaceutical agent.

It has been pointed out that, as far as herbal medicine is concerned, it is not unusual to find that correlation does not exist between laboratory research and clinical trials. When studies on the pharmacology, pharmacodynamics and pharmacokinetics are carried out after the clinical trials, positive values in support of the clinical observations may not be impressive.

The possible explanation to this observation may lie in the fact that the clinical consumption of the herbal preparations involves multiple, complex *in vivo* biological interactions, whereas laboratory tests consist of only simple unidirectional biological interactions.

11.4 How Do Concepts of Traditional Healing Affect Clinical Trials on Chinese Medicine?

The application of modern concepts in the direction of clinical trials leads to the inevitable sacrifice of some of the fundamental principles. Experienced herbal experts may therefore have doubts about participating.

The following paragraphs list out the important concepts in Chinese medicine practice being sacrificed in the modern evidence-based clinical trials.

Symptom identification principle

Following this principle, the herbal expert adjusts details of his treatment according to observations on the day-by-day changes of symptomatology. He may then use different drugs for the same symptoms or use the same drug for different symptoms. Proper clinical trials can only use a uniform choice of treatment modality. This violates the symptom identification principle.

Holistic approach

Chinese medicine emphasises on holistic care and response, whereas clinical trials prefer objective, specific data as end-points.

The inclusion of specific data into herbal research probably does not invite objection from the herbal expert, as long as general data like different aspects of well-being (i.e. quality of life) are included.

Response to pathological processes

Chinese medicine emphasises on the responses of healthy organs to diseases. The ability of the healthy organs to respond to pathological changes ensures that the individual would be able to better resist adversities. Modern clinical trials aim mostly at diseased organs.

Old system of clinical observation

Herbal experts utilise a system of clinical observations which, today might be considered obsolete and over-subjective. This system of clinical signs include tongue observation, pulse detection and a collection of subjective feelings (Cheng, 1996). Modern clinical trials insist on objective data that can be monitored. We therefore have to either develop means to objectively assess the subjective signs in the tongue and the pulse or we sacrifice the whole system of observations. Herbal experts might not appreciate either choice.

Strong tradition

Herbal experts place genuine confidence on anecdotal observations and experience of individual patients. Insisting on the need to investigate collective observations and condemning single case experience would not be welcome by herbal experts. This conceptual difference directly affects the participation and cooperation of the traditional and modern experts.

While thoroughly recognising the unique nature of Chinese medicine and having pointed out the lack of harmony between the old tradition and modern science, one realises that the current compromise adopted is to insist on a modern scientific approach as far as possible. Hence, the following are advocated (Leung, 2001), as standard instructions for clinical trials:

- Use the principles of randomisation, blinding and repetition.
- Adopt good protocols for clinical trials.
- Avoid bias at all cost.
- Eliminate chance factors.
- Establish new standards of clinical assessment.
- Establish unique outcome studies.
- Establish unique quality of life assessments.
- Insist on using modern statistics.

11.4.1 *Adverse effects*

Historically, in the ancient days, the great herbal masters of China had produced records on adverse effects and toxic problems of some herbs. As early as during the Han dynasty (2nd century), documents on herbs that should only be used extreme caution were produced (Chang, 220). This tradition was followed closely in the subsequent centuries.

More reports on methods and means with which toxicities and adverse effects could be reduced (Suen *et al.*, 1998) were available. Despite the incriminating data obtained in the past, the prevalent belief is that Chinese medicinal herbs are safe. On the other hand, however, an increasing number of reports on adverse effects and toxicities, with slight exaggeration from the non-users, have appeared.

When new preparations come onto the market, the innovative processes of extraction and/or production may have produced or initiated new possibilities of adverse affects or toxicity. This experience is already well recorded in a number of modernised preparations, particularly those for injection (Lai, 2001). Among the adverse effects, allergic reactions are the most common.

To date, standard instructions on clinical trials for Chinese medicine define adverse drug reaction in exactly the same way as modern scientific clinical trials, and explanation to the reactions have been similarly identified (Lai, 2001).

Categories of adverse reactions include the following:

(1) *Reactions to herbs*

Reactions are defined as harmful and unexpected effects while the standard dosages are used in certain drug trials. It is specially pointed out that for Chinese medicine, the harmful reactions can be due to the quality of the herb and poor choice of indication. These reactions do not include allergic responses.

(2) *Dosage-related adverse effects*

Using an unnecessarily high dose can induce excessive effects, side effects or even toxic effects. Secondary effects like electrolyte imbalance may also be observed.

(3) *Dosage-unrelated adverse effects*

These adverse effects can be the result of unfavourable preparation, contaminants in the herbs, sensitivity of the consumer, allergic reactions or specific inductive effects of the herb.

(4) *Drug interactions*

Classically, records are available in old Chinese medicinal literature on combined effects of herbs, their facilitatory and antagonistic effects. Nowadays, not only drug interactions between herbs are important, but possible interactions between herbs and commonly used pharmaceutical preparations are becoming issues of great concern since users of herbal preparations are greatly increasing.

In the area of anaesthesia, drug interactions between herbs and modern medicine can induce life-threatening reactions. Special attention and studies are recommended.

(5) *Delayed adverse effects*
Adverse effects of delayed nature include induction to cancer formation, foetal abnormalities and even blockage of bacterial sensitivities.

(6) *Drug dependence*
There are suspicions that herbal preparations may lead to drug dependence. Apart from a few opium-related herbs, Chinese herbs, in fact are well known to be non-addictive because of their gross lack of specificities.

From the above account, it appears obvious that adverse effects in clinical trials using Chinese medicine in fact follow closely the experience encountered in other drug trials. As far as the grading of adverse effects is concerned, it would be appropriate to categorise the effects as mild, moderate and severe (De Smet and A'Arcy, 1996).

Whatever the situation, detection of adverse effects should include both clinical observations and laboratory data, and detection should be acompanied with follow-up observations. The summation of observations should be thoroughly analysed so that explanations to the adverse effects may be eventually worked out. All adverse effects should be properly recorded and stored up for proper reporting when required (Sackett, 1991; WHO, 2000).

11.4.2 *Quality of life*

While clinical trials aim at a thorough scientific understanding of the effectiveness of specific forms of treatment, end-points of measurement are set to give objective standards of evaluation. Primary end-points are unique, focused, specific criteria which indicate the situation of the target against which the trial is directed. Changes of primary end-points illustrate the efficacy directly. Secondary end-points are supplementary criteria created to support observations on changes and efficacy. Secondary end-points become more important when predictably, primary end-points do not give clear-cut, impressive results. Secondary end-points become more important when primary end-points are expected to change slowly and would be particularly important when chronic problems are being faced.

Since Chinese medicine, under most circumstances, does not operate via a direct, confrontation route but rather, acts indirectly to support the healthy organs and helps to maintain vitality and prevent functional deterioration, critical and detailed assessment of the secondary end-points are therefore of utmost importance.

Quality of life is an important aspect on the assessment of care given to the chronically ill. It often measures the competency of the care and the ethical standard of the society in mental disorders and other disorders that demonstrate strong social orientations. Not infrequently, using technical end-points as results of clinical trials, reasonable outcome is observed, and yet, patients may not be satisfied with their quality of life. It is therefore multifocal: differing between developed and under-developed areas, and also under different cultural circles (Jaeschke and Singer, 1989). Different countries and regions therefore try to develop their own data to be included within their own studies on quality of life (Wyrwick and Nienaber, 1999), while global, generally acceptable quality of life charts are also being planned, examined and validated.

Before an acceptable general data chart is ready, one has to accept the achievements already revealed in different fields. Generally speaking quality of life data sheets take in information about physiological well-being, psychological well-being, social well-being and the individuals' subjective feeling on the treatment received and the rehabilitation under-way. Different specialties and special areas of concern have created charts of their own and all these are valuable information when equivalent studies come up. Usually they are adopted right away or after validation. Hence, there are charts already developed for children and elderlies, and different medical specialties and sub-specialties likewise have created their own charts. Just to mention a few, special quality of life charts are available for the mentally ill, cardiovascular diseases, rheumatological disease respiratory problems, gynaecological problems, and special infections (Keinginger, 1999).

What are the recommendations for clinical trials of Chinese medicine?

The simple thing to do is to take reference to the available charts in whichever clinical trial is being conducted and think about possible improvements to make them even more suitable.

Are there unique features that need to be observed?

There are features related to health which are derived from the philosophy of Chinese medicine ever since its initial development. Chinese people from all walks of life are influenced by this philosophy without being aware of it at all stages of their life. The belief that health depends on a harmony between contrasting forces prompts the individual to feel either "hot or cold", "light" or "heavy", "sick inside" or "sick outside". After treatment, the feeling may remain, reverse or get balanced. Though the feeling is subjective, one cannot ignore the outcome of the philosophical influence affecting the whole system of healing in any clinical trial (including the data on quality of life).

Henceforth, it is obvious the quality of life studies are particularly important for clinical trials of Chinese medicine and research should be done on special inclusions of data which are unique fo Chinese medicine (Farquhar, 1994).

11.5 A Complex Trial of Chinese Medicine

What has been discussed could be further illustrated by reference to a complex trial of Chinese medicine, currently taking place in Hong Kong.

Trial: Use of a triple herb formula for the treatment of osteoporosis among the post-menopausal women

The design of the trial is to choose a difficult, unsolved medical problem and to try solving it with a promising Chinese herbal formula. Osteoporosis is chosen as the problem because it is common and, although factors affecting the problem are known and means to control it are available and being trialled, uncertainties are still plentiful. Uncertainties about the absolute indications for treatment, the choice of treatment modalities, the duration of treatment and the possible adverse effects.

Since osteoporosis affects all human beings towards ageing, preventive measures become important.

Osteoporosis has never been a documented symptom in conventional Chinese medicine reports, possibly because of two reasons: people in ancient days succumb before the development of osteoporosis and the mechanisms leading to the pathology and the pathology itself are unknown.

However, elderly people with back pain and progressive spinal deformities were described and correlated with "kidney deficiency", a common understanding in the Chinese medicine literature. Hence, many methods of dealing with "kidney deficiency" have been described and further treatment and prevention of this condition have been documented. When osteoporosis became known, preparations and formulae for "kidney deficiency" were tried and a satisfactory outcome was observed.

Assuming that herbal remedies carry little long-term adverse effects and that herbal choices can be indicated for preventive means, the trial "Use of a triple herb formula for the treatment of osteoporosis among postmenopausal women" was designed. The triple formula is created from a variety of herbs, all of which have shown promise in the treatment of "kidney deficiency", and some of which have been subjected to animal studies and demonstrated abilities to improve bone density.

We are therefore looking for a herbal solution to a yet unsolved problem, viz. osteoporosis. Once proven, there is potential for development of a safe and effective product for prevention of osteoporosis.

The trial needs to be complex as it is required to prove the formula's efficacy and subsequently develop the formula as a drug.

The procedures required include the following:

Literature search

Herbs documented to be useful for "kidney deficiency" are identified and a basic review of their mode of action, adversities and indications is carefully carried out. Toxic varieties are excluded. Reports on their clinical results are collected and analysed. Three supposedly most promising herbs are chosen. More details about their source of production and pharmacological properties are searched. Over the past decades, a large amount of herbs have been studied for their LD50 data, basic pharmacological nature, and their effects on different physiological functions.

Selecting three herbs from a wide range of different varieties requires extensive discussions with experienced herbalists and clinical scientists. The same group of experts are responsible for the relative proportion of the herbs to be used.

Design of study

A two-pronged approach is the standard direction. A properly designed evidence-based clinical trial aims to prove the efficacy of the herbal formula used. In parallel with the clinical trial, work is conducted in the laboratory under both *in vitro* and *in vivo* conditions, to investigate the effect of herbs on special cell growth in cultures and their direct and indirect influence on the bone metabolism of special animals.

(A) Clinical trial

A summary of a stage 2 clinical trial is included as follows:

(Title: A Randomized, Double-blind, Placebo-controlled Clinical Trial on the Effects of a Herbal Capsule in Post-menopausal Osteoporosis)

(1) Composition of the herbal formula:

Herba Epimedii
Fructus Ligustri Lucidi
Fructus Psoraleae

(2) Preparation of the medication

(i) Herb capsule: These contain herbal extracts and calcium (100 mg/capsule). The subjects will take six capsules a day for 12 months.

$$\text{(Herbal capsule} = 6 \times 365 \times 70 = 153{,}300)$$

(ii) Placebo capsule: These will be filled with starch only and coloured to the same colour as the herbal extract. Placebo capsule contains calcium 100 mg/capsule. Subjects in the placebo group will take six of these capsules a day for 12 months.

$$(\text{Placebo capsule} = 6 \times 365 \times 70 = 153{,}300)$$

(3) Subjects

One hundred and forty subjects will be randomised and divided into two groups (group herb and placebo, 70 subjects per group). These women will only be allowed to enter the study after signing an informed consent form approved by the Ethics Committee of the Chinese University of Hong Kong at the Prince of Wales Hospital.

(4) Inclusion criteria

(i) The subjects must be at least one year post-menopausal.
(ii) The subjects must be aged between 45 to 60 years old.
(iii) The lumber BMD (L1–L4) value must be lower than 0.891 g/cm^2, as reported by Hologic DEXA scanning.

(The peak value of bone mass of mean lumbar spine (L1–L4) BMD for Oriental females offered by the Hologic Co. manufacturer is 1.006 ±0.115; thus any BMD value below 0.891, i.e. the mean of peak value minus 1SD is indicative of osteopenia in Chinese post-menopausal women.)

(5) Exclusion criteria

(i) Subjects on active treatment for bone pathology including TCM medication.
(ii) Subjects with serious concomitant diseases (including liver and kidney dysfunctions and haematological disorders). Subjects with mild stable hypertension will not be excluded providing their medication does not change.
(iii) Subjects with psychiatric or addictive disorders.
(iv) Subjects who are pregnant or are nursing.
(v) Subjects who were previously consuming more than 500 mg calcium daily. Subjects consuming less may enter the study providing the dosage does not change during the study.

(6) Randomisation

This will be done by block randomisation for 30 subjects (15 per group) for five blocks. Once the study number has been assigned, the subject will attend the Clinical Trial Center at the Prince Wales Hospital, Chinese University of Hong Kong. At the Clinical Trial Center, the previously prepared randomisation envelope will be opened and the correct medication dispensed. Neither the study personnel (doctors and nurses) nor the subject will be informed of the medication group. If there are clinical or safety grounds for knowing the treatment of a particular subject, only the doctor in charge of the study may release the treatment category for that subject.

(7) End-points and data collection

(i) Bone density testing

The spine bone density (L1–L4) and global bone density will be determined once at baseline, four-, eight- and 12-month time points using a Hologic 4500 DEXA bone densitometer available at the Prince of Wales Hospital. Also, the upper and lower limb bone density will be determined by p-QCT. The bone densitometer will have a QC quality control standard measured before each patient measurement.

(ii) Questionnaire investigation

Baseline data collection will consist of a record of current medical problems and medication. In addition, a questionnaire for quality of life (SF-36) will be completed. A follow-up questionnaire will be completed at four, eight and 12 months. This will include the baseline questionnaires and an adverse event questionnaire.

(iii) Biochemical testing

Fasting resting blood and urine samples will be collected at baseline, four, eight and 12 months. The urine sample collected will be the second voided sample after consumption of four glasses of water. These samples will be analysed for the following:

Efficacy
- Urine deoxypyridinoline (Dpd)/creatinine (Cr) ratio
- Urine calcium (Ca) creatinine (Ce) ratio
- Serum carboxyterminal telopeptide of type 1 collagen (ICTP)
- Serum bone-specific alkaline phosphatase (ALP), osteocalcin (OC)
- Serum triglyceride (TG), cholesterol (CHO), high-density lipoprotein cholesterol (HDL), low-density lipoprotein cholesterol (LDL)
- Serum estrogen (E2), follicle-stimulating hormone (FSH)

Safety
- Full blood count
- Serum GPT (liver function test)
- Serum Cr (kidney function test)

(vi) Examination

A medical examination will be carried out at baseline. This will include blood pressure testing after the subject has been resting for ten minutes, and will be repeated at four-, eight- and 12-month time points.

The target population for the clinical trial is limited to women. This design has been accepted as a standard approach in many of the completed drug trials for osteoporosis. The results of our herbal formula, therefore offers better comparative value to the previous completed trials.

A second clinical trial targeted towards a much older group of patients who actually suffer from bone pain as a result of osteoporotic fractures is already underway. This is the group of our equal concern who requires attention and treatment, perhaps for a long period until life termination.

(B) Laboratory study

A summary of the laboratory study is given as follows:

(Title: Oral Dose-response Experiment of Herbal Extraction (YYH/BGZ) in OVX Aged Rats with Established Bone Loss)

(1) Purpose
In this study, we will compare the effect of high, middle and low dose of herbal extraction YYH/BGZ(YB) in OVX aged rats, and compare the difference between YB and raloxifene on bone and lipid metabolism.

(2) Animal groups (15 rats/group, total number of rats = 90)

(i) OVX (Ovariectomized and treated with vehicle)
(ii) OVX-L (OVX and treated with low dose YB)
(iii) OVX-M (OVX and treated with middle dose YB)
(iv) OVX-H (OVX and treated with high dose YB)
(v) OVX-R (OVX and treated with raloxifene)
(vi) Sham (Sham-OVX and treated with vehicle)

(3) Time course

(i) Week 1 → 8 (eight weeks):

- Rats will be fed with 15 g/day food containing 0.1% Ca and 0.3% P, and de-ionic water

(ii) Week 9 → 16 (eight weeks):

- OVX or sham operation will be conducted in six groups of rats
- Rats will be fed with 15 g/day food containing 0.1% Ca and 0.3% P, and de-ionic water

(iii) Week 17 → 28 (12 weeks):

- Rats will be treated with YB (three doses), raloxifene (one dose) or vehicle (de-ionic water)
- Rats will be fed with 15 g/day food containing 0.1% Ca and 0.3% P, and de-ionic water

(4) End-point

(i) Bone density (week 1 → 8 → 16 → 22 → 28)
DEXA
(ii) Blood sample (week 1 → 8 → 16 → 22 → 28)
Efficacy: serum bone-specific alkaline phosphatase (ALP), osteocalcin (OC), estrogen (E2), follicle-stimulating hormone (FSH), cholesterol (CHO), triglyceride (TG)

Safety: serum GPT, creatinine (Cr)

(iii) Bone samples (week 28)
Micro Ct, bone histomorphometry, biochemical test

(iv) Uterine, liver, kidney, brain, heart, lung, spleen sample (week 28)
Histopathological examination

(5) Triplo herb formula

In view of the absence of Good Agricultural Practice (GAP) and Good Manufacture Practice (GMP), one has to make basic assumptions on when the triplo formula was acquired.

It is assumed that what is available on the herb market is optimum best for the triplo formula. One way to guarantee the quality of the preparation is to calculate the amount of drugs required for both the clinical trial and laboratory work, so that one batch fulfills the overall requirements, to ensure uniformity of raw material.

Manufacture of convenient preparation is necessary to ensure simplicity of consumption and absorption. The innovative triplo formula created has not appeared on the market. Hence, the GMP has to be totally created and no practical procedures are available as reference. Once more, to maintain uniformity, a single batch of product is used. Sufficient extracts must be stored for the laboratory tests.

(6) Placebo

Herbal preparation placebo has always been a difficult challenge for clinical trials involving Chinese medicine. Difficulties lie in not only the colour, taste and appearance, but also the characteristic odour unique to special herbal items.

With experience, the common problems can be easily solved. Of the two forms of preparation, either raw powder mixture or decortion condensation, we prefer the latter as it may be more consistent with the classic decortion (unlike mixed powders which lack the brothing process). The condensation makes colour and texture matching easier. Taste is still a problem while odour can be partially overcome by keeping the finished product in an enclosed environment together with the placebo. Or alternatively, an odour-absorbing cotton wool spacer can be kept together with the strong-smelling component herbs, and later removed to accompany the placebo.

(5) Further studies
Unless the clinical trial shows negative results, otherwise further studies are indicated.

Optimisation of the formula

The early laboratory tests on the triplo formula and individual herbal actions should be able to guide the subsequent planning on the optimisation of the formula. Pharmocodynamic and pharmacokinetic studies on the formula and on the individual herbs (investigating their absorption, distribution, metabolism and excretion) will eventually mature into practical recommendations on variations of the original formulation.

Basically, the clinical trial is of a Phase 2 nature. With success of the early results demonstrated, larger scale trials with modification of the original formula can be started. This subsequent trial would be of Phase 3 nature.

Optimisation of the triplo formula is a logical outcome that will probably enhance the efficacy of the formula. Whether more research is justified depends on whether pharmaceutical companies find the project attractive, and hence are willing to invest in it. If such interest and investment are consolidated, one expects the chemical formula to make its appearance in the pharmaceutical industry (WHO, 2000).

11.6 Conclusion

Complementary medicine does not have its own history of scientific development. The knowledge was built on observations and experience. In order to integrate this unscientific stream of medicine into a scientific world, we must first explain why it works in the area of our concern. We choose those areas that are not well served by scientific medicine as our targets. This makes the scientific explanations even more important.

Providing scientific explanations to healing processes involves the application of methodologies that are well known and accepted by all clinical scientists. The standard way to start a scientific approach to clinical trials using traditional Chinese medicine is just an application of the same methodologies. However, this approach is not feasible if we are not willing to bend our principles. We are barred from a smooth application of the scientific methodology, basically because of the different philosophy behind the traditional Chinese way of healing. Moreover, the lack of knowledge about the exact chemistry of the active component of the herbal remedy when herbal drug trials are being done, further jeopardises the validity of the clinical trials carried out (Richardson, 2001).

Evidence-based medicine takes many forms. Following the practice of an experienced authority is evidence-based, as long as the authority is trustworthy and honoured and there is no better evidence available. In a scientific world, taking an authority's words alone is no longer acceptable support for one's behaviour and practice.

Depending on one's own experience, if well supported by authority, will form the next level of evidence. Such personal experience, though valuable, is limited to only case reports, short of more convincing value.

Grouping together a series of cases and observations will offer more objective data as long as the collaborators are not biased. Cohort studies of this nature are plentiful, including those involving Chinese medicine. We should treat them with respect. Nevertheless in today's clinical medicine, ways to control the frequently occurring biases are already available. That is why randomisation, double-blinding with placebo control are essentials for good clinical practice. No other methodology can substitute these requirements.

It is therefore good to know that in spite of the fundamental difficulties, efficacy-driven trials, utilising principles of evidence-based-medicine, are still carried out. As long as the scientific gap is successfully narrowed, the practical use of complementary medicine will become safer, more logical and will deserve wider applications. Lastly, those who consistently oppose alternative medicine should realise that even in our scientific mainstream practice, a large number of treatment protocols are still short of evidence-based (Nachemson, 1989).

References

Bensky, D. and Gamble, A. (1993) *Chinese Herbal Medicine Materia Medica.* Eastland Press, Seattle.

Chalmers, I. (1993) The Cochrane Collaboration: preparing, maintaining and disseminating systemic reviews of the effects of health care. *Ann. N.Y. Acad. Sci.* **203**, 166–172.

Chang, C.K. (Han Dynasty) (220) *Discussions of Fever.* Classics.

Cheng, K.C. *Research in Chinese Medicine.* China Health Publisher, Beijing.

De Smet, P. and A'Arcy, P.F. (ed) (1996) Drug interactions with herbal and other non-toxic remedies. In: *Mechanisms of Drug Interactions.* Springer-Verlag, Berlin.

Eisenberg, D.M., Kessler, R.C. and Foster, C. (1993) Unconventional medicine in the USA — Prevalence, costs and patterns of use. *New Engl. J. Med.* **328**(4), 246–252.

Fair, W.R. (1999) The role of complementary medicine in urology. *J. Urol.* **162**, 411–420.

Farquhar, J. (1994) *Knowing Practice — The Clinical Encounter of Chinese Medicine.* West View Press, San Francisco.

Jaeschke, R. and Singer, J. (1989) Measurement of health status. Ascertaining the minimally important difference. *Control Clin. Trials* **10**, 407–415.

Kaptchuk, T.J. and Eisenberg, D.M. (1998) The persuasive appeal of alternative medicine. *Ann. Intern. Med.* **129**(12), 1061–1065.

Keinginger, D.L. (1999) Why develop IQOD? International health related quality of life outcome database. *QoL Newslett.* September–December, (23)2.

Kong, Y.C. (1998) *Formulations from South-West Asia.* Chinese University Press, Hong Kong.

Lai, S.L. (2001a) *Clinical Trials of Traditional Chinese Materia Medica.* Guangdong People's Publishing House, China, Chap. 1.

Lai, S.L. (ed.) (2001b) *Clinical Trials of Traditional Chinese Materia Medica.* Guangdong People's Publishing House, China, Chaps. 2–4.

Leung, P.C. (2001) Editorial-seminar series on evidence-based alternative medicine. *Hong Kong Med. J.* **7**(4), 332–334.

Leung, P.C. (2001) *Traditional Chinese Medicine in China: Seminar on Health Care in Modern China.* Yale-China Association.

Leung, P.C. *Clinical Trials in Chinese Medicine — The Efficacy Driven Approach.* Hospital Authority Convention, Hong Kong.

McGuire, M.B. (1988) *Ritual Healing in Suburban America.* Rutgers University Press, Newbrunswick and London.

Nachemson, E. (1989) *Causes and Treatment of Low Back Pain.* American Academy of Orthopaedic Surgery Lecture Series.

Ng, B. (1986) *Herbal Drugs and Phytopharmaceuticals.* Medpharm Scientific Publisher, BocaRaton.

NIH (2001) *National Centre for Complementary and Alternative Medicine Five Year Strategic Plan 2001–2005.* NIH Document.

NIH (1997) *Acupuncture.* NIH Consensus Statement **15**(5), 1–34 (November 3–5).

Richardson, W. (2001) *Crossing the Quality Chasm: A New Health System for the 21st Century.* The National Academic News.

Sackett, D.L. (1991) *Clinical Epidemiology*, 2nd Ed. Little, Brown & Co., Boston, pp. 297–299.

Stewart, A.L., Greenfield, E.R. and Hayo, R.D. (1989) Functional status and well-being of patients with chronic conditions. *JAMA* **262**, 907–913.

Su, W.T. (1992) *History of Drugs.* United Medical University Press, Beijing.

Suen, T.Y., Wang, S.F. and Wang, K.L. *Adverse Effects of Drug Treatment.* People's Health Press, China.

Tang, W. and Eisenberg, G. (1992) *Chinese Drugs of Plant Origin: Chemistry, Pharmacology and Use in Traditional and Modern Medicine.* Springer-Verlag, Berlin, New York.

Uppsala Monitoring Centre (WHO) (2000) *Safety Monitoring of Medicinal Products: Guidelines for Setting Up and Running a Pharmaco Vigilance Centre.*

Wang, P.Y. (1995) *New Chinese Medicine: Research Production and Registration.* Chinese Medicine Press, China.

World Health Organization (2000) *General Guidelines for Methodologies on Research and Evaluation of Traditional Medicine.* World Health Organization Publisher, Geneva.

Wyrwick, K.W. and Nienaber, N.A. (1999) Linking clinical relevance and statistical significance in health related quality of life. *Med. Care* **37**, 469–478.

Chapter 12

Modernisation of Chinese Medicine: An Anthropologist's View

Ting Hor

12.1 Introduction

As a part of traditional Chinese culture, Chinese medicine is also called traditional medicine. In China, since the transformation of traditional society, Chinese medicine has been modernised from its traditional aspects. For most contemporaneous Chinese, as for the author, the modernisation of Chinese medicine seems quite natural and uncontested. In fact, this view is formed *a priori* on three assumptions:

(1) Chinese medicine has to change from its ancient form to a new form.
(2) Chinese medicine has to complete its evolution from its present primitive level to a higher level.
(3) Chinese medicine has to be transformed from an unscientific practice to a scientific practice.

Our debate starts by examining these three assumptions through an anthropological approach.

12.2 Modernisation of Chinese Society: Cultural Background

The definition of modernisation varies according to different dictionaries. A simple one would read, "Giving to something a form according to the current techniques". These current techniques do not refer to the time sequence alone. Otherwise, today's Chinese medicine would already be modern as opposed to the past; and in that sense modern Western medicine would still require further modernisation. Why is it that nowadays Chinese medicine has become an object of modernisation, made to assume a new form?

Indeed, modernisation as we understand it, does not only refer to a chronological order, but involves geographical and cultural concepts as well. It consists of the development and the diffusion of industrial civilisation, tracing back from the European Renaissance and the discovery of the "New World", including rational thinking, experimental science and technology, modern socio-political systems and even European cultural tastes. The West became, and is still becoming, the original centre of modernisation. For non-western societies, modernisation refers to a gradual process of Westernisation during which their own traditional culture has become marginal.

For the Chinese of the Celestial Dynasties, the Europeans were always looked upon as barbarians and their ridiculous techniques, including Western medicine, were considered useless. But starting from 1840, during the Opium War, the Chinese began to feel the strength and the efficiency of these barbarian techniques, and the process of Westernisation actively spread throughout China.

The last Qing Dynasty collapsed in the early 20th century, bringing down the self-confidence of the Chinese people in their own culture. After the May 4th movement in 1919, almost everything traditional, from Confucianism to customs, language and clothing, were all condemned. The Western way became the desirable new way as opposed to the traditional Chinese way, which was then labelled ancient. For example, the Western schools were called "new schools" (*xin xue tang*) while the traditional ones were called "ancient schools" (*jiu xue tang*). According to the same logic, Western medicine became the "new medicine" (*xin yi*) while traditional medicine was called the "ancient medicine" (*jiu yi*).

This contrasted view opposing the Western *new* way and the Chinese *ancient* way, led Chinese tradition to be marginalised. Thus, traditional cultural activities like music, painting, sports, etc. became estranged in the eyes of the Chinese people, and had to be prefixed with "*Guo*",[1]

[1]"*Guo*" (國) means national.

"*Zhong*",[2] "*Tang*"[3] or "*Min Zu*",[4] in order to differentiate them from the mainstream — "normal" music, painting and sports — imported from the West. In the same way, traditional medicine was labelled "National medicine" (*Guo Yi*) or "Chinese medicine" (*Zhong Yi*), in opposition to modern Western medicine, which is referred to in China as "the" medicine.

It has only since been then that Chinese medicine has become an ancient and strange therapy in China. To most Chinese, it is only through modernisation that their traditional medicine can be saved from its marginal situation, always in reference to a current therapy introduced from outside China, i.e. modern Western medicine. Hence, at the end of the 19th century, a movement aimed at "intermingling Chinese and Western medicine" (中西匯通) was launched. In 1929 during the Republic, there was a movement of "removing traditional medical care but retaining its pharmaceutical materials" (廢醫存葯). And, after the Chinese communist takeover in 1949, a movement of "reforming Chinese medicine" (改造中醫) and another of "integrating Chinese and Western medicine" (中西醫結合) have spread over the mainland of China. In these movements, Chinese medicine was always required to assume a new form, copied from modern Western medicine, in order to restore its rationality and legitimacy in a new society.

Nowadays, we are witnessing an interesting phenomenon: while in China modernisation is spreading rapidly, in the West where modernisation originated, is emerging a genuine interest for traditional Chinese culture. Indeed, Western countries have experienced a similar history of rush towards modernisation and their own traditions were also downgraded. But now the appreciation of the traditional culture of non-western societies has become a modern cultural trend in Western countries. Of course, Chinese medicine is far from being validated as a common therapy by the authorities of Western countries, and its ancient and Oriental form looks twice as strange to Western people than to Chinese people. Nevertheless, Chinese medicine in its most ancient form is largely

---

[2]"*Zhong*" (中) means Chinese.

[3]"*Tang*" (唐) means Tang Dynasty.

[4]"*Min Zu*" (民族) means folk, ethnical.

preferred by the Western public: it has even been referred to as the "medicine of the future". Ironically in Chinese society, traditional culture including medical practices is still considered an obstacle to modernisation.

Hence, the so-called "new form" is not the only possible future for Chinese medicine, but just a specific choice resulting from the cultural tastes stemming from the Westernisation complex in China during its transformation. Outside this given space and time, Chinese medicine does not need to have a "new form". By studying this cultural background, we now prove wrong the first assumption about the modernisation of Chinese medicine. The discussion on the two other assumptions requires a greater understanding of Chinese medicine.

12.3 Understanding Chinese Medicine Through an Anthropological Approach

As Chinese medicine, along with other alternative medicines, is getting quite popular these days, there is hardly anyone who has not heard about acupuncture or *Qigong*. People familiar with complementary medicines would even talk about Chinese pharmacopoeia, moxibustion, cupping therapy (拔火罐), Chinese massage (推拿), bone-setting and fracture stabilisation (正骨-跌打), treatment for ulcers and carbuncles (瘡瘍科), nutritional therapy (食療), etc. As a matter of fact, these treatment modalities as well as other diagnostic means like pulse detection and tongue observation are very particular procedures, forming the visible characteristics of Chinese medicine.

Nevertheless, behind the complexity and diversity of diagnosis and treatment, there is one philosophy guiding the different aspects. To understand the essence of Chinese medicine, we should concentrate on its philosophical theories.

Broadly speaking, Chinese medicine bases its clinical practices on the Taoist philosophy of *Yin-Yang and Five Elements* (陰陽五行). These theories took the view that the human body, like everything in the Universe, is formed and controlled by an invisible *Qi* (氣). The *Qi* circulates through the *meridians*, connecting the *Viscera* and the *Bowels* according to the law of the *Five Elements*, and keeping a good balance between *Yin* and *Yang*. When the *Qi* loses its balance while facing the

Evil Forces (邪) — the *six external excesses* (六淫), the *seven internal emotions* (七情) or improper living habits — sickness is likely to set in.

The physician's duty is to help to maintain and restore the balance by using the various means already described. On the practical side, Chinese medicine healers have developed a unique system of diagnosis and treatment. It is called "*treatment based on the differentiation of Syndromes*" (辯証論治).

The diagnostic techniques include a process of inspecting, listening, enquiring, pulse-taking and palpation (望聞問切), the findings of which are integrated into a proper diagnosis in order to differentiate one *Syndrome* (証) from the others. The method of integration varies depending on the nature of affections; and one affection can be analysed by the combination of several methods. Once this diagnosis is established, management follows with ease.

For example, if a patient complains of weakness and weight loss, the following procedures are undertaken: the physician identifies his red tongue; listens to his weak voice; enquires about his general situation: whether there is night sweating, semen discharge, afternoon fever, lower-back pain or knee pain, tinnitus, etc. During palpations he might identify a weak *Kidney pulse* appearing at both wrists. The diagnosis is therefore the syndrome of *Yin deficiency of Kidney* (腎陰虛). The *Yin deficiency* is derived from the method using the *Eight Principles* (八綱辨証), because when the *Yin* is down, the *Yang* (fever, night sweating, red tongue) becomes too strong. Apart from indications identified during pulse-taking, the identification of the *Kidney* (腎) as the problematic organ is based on another method, namely the "*differential diagnosis of Viscera and Bowels*" (臟腑辨証), since in the Classics Chinese ancestors wrote that the *Kidney* "controls the bones", "preserves the male vitality" and "has its openings at the ears". So, in the case of dysfunction, symptoms like lower-back pain, semen discharge and tinnitus will appear.

Following the diagnostic deduction, the prescription is likely to be: *Kidney's Yin* tonics, for example *Liu Wei Di Huang Wan* pills (pills combining six ingredients based on *Radix rehmannae*) (六味地黃丸) In the formula, some ingredients *nourish the Yin* (補陰), some carry the therapeutic effects into the *Kidney meridian* (入腎經) and some *harmonize* the relationship between the ingredients (和味). The choice of treatment can also be acupuncture so that the points on the *Kidney meridian* will be stimulated, by "supplying action" (補法) of course.

Modern clinicians and scientists may feel rather sceptical about Chinese medicine: for each *Syndrome*, there are always one or several formulas already determined. However, we will see later that in the evolution of medicine, treatment ahead of diagnosis is a common occurrence. As far as Chinese medicine is concerned, means of treatment have been observed to be effective against groups of symptoms, before the symptoms and signs were grouped to form a *Syndrome*. In other words, the healers were not interested in giving the name of a *Syndrome* to a group of symptoms and signs for which they had not yet found a treatment.

So we have seen the essence of Chinese medicine: a careful prescription should be based on one or several identified *Syndromes*. Actually, the practice of this diagnostic approach differs from specialty to specialty. However, strictly speaking, Chinese medicine should be confined to practices where a *Syndrome* is established and subsequently an adequate treatment deduced. Other non-diagnostic based practices should just be considered as empirical treatment forms, and need to be further integrated into Chinese medicine (or into other medical systems). We can now determine what Chinese medicine is. But to find out whether it has achieved its evolution, we need to see what kind of a medicine it is.

Medical practices can assume either a supernatural form or a natural form. The former communicate with mythical forces like divine or ghostly media, which are expected to remove the illness directly or provide an effective formula to treat it. In the early days of Chinese medicine, supernatural healing was used widely. But obviously, supernatural healing stopped being a mainline practice a long time ago.

Natural healing on the other hand, includes both psychical and material methods. In the first case, Christian scientists, for example, believe that the healing follows a strong conviction that the illness never existed. Although Chinese medicine may sometimes adopt psychical treatments, the major part of Chinese medicine is still material.

Material therapies can be based on effects at a distance, as in the case of the school of Paracelsus which was interested in celestial movements and in their influence on the human body. Then in the case of Chinese medicine, therapy is based essentially on material effects that influence the body directly, as we have indicated such as using herbs, acupuncture, moxibustion and massages, etc. These therapeutic skills, used in Chinese medicine for several thousand years, are indeed technically primitive.

From this viewpoint, the therapeutic effects of Chinese medicine — or at least most of them — are related to direct interactions between materials in Nature. So these interactions can be researched and interpreted with experimental methods of modern science and can be served by modern technology. Which means that the traditional techniques of Chinese medicine can "evolve" into a more efficient level.

However, Chinese medicine is by no means a mere chaotic mass of therapeutic solutions derived from empirical practices. Chinese medicine is, as we have seen, a well-established system of knowledge and skills. Within this system, the explanations of the human body, illnesses and treatment have all been logically linked with Taoist theories. The singular "*treatment based on the differentiation of Syndromes*" is an extremely sophisticated deduction. The clinical processes of "*Li*, *Fa*, *Fang*, *Yao*"[5] indicate that Chinese medicine has become a complete medical system. Anthropologically speaking, Chinese medicine is an empiric-speculative medicine, developed into its full maturity.

For this reason, Chinese medicine, taken as a whole, should not be considered as a primitive therapy, needing to complete its evolution with some help from, for example, modern technology. And there is no necessity either for it to evolve into another more modern medical system, for, as we will see, hierarchy between the different medicines is an illusion. The second assumption in which Chinese medicine is considered primitive should thus be disqualified.

Nevertheless, these attempted descriptions of the human body, diseases and treatments, are far from being similar to the concepts derived from modern anatomy, physiology and pathology. The metaphysical terms like *Qi*, *Yin deficiency*, *meridians*, etc. seem mythical for our contemporaries. There is no definite cause/effect correlation between the pulse/tongue signs and the diseases indicated. Principles used as treatment modalities like *nourishing the Yin* and *stimulating the meridian*, are likewise

[5]"*Li*, *Fa*, *Fang*, *Yao*" (理法方药) meaning explanation of illness, principle of treatment, determining the fomula and choosing pharmaceutical materials.

over-simplistic. From the scientist viewpoint, there is no room for such superstitions, and it is uncontested that Chinese medicine has to rebuild its total system in the light of modern physiology and pathology.

Challenged by these criticisms, the fervent users and practitioners of Chinese medicine are fighting hard today to protect their system of healing. A common argument states that the Chinese ancestors in their wisdom discovered subtle body elements like *Qi*, *meridians*, etc. which are still too complicated to be accounted for by modern science. Sometime in the future, thanks to further developments of technology, their existence will be proved. Chinese medicine is thus given a "scientific form of the future" which refuse any control from a contemporary scientific discipline.

However, we find that supporters or detractors both base their arguments on the same conviction: a true medicine is necessarily scientific, based on physical objectivity. We need to adopt once more a neutral anthropological standpoint to look at the origin and the development of medicines, in order to see if Chinese medicine is scientific, and if it is necessary for it to be scientific.

12.4 Medicines and Science

As of the very first day of existence of human beings, "illnesses" occurred. As opposed to "health", illness led to suffering and an early death. The urgent need for mankind was to find ways to relieve the illnesses and restore health: "cure". This quest for a cure was purely empirical. The accumulation of both successes and failures revealed the specificity of the cure: generally, one given cure was only good for one given illness. Hence, the decision to resort to a specific cure to treat a particular individual required determining which illness he suffered from — "diagnosis". The people who proved the most capable of making the diagnosis and choosing the appropriate treatment became "healers". Then their knowledge and skills became "medicine". All systems of medicine must have developed in this common way. We can identify here two ultimate purposes of medicine: to find an efficient cure for a given illness; and to recognise this illness each time in order to treat it with the appropriate cure. We call medical systems that required just empirical practices "primitive medicine" or "folk medicine".

Later on, the healers belonging to early-developed civilisations tended to integrate their empirical practices into their own general law of the Universe. These explanations about the human body, the illnesses and treatments did improve the empirical medical practices: they gave a direction to the exploration of new cures, and organised diagnosis and treatments in a logical system. Although explanations vary between these "savant" medicines — Greek-Roman, Indian, Arabian, Chinese, etc., their methodology remains the same: a philosophical speculation based on clinical observation. Causes of illnesses, abnormal processes and effects of treatments were all explained by metaphysical expressions and philosophies. What happens inside the human body — its structure, functions, situation when it becomes dysfunctional or reverts to normal — therefore remains obscure.

Meanwhile, from an early date, the healers of traditional Western medicine — Greek-Roman medicine — were not satisfied by their external observations and speculations. The Greek philosophy based on the atomic theory postulated that all things originated from *atoms* which interacted by direct contact with one another. These philosophers assumed that an in-depth investigation of these *atoms* would lead to a genuine understanding and control of the Universe. The pioneers of Western medicine were thus called the "mechanists"; they firmly believed that the observation and the manipulation of *atoms* in the human body is the best approach to medical practice.

This idea may seem natural nowadays. However, during the pre-industrial era, the therapeutic results of empirical or speculative practices were far better than the ones obtained by the "mechanists" whose instruments were not efficient enough to observe detail of the *atoms*. For a long time, the mechanists were therefore considered as "quacks". Their situation was certainly as miserable as that of the present day folk healers.

With the Industrial Revolution, technology enjoyed a breakthrough, which led to a brilliant victory for the mechanist practitioners. Gradually, the structures of the human being (such as organs, tissues, cells, molecules and genes), its functions (physiological, biochemical, immunological and genetic), and aetiologies of diseases, including reactions to pathological and therapeutic changes, were unveiled in the laboratories. The understanding of the objective realities of the human body, diseases and treatments naturally led to more and better clinical solutions.

Western medicine has thus conquered the world as a "scientific medicine", because it is based on physical objectivity. Using experimental methodology, Western medicine explains objectively the causes of pathological changes in the organs, tissues and molecules. It gives objective justifications for a treatment. Diagnosis and treatment are now based on the objective reality of material changes, no longer on vague and variable clinical behaviours. Although clinical observations are not totally ignored today, Western medicine relies more and more on laboratory investigations.

Thus we have shown that Western medicine is not more mature in the course of medical evolution than the others. The clinical advantages of Western medicine derive from recent technological developments independent from its medical system. In fact, its supremacy today relies essentially on the cultural dominance of a rationalist mentality, which considers physical objectivity as the unique parameter of truth. Although nowadays Western medicine has become the mainstream medicine all over the world, in the light of our anthropological studies, it is Western medicine and not Chinese medicine which should be considered as strange, since its experimental methodology is very different from all other medical systems. The application of scientific methods in the medical practice is, in fact, an isolated case in medical history.

As opposed to the "mechanists", Chinese healers insist that it is the *Qi* and not the *atoms* that is the basis of the human body, of illnesses and of treatments. Although considered as "material", the *Qi* cannot be seen under any circumstances. All the healer can do is observe the clinical behaviour and deduce what happened inside the body, and then formulate his diagnosis and treatment strategy. Thus, in Chinese medicine, clinical observation and philosophical speculation are fundamental methodologies which have remained unchanged from the very early ages until now. This is the real reason why Chinese medicine is called traditional medicine, and why compared with Western medicine, it looks unscientific and needs to be modernised.

Nevertheless, we now know that the ultimate purposes of medicine have to do with the keyword "how": how to cure a given disease, and how to keep these findings at the disposition of practitioners. If we have to deal with a simple and straightforward problem, we do not have to ask the question "why". It is only when the problems become more complicated, that further understanding of the human body and illnesses are required so that diagnosis and treatment can follow logical categories. So, for medical systems, the reason for asking the question "why", is just to answer more efficiently the question "how": a system regulating logically the clinical behaviours and the therapies allows practitioners to find a solution for each case, more quickly and more precisely than by just using empirical practices.

As we have seen, the ways to establish such a system can be different. The experimental methodology explored by modern science is just one way by which Western medicine has established its diagnostic-therapeutic system. Because of the positivist nature of this method, the answers to the question "why" given by modern Western medicine — explanations concerning the human body, diseases and therapeutic effects — are not just aimed at providing an answer to the question "how", but they account for objective realities, which are independent of clinical interests. Therefore, modern Western medicine validates diagnosis and treatment according to their scientific value only — objectivity. Anything considered unscientific, will be automatically disqualified.

On the contrary, other systems of healing, including Chinese medicine, do not pay any attention to the scientific value. For example, considerations on *Qi*, *meridians*, *Viscera* and *Bowels*, etc. do not depend on their objectivity, but on their clinical value: to achieve more easily the *differentiation of Syndromes*. In these systems, the scientific value and clinical value do not necessarily co-exist; and it is only the clinical value which validates each specific concept, logic and practice.

Now, when we look again into the *Yin deficiency of the Kidney*, we realise that in the course of their empirical practices, ancient Chinese healers have observed two sets of "realities": first, collections of certain symptoms and signs usually appearing together in some common conditions; and second, the fact that these symptoms and signs can be improved with certain cures. And then the healers would need to organise these two findings into a system of classification, in order to extract them quickly from numerous other findings, in case they may encounter a similar case one day. The logical system of *Yin-Yang and Five Elements* was chosen, since it was the most comprehensive explanatory system achieved by the Chinese ancestors who thought that the human body should function in the same way as all other visible phenomena in Nature. When the concepts and deductions derived from the observation of Nature, like *Yin-Yang*, *Deficiency-Excess*, etc. were used in Chinese medicine, their new meaning was determined only by their clinical value — which emphasises the healer's practices — and not by their physical objectivity in relation to Nature or the human body.

So, it is useless to try to establish if a patient's *Yin* is really *deficient*, or if his *Kidney* is actually infected. The *Yin deficiency of Kidney* is nothing else but a combination of symptoms such as fatigue, weight loss, sweating, fever, abnormal seminal discharges, joint pains and tinnitus, etc. The reason why they were given such a name as *Yin deficiency of Kidney* is just to help the healer to memorise a complex collection of symptoms and signs. Also, it is pointless to argue if, in the *Liu Wei Di Huang Wan* pills, some ingredients can really *nourish the Yin*, and if others can carry the therapeutic effects into the *meridian of the Kidney*. To understand and to evaluate the concepts and deductions used in Chinese medicine, we should not debate whether they are objectively true, but whether they are clinically useful to achieve the *differentiation of Syndromes*.

Since its deductions and explanations of the human body, illnesses and treatments do not rely on physical objective evidence, which is the essence of experimental science, Chinese medicine is indeed not scientific. The objective or scientific nature of its deductions and its concepts, even if they may occasionally exist, cannot turn Chinese medicine into scientific — it is the experimental research on Chinese medicine but not Chinese medicine itself which will be scientific. However, the lack of a scientific approach did not prevent Chinese medicine from completing the ultimate purposes of medicine. Using their unscientific deductions and explanations, healers categorised clinical observations into a logical matching system of diagnoses and treatments, which can improve their practices. Therefore, clinically speaking, there is no need for Chinese medicine to become scientific.

This viewpoint of the author, who considers that Chinese medicine is not scientific, naturally irritates the Chinese medicine's zealots: since nowadays, being unscientific means being wrong or false. In fact, this emotional reaction comes from the confusion between two different judgments. To be considered as scientific or not is a judgment of *fact*:

used to evaluate whether a methodology is experimental, and whether findings are objective. In the domain of scientific research, this judgment of fact is also a judgment of *value*: used to evaluate if a methodology is right or wrong, if findings are true or false. But obviously, to be scientific or not cannot be systematically used as a judgment of value in the other domains of human activity, like the arts, literature, music, etc.

As far as Chinese medicine is concerned, traditional healers did organise their clinical findings into some logical classifications, then turned their practice into a science in a wide conception of the term. Chinese medicine can also have some scientific natures: as it operates in a material way, experimental methods can prove the objective mechanism of its therapeutic effects. We can even imagine that some wisdom of this ancestral system might exceed the domain of scientific research — this may comfort the zealots insulted by the author's sacrilege, namely considering Chinese medicine as a mere matching tool. Nevertheless, if we accept that deductions of Chinese medicine are not based on experimental method, and its concepts are not based on objectivity, then Chinese medicine is definitively not scientific; and most of its explanations concerning the human body, diseases and treatments can be wrong and false in the light of a scientific approach. But Chinese medicine can still be a right and true *Medicine*, which is qualified by its capacity to find effective cures and to classify them into a logical system.

We see now that the third assumption, i.e. the Chinese medicine must be transformed to a scientific practice, proves also to be incorrect. It is true that the skills of the ancient healers can never exist as a universal and independent field of knowledge, like human anatomy and physiology in modern medicine. Instead, their conceptions are meaningful only when applied within their own medical system. This may mean that Chinese medicine remains a strict healing discipline whereas modern Western medicine, built on independent knowledge, has gone beyond the healing area of experimental science.

Through our debate on the three assumptions, we know that modernisation is not as necessary for Chinese medicine as we thought. But we can still wonder if Chinese medicine can benefit from modernisation. Would modernisation help to improve its clinical practices? Would the modernisation of Chinese medicine help with economic and ecological development? Before we engage in such a discussion, it is necessary to have a general view of this modernisation, specially as it has developed in China where it is the most representative.

12.5 Panorama of the Modernisation of Chinese Medicine

12.5.1 *Medical techniques*

(1) The development of acupuncture and moxibustion

Traditional acupuncture refers to the introduction of a needle into an acupuncture point in some part of the body. The needles used in traditional China can be made of bamboo, stone, gold or silver. When burnt herbs (Armoise) are used to heat the same point, the technique is referred to as moxibustion.

Though modernisation of acupuncture began 70 years ago with the introduction of stainless steel needles, it was the introduction of electrical acupuncture in the 1950s which was regarded as the true revolutionary breakthrough. More technological applications followed, such as the use of laser, microwave, infra-red rays and electronic acupuncture point detectors, linkages with computers, etc.

(2) Changes in the forms of pharmaceutical materials

The traditional formulae were prepared in the form of broth (湯), pill (丸), granules (散) and paste (膏), etc. which were processed from a mixture of herbs, animal products and sometimes minerals. Broth or decoctions required lengthy steaming. In the recent two decades, new forms of preparations appeared. These came in the form of mixed powder for instant drinks with the adjunction of hot water, precooked concentrates, or extracted preparations kept in ampoules for injection use. Other rare means of administration include transcutanious introduction through electrical means.

(3) The application of new techniques already in use in modern Western medicine

The most remarkable example of this is the use of antiseptic techniques in acupuncture, from the simple application of alcohol swabs to boiling and autoclaving equipment. There is a full range of basic modern techniques in use: not only is equipment for sterilisation widely used, but the antiseptic handling procedures are also strict adaptations derived from practices in modern Western hospitals.

The invention of so-called "water-needle" — injecting different solutions, like physiological saline, vitamins, pain removers or local anaesthetics, into the acupoints — is another good example of the transfer of modern medical techniques into traditional practices. Other examples include the use of radiography and other laboratory studies as means of investigation.

(4) Introduction of traditional techniques in modern medical practice

"Acupuncture anaesthesia" (correctly acupuncture analgesia) in the early 1970s was a show-case example, which made Chinese medicine famous throughout the world. Not only has acupuncture been well accepted among modern practitioners as a valid means of treatment, but the mechanisms responsible for acupuncture's therapeutic effects were also considered as an important object for scientific research.

(5) Creation of new clinical instruments

Equipment like the pulse differentiator and the tongue analyser have been designed in an attempt to replace traditional practices. The current computer-driven diagnostic equipment illustrates another effort to make Chinese medicine's diagnostic more automatic. Instead of being used in limited applications of this sophisticated equipment, the acupuncture point detector has enjoyed wide popular use, from the hospital environment to ordinary households.

12.5.2 *Pathways of practice*

Although *Guan Zi* (管子, ?-645 BC) already built a first primitive hospital, and in spite of the existence of official pharmacy-clinics from the Song Dynasty (1076) onward, early Chinese medicine practitioners normally worked as individuals in private clinics and pharmacies or as itinerant practitioners.

In today's China, with the movement of collectivisation in the 1950s, Chinese medicine practitioners have gradually moved into the hospitals. These Chinese medicine hospitals are built on the model of modern Western hospitals, both in terms of architectural structure and management. Attending practitioners serve in outpatient clinics or in the wards. The staff hierarchy follows exactly the same pattern as in modern Western hospitals. Patients coming for medical advice undergo the same procedures as in modern hospitals. The standard practices of morning rounds and evening case studies are not different from modern Western medicine. Anthropologists are also watching out for symbolic items like uniforms, signs and environmental set-ups. All these symbols, typical of modern Western medicine, have been adapted in Chinese medicine hospitals. While young Chinese medicine practitioners practice today in that way, they take it for granted, and are not aware that it is the result of real modernisation.

Nevertheless, within the rural areas, some individual Chinese herbalists are still active. These healers take care of their neighbours' health, using only traditional medical tools. They can be considered marginal outcasts of the modernisation process. The situation in Hong Kong is also rather traditional. Many Chinese medicine practitioners still work within herbal pharmacies. The bone-setters, likewise, maintain their working tradition. However, practitioners who emigrated from Mainland China tend to provide a modern image to their clinic. For example, they will naturally choose Western white gowns as their work uniforms.

12.5.3 *Teaching and training*

From the Southern-Northern Dynasties (443) onward, each dynasty has established its empire medical schools for a very limited number of practitioners. Most of the traditional practitioners were trained through individual apprenticeship. Apprentices were often the direct offspring of their masters. There was actually an old saying that went "avoid a healer who is not third generation". Some healers were originally scholars who failed the examinations for mandarinate.

Modern training in Chinese medicine started only after the fall of the Qing Dynasty (1911). National level Chinese medicine colleges were built in the 1950s. These colleges have become the main training institutions for Mainland China ever since. The education system and college administration follow closely those of modern medical schools. In their curricula, one finds a mixture of natural sciences, modern Western medicine and Chinese medicine. Most of teaching material for Chinese medicine consists of modern Chinese documents. Old Classics and classical Chinese documents are also used, but in relatively small proportions.

The teaching environment (including classrooms and teaching aids, and also teachers' gowns) is quite similar to modern Western education systems. Academic positions and titles (professors, lecturers, tutors, etc.) and conferrment of degrees (bachelor, master, doctor, etc.) are inspired from the Western pattern. Graduation ceremonies in full Western taste have become popular since the 1990s for both Western and Chinese medical colleges.

12.5.4 *Scientific research*

Chinese medicine has relied on the success of clinical experiences, which just needed to be accounted for with classical concepts formulated in ancient medical works like the "*Treatise on Febrile Diseases*" (傷寒論) and the "*Prescriptions Worth a Thousand Gold Pieces*" (千金方) etc.

In 1951, a French researcher *Niboyet* started to use a scientific approach to study the electrical nature of acupuncture points and *meridians*. Ever since then, more research has been performed with experimental methods. No matter what technique is used and how much expansion of scope of interest is observed, two major lines are followed. The first one involves clinical trials using randomisation, with double-blind placebo control which requires statistical analysis and meta analysis. The second one is related to basic research aimed at proving or replacing classical theories by scientific explanations. Different centres in China are investing a lot of effort on both targets.

Now we can assess the modernisation of Chinese medicine in the light of our one valid parameter — the clinical value. Is it affecting medical practice? Can it improve the procedure of the "*differentiation of Syndromes*" or provide alternative and better methods?

12.6 Evaluation of the Modernisation of Chinese Medicine

12.6.1 *Modernisation expressed by "cultural taste"*

Obviously, most of this modernisation of Chinese medicine stems largely from a preference for Western products, particularly for modern Western medicine. Looking at the design of Chinese medicine hospitals, the organisation of practice, the teaching curriculum, the uniform and the behaviour of practitioners, etc. we find that they all follow the pattern of modern Western medicine. Actually, such superficial changes in Chinese medicine do not necessarily indicate any progress in its clinical practices.

Outside of China, Chinese medicine takes more diversified forms. The oldest traditional appearance can become important for Chinese medicine in Western countries. When a Chinese medicine hospital in Germany puts a pair of stone lions at its gate, we easily get an impression of the conception that Western people have of Chinese culture: China and its products should hold on to their authentic look of "Celestial Dynasties".

Facing such divergent views on Chinese medicine in the West and in China, the anthropologist's task is to analyse the reasoning attached to the different cultural backgrounds. In China, the modern or Western format does help Chinese medicine practitioners to liberate themselves from their old habits of thinking and behaviour patterns. As to the taste for traditional props in Chinese medicine in Western countries, one has to realise that it has to do less with tradition than with a fashionable trend. Nevertheless, this tendency to follow the oldest looking forms of Chinese medicine may somehow preserve its specific characters from the influence of its new cultural environment.

Anthropologists can also emphasise the following points:

(1) The two contradictory attitudes towards Chinese medicine — the modern form trend in China and the preservation of the traditional form in the West — should best be kept within each separate cultural area and not generalised as politically correct ideologies. Otherwise, in the current situation of Western dominance, there may be a cultural supremacy of "traditional Chinese medicine" as defined by the Western taste.

(2) Even when these two forms of Chinese medicine are limited within their own cultural area, the "modern look" or "traditional look" should be kept under proper control. Failing this, Chinese medicine will lose its specific character in China; while in Western countries, it may turn into some kind of religious conviction or esoteric practice.

12.6.2 *Modernisation as realised by the new technology*

As we have seen in China, many new techniques and instruments have been introduced in traditional diagnosis and treatment. Although this equipment has given Chinese medicine's clinical activities a very modern look, they still have not changed its traditional essence: "*treatment based on the differentiation of Syndromes*". Our evaluation should be based on the clinical benefits derived from these techniques.

The first group of techniques consists of the ones which do not alter traditional practices in any way, but make them look modern; for example, the use of antiseptic techniques in acupuncture. Although such techniques involve knowledge of bacteriology, antiseptic agents and perhaps disposable agents, their application does not affect the traditional diagnosis or treatment. Nevertheless, because of the value of these techniques in the prevention of infection, they should be routinely used in traditional practices like acupuncture.

The second group consists of the techniques which just modify traditional instruments, like acupuncture needles. Stainless steel needles have replaced traditional needles, so that the puncturing is safer and more convenient. As a result, these new needles are so widely and so naturally used in traditional practice today, that not many people remember that they have actually benefited from modern metallurgy.

The third group refers to instrumental techniques which try to make traditional practices (diagnosis and treatment) data visible, standardised, quantified and automatic. They can be applied to tongue examination, pulse detection and acupoint detection, and include the use of computers. This equipment is certainly the result of new advanced technology. But its application may not necessarily improve the process of diagnosis and treatment in Chinese medicine. Facial appearance, for example, is not only related to haemoglobin contents, but is affected also by more complicated elements, like luster, humidity, etc. In such intricate cases, compared with the results obtained through the traditional "crude" approach, the results obtained through exact instrumental analysis are not always more useful for the practitioner. The issue of automation is another area of controversy. When an electrical stimulator is used for acupuncture, the operator does not need to resort to manual stimulations. When an acupoint detector is used, even less human effort is required for the diagnosis. Nevertheless, this type of industrialised automation induces a loss of humanity in the medical practice, which happens to be the main drawback in Western medicine. Anyway, the modern equipment applied to acupuncture still lacks the complexity and sophistication that may affect the humanity of traditional practices. However, the author does spot a potential danger behind this ideology of automation.

In the field of the preparation of herbal drugs, the use of modern technology appears to be more successful. For example, the use of mechanised equipment reduces the need for human labour and increases production; the new form of pharmaceutical materials makes their administration more comfortable. Nevertheless, we should adapt these modern processes to the other aspects of Chinese medicine which are still very traditional. Otherwise, the application of any given new technique, even if very efficient in itself, can impair the general efficiency of clinical practices.

12.6.3 *Modernisation attempted by scientific rationalisation*

Scientists try to replace the philosophical approach of Chinese medicine by an experimental approach like explorations on the scientific meaning of *Yin-Yang*, electrical studies on *meridians*, etc. This may prove to be the most thorough modernisation of Chinese medicine through which Chinese experts hope to put Chinese medicine on the international standardised way of development.

It is encouraging to realise that scientific attempts may well provide objective data on Chinese medicine, and thus control the quack's practices which infect all traditional medicines. Nevertheless, the clinical outcome from these scientific methods may not always be superior to that obtained from the traditional ones.

As in the case of the *Yin deficiency of Kidney*, assuming that all symptoms and signs decrypted in the *Yin deficiency of the Kidney* can be objectively measured at different levels (organ, tissue, cell, molecule and genes) according to pathological changes inside the human body (structural, functional, metabolic or congenital), and that all therapeutic effects produced by the *Liu Wei Di Huang Wan* pills can be accounted for by molecular research, the treatment will thus rely on factual analysis instead of speculations. The expected advantages are that the diagnosis can become more accurate and the treatment more certain. It appears therefore that experimental practice should further enhance the efficiency of Chinese medicine. Numerous questions to challenge this optimistic deduction can be asked.

Firstly, a question on a philosophical level: Are all symptoms traceable to material changes? — Are there always *atoms* to observe? The symptoms of tinnitus, night sweating and lower-back pain, etc. may be unveiled by experimental methods only after the occurrence of real pathological changes. However, if some symptoms are not related to structural or functional changes, nothing more can be found behind the traditional description of the *Yin deficiency of the Kidney*, even by using the most effective equipment.

Secondly, a question on a technical level: Is it possible for scientific investigation to reveal all structural and functional changes? — Can all *atoms* be observed? We know that the quantum theory marks the limit of experimental methodology. Furthermore, our assumption that scientific progress is unlimited implies that no matter how advanced the equipment we use, there will always remain new areas to explore. (This may help our contemporaries understand why the ancient Chinese philosophers considered that their *Qi* is invisible.) Therefore, even if all of the symptoms and signs in the *Yin deficiency of the Kidney* had a material foundation, it may however never be totally revealed by experimental method.

Finally, a question on the clinical level: Are these scientific methods more efficient than the traditional ones for diagnosis and treatment? — Is observing *atoms* better than speculating on the *Qi*? The scientific approach concentrates on a thorough revelation of the course of each event. We need to answer whether the detailed revelation of all the individual mechanisms behind the *Yin deficiency of the Kidney*, if possible at all, will provide us with a better global understanding of the patient. Chinese medicine takes into account the global sum of all the disorders, and does not target individual ailments. Because of the opposition of these two strategies, we cannot be certain that the *Yin deficiency of the Kidney* as identified by scientific approaches will indicate the same clinical case that had been decrypted by traditional diagnosis; and neither can we be certain that the ingredients selected by scientific research would treat the patient as well as the *Liu Wei Di Huang Wan* pills.

Apart from theoretical arguments, there is still the economic barrier to consider. If these complicated modern processes of investigation demand a greater investment in effort, time and money, they cannot replace the traditional approach in the clinical practice.

12.7 Conclusion

Although the author has adopted a critical attitude to this article, it is obvious that Chinese medicine has already benefited greatly from modernisation. It is also apparent that this modernisation is as yet insufficient. The aim of this article is to reveal the danger when the concept of modernisation turns into an ideology. By our anthropological approach, we know that the validation of a therapy should depend on whether it is capable of giving an accurate diagnosis and an effective treatment for a given case, and not whether it is scientific or modern.

Any judgment passed on Chinese medicine should be based on a neutral understanding of this therapy. The anthropological approach is one of the ways to understand Chinese medicine. The author's viewpoint may not satisfy the Chinese medicine's zealots nor the scientists, but may lead these two opposite parties to an agreement. Whether Chinese medicine is scientific, "scientific to be" or even "supernatural", it does open a specific path in human medical practices. Mythical or not, its traditional methods can still provide therapeutic solutions today, even more efficiently than modern methods in some cases.

In a time when the understanding of diseases becomes more sophisticated and when concepts of health are changing, we should not focus on reducing systems of healing into a unique pattern, but on enriching them. So, today, it seems better that Chinese medicine takes multiple and divergent forms, rather than confining itself to the uniform pathway of modernisation. Chinese medicine practitioners — whether traditional, modern or even "post-modern" — and other medicine practitioners should work together to define their own areas of concern and expertise, so as to determine the most efficient healing services for each case. This spirit of cooperation with other medicines can be considered as one of the real modern aspects of Chinese medicine today.

Another modern aspect could be the exchange with other medicines. For example, we do not need to insist on the Chinese origin of some traditional drugs used in modern Western medicine: in prescriptions based on scientific logic, they have become modern drugs and have no more relation to the traditional practice. On the other hand, some modern drugs can be used in Chinese medicine in a traditional way. For example, we should not be shocked if antibiotics are differentiated by their *Yin* and *Yang*, or cold and hot natures: since we know that these "natures" are not accounted for by physical facts, but by clinical experiences from Chinese healer's practices.

The author was trained as a practitioner of modern Western medicine and has grown up in a Chinese society estranged from its tradition, he feels the need to express more respect for Chinese medicine and other traditional skills. It may be appropriate here to quote a story from *Zhuang Zi* (莊子, 369 BC–286 BC) about *Hun Tun* (渾沌) (which means turbid and chaotic):

> "*Hun Tun* was an emperor of the Central Territory born without eyes, ears, nose and mouth. Those concerned tried to restore the missing parts, one hole a day… After seven days, Hun-Tun lived no more".

Be careful that modernisation does not result in Chinese medicine's deadly holes.

Acknowledgements

This chapter was translated by Prof. Ping-Chung Leung.

Chapter 13

Information Systems in Chinese Medicine

Pak Kwan Hui & Esther Ma

13.1 Introduction

Medical informatics is a dynamic discipline based on the medical sciences, information sciences and cognitive sciences (McGinnis, 2002). The modern medical information system is an integration of clinical information systems and knowledge management systems (Cross, 1990; Muller *et al.*, 2000). This chapter outlines the author's experience in the design and applications of medical information systems actually running in a Chinese medicine clinic in Hong Kong. Listings of useful Internet and web-teaching resources for Chinese medicine is also included. As articles published in Chinese-language journals are not generally available, priority of literature citation is given to articles indexed in Medline.

13.2 New Breed of Clinics, New Breed of Patients

Up to now, Western medicine is the conventional medicine in Hong Kong. After the Chinese Medicine Ordinance became effective in 1999, a new breed of Chinese Medicine clinics began to emerge in conventional medical settings in Hong Kong. (Hong Kong Hospital Authority Annual Plan, 2002; Tung Wah Group of Hospitals Annual Report, 2002). These new Chinese medicine clinics are often run by reputable organisations experienced in managing Western medicine services. As Chinese medicine is not subsidised, patients have to pay more to access Chinese medicine services located inside public hospitals. Users of this new breed of

Chinese medicine clinics are typically young and better educated. At Kwong Wah Hospital, for example, over 75% of Chinese medicine patients are younger than 60 years old and 28% of them attained University education. Eighty-five per cent of patients who use Chinese medicine services at Kwong Wah Hospital are concurrently under Western medical care (Hui and Chan, 2003). The peer environment within which these new clinics operate is a mixture of supportiveness and negativism. Expectation from peers and healthcare authorities is extremely high and frequently out of proportion to the support therefrom. To ensure safety and accountability, it becomes advantageous to Chinese medicine administrators to align to conventional medicine by adopting modern healthcare administrative methodologies, including information technology.

13.3 Scope and Components of Information Systems in Chinese Medicine

Clinical information systems in Chinese Medicine are largely similar to their counterparts in Western medicine although there is a special kind of logic indigenous to Chinese medicine, namely syndrome-based therapy, that needs to be addressed and preserved (Kapchuk, 1982; Zhong and Shi, 2000; Li *et al.*, 1995; Zhou and Li, 1999). Pharmacy systems in Chinese medicine are interfaced with clinical information systems, and accommodate the prescription of formulas rather than single herbs. As it is a syndrome-based form of therapy, there is a special need to document the therapeutic principle, because the same formula may be used to treat different diseases or different formulae may be used to treat the same disease (Zhu, 1982; Lin, 1994; Zhou *et al.*, 2001). Robotic assemblers of herbal granules are now commercially available and a modern pharmacy system in Chinese medicine should be able to interact with robotics to enhance efficiency and accuracy of pharmacy practice (Lee, 1995; Marietti, 1997). Knowledge bases assist and enhance reproducibility of decision making (Zhao *et al.*, 1994). For individuals learning or practicing Chinese medicine, a list of Internet resources, including web-teaching is also included in this chapter.

13.4 Why Implement an Information System?

To run a group practice that delivers Chinese medicine services to a population, it is necessary for healthcare administrators to actively control all processes that lead to diagnosis and treatment. Information systems are excellent tools for process control, that can also ensure a high degree of uniformity of practice. Information systems can quickly accumulate evidence for research and development (Schwid *et al.*, 1990; Wong and Abendroth, 1996). At Kwong Wah Hospital, for example, the clinical database for Chinese medicine is growing at a monthly rate of 1000 new patients, 4000 visits and 2800 formulas prescribed. Although speediness is not the major objective, information systems can greatly speed up the retrieval of old records, entering generic structured data and prescription of self pre-set formulas. It is realistic to assume that speediness is not always associated with the use of information systems, particularly for senior and distinguished Chinese medicine physicians who are more accustomed to using paper records.

13.5 Information Systems to Preserve Logic of Chinese Medicine

There is no practical need to use a separate Chinese medicine clinical information system if physicians make Western medical diagnoses and prescribe Chinese medicinal products like ordinary drugs. To preserve the logic of Chinese medicine, the clinical information system should contain data fields to accommodate two diagnoses, namely the illness diagnosis and the syndrome diagnosis. In the context of Chinese medicine, common cold and menstrual disorders are examples of illnesses, whereas damp-heat and wind-cold are examples of syndromes. To arrive at the illness and syndrome diagnoses, the physician must collect relevant clinical data, which include the chief complaint, history of present illness, relevant clinical signs, and the pulse and tongue findings (anonymous, 1983; Yu *et al.*, 1990; Yu, 1998). To enhance ease of use, many of the mentioned data fields can be designed to accept structured data entry, meaning that pre-defined lists of choices are available for physicians to point and click. For example, in Kwong Wah Hospital, structure data entry is available for tongue findings, pulse findings, illness diagnosis and syndrome diagnosis

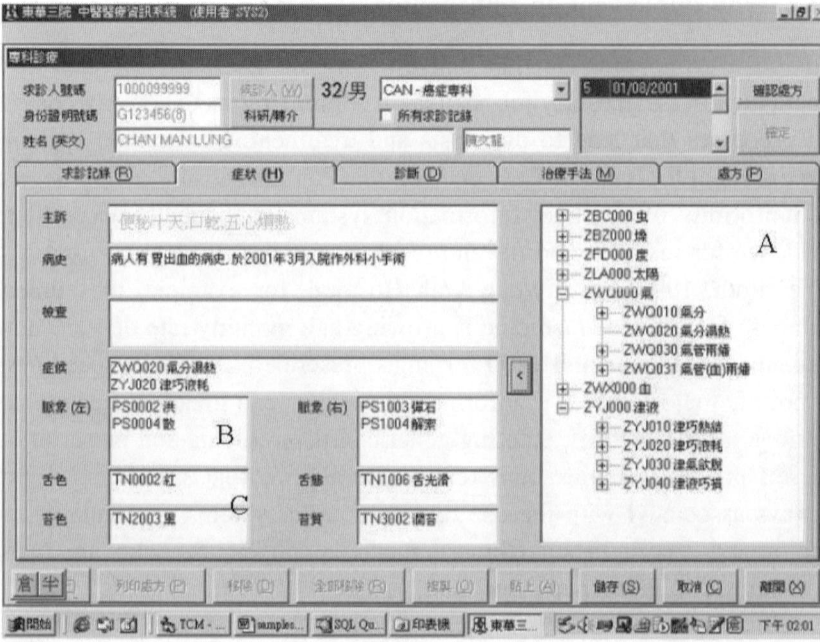

Figure 13.1. A representative screen shot to illustrate point-and-click type of structured data entry panel (A); pulse finding panel (B); and the tongue finding panel (C). This Chinese medicine clinical information system is developed by the Tung Wah Group of Hospitals, Hong Kong.

(Fig. 13.1). For chief complaint and history of present illness, free text entry is allowed.

Another mandatory data field in a Chinese medicine clinical information system is the therapeutic principle (see examples below). Because choice of therapy is based on the syndrome diagnosis, specifying the therapeutic principle not only reinforces the logic of Chinese medicine but also adds accountability to subsequent prescription, thereby containing risk for patients as well as for the clinic. For example, a patient with the *common cold* presents with *signs and symptoms* of a *heat-excess syndrome*. The logical *therapeutic principle* will therefore be clearing of heat and the subsequent *prescription* will be a heat-clearing formula. The words in italics represent different data fields. It is obvious that if the system is implemented, all steps will be controlled and decisions logically related.

The following is a hypothetical example. A physician diagnoses a patient with cold-excess syndrome, but enters "clearing of heat" as the therapeutic principle, which is obviously illogical. If designed with build-in logic, the clinical information system can flag alerts to the physician, thereby preventing the clinic from making errors and protecting patients from receiving inappropriate therapy. It is well known that prescriptions based on wrong syndrome diagnosis or wrong therapeutic principle will be ineffective or even cause discomfort to patients (Chen and Hou, 1988; Wang *et al.*, 2001).

13.6 Information Systems for Prescriptions in Chinese Medicine

Prescriptions in Chinese medicine can be an array of herbs that constitute a formula or a set of acupoints. Very seldom does a Chinese physician prescribe a single herb or a single acupoint. In addition to the ingredients of formulas, the method of decoction must also be recorded in the database. For herbs, there are different preparations and brands. For example, the two major preparations used at Kwong Wah Hospital are the processed raw herbs and herbal extracts in granular forms (Fig. 13.2). Raw herbs need decoction before use. Granular herbal extractions can be used after reconstituting them with hot water.

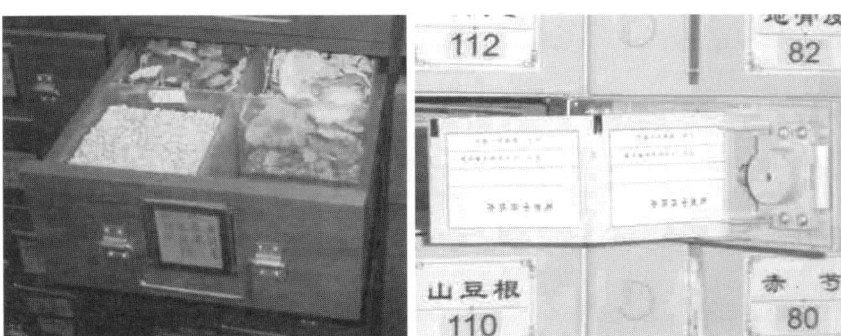

Figure 13.2. The left panel shows raw herbs stored in wooden drawers. The right panel shows packets of herbal granules stored inside compartments of an automatic assemble like a chain of stamps (source: Pharmacy of the Chinese Medicine Research and Services Centre at Kwong Wah Hospital, Hong Kong).

In an information system, the different preparations must be accordingly encoded. For ease of use, all available herbs should be pre-typed for the physician to choose by point-and-click. Physicians should also be given the functionality to pre-set their commonly prescribed formulas for repetitive use. Generating a neat prescription printout, with SI and traditional Chinese units of weight, method of decoction, patient's identity and physician's identity, is an important function of the information system. A well-designed prescription printout will not only help patients assemble the formulas in any herbal shops, but will also enhance the image of your clinic. Table 13.1 shows data fields useful for building database-driven information systems for Chinese medicine.

Table 13.1. Minimum data fields that must be included when building clinical information systems for Chinese medicine.

Data fields	Explanation
Demographics	Usually include name, gender, age, identity numbers, and patient serial numbers. Conformance to conventional medicine recommended.
Chief complaint	Can use free-text or structured data entry. In Chinese medicine, many illnesses are actually based on the chief complaints.
History of present illness	Free text entry.
Clinical signs other than tongues and pulse	Can use free text or structured data entry.
Tongue findings	Structured data entry.
Pulse findings	Structured data entry. Can have different fields for left- and right-sided pulse findings.
Syndrome diagnosis	Mandatory entry. This is the parameter that determines therapy. Can use structured data entry.
Illness diagnosis	Can use structured data entry.
Therapeutic principle	Mandatory entry before prescribing. Can use structured data entry.
Prescription	Use structured data entry and must accommodate formulas rather than single herbs. Leave a socket for robotics here.

13.7 Interacting with Robotics

Granules are extraction of herbs that can be reconstituted by simply mixing them with hot water. At Kwong Wah Hospital, patients can choose herbs or granules. The latter is now the more popular form of herbal preparation. Dosage of granules are expressed as weight-equivalent of their herbal counterparts. For example, a 10 g equivalent of herb A means that the granules represent an extraction from 10 g of herbs; it does not mean that the granules should weigh 10 g. While herbs are irregular in shapes and sizes, granules are available in remarkably regular packages highly suitable for robotic assembling. The Chinese medicine clinic at Kwong Wah Hospital uses a brand of granule manufactured by Sanjiu Medical and Pharmaceutical Company (Access Asia Company Profile, 2001), in which the granules are packed in small, labelled aluminium bags linked together like a chain of stamps. These chains of bags of granules are allocated to unique compartments of robotic assemblys, so that each type of granule will have its own positioning value along the x and y coordinates. When physicians prescribe Sanjiu granules, the prescriptions initially stored in database will be transformed to computer commands that drive the robotics to assemble the formula with remarkable speed and accuracy.

13.8 Obtaining Knowledge from the Internet

There is an immense volume of information relating to Chinese medicine on the Internet. There are websites that levee charges, which can be quite expensive, on users. These sites are undeniably better than free sites, which may not be up and running all the time. The advice is therefore that if one encounters useful information on free sites, one should consider downloading it straight away as it may soon be unavailable. Websites serving laws and regulations on Chinese medicine are usually free. University, hospital and pharmaceutical websites are also useful sources of free information, but the information provided is usually piecemeal and less comprehensive than paid websites. The following table (Table 13.2) is a list of websites that are up and running in April 2003 (browsed by author). The list is obviously not exhaustive. The first four listed sites are most useful to researchers in Chinese medicine.

Table 13.2. Obtaining information on Chinese medicine from the Internet.

Website	Contents
Cnki.net	Full-text Chinese-language journal papers on Chinese medicine for about RMB2000 year. Non-Chinese may need to pay more. Also sells DVDs of Chinese medicine journal papers.
cintcm.com	Access abstracts of Chinese medicine papers and several databases on herbs and clinical Chinese medicine. Costs about RMB2000 year for the Chinese.
Nstl.gov.cn	Dissertations from universities in China. Need to pre-pay in advance for paper to be mailed to you.
jy.ssreader.com.cn	Full-text Chinese medicine books and dictionaries. Need to install reader software, and require payment for id and password at RMB100 per year. You can download and print unlimited number of books.
wanfangdata.com.cn	Full-text journals online. Annual subscription is about RMB1000 per user.
theqi.com	Free. Basic theories and clinical Chinese medicine information in text and tables. Good for students.
okbuy.com.tw	Free. Historical books and examination questions on Chinese medicine to download.
twghkwhcrsc.org	Free. Chinese medicine software for downloading onto Palm PDA.
netcity2.web.hinet.net/UserData/p1200729/New-messages.htm	Free. Chinese medicine software and historical books to download. Server slow.
sdb.ac.cn/chinesedrugs/chinesedrug2.html	Free databases on Chinese herbs, formulas and proprietary medicine. Also has an English database on Chinese herbs.
yaoxue.net/search/001/	Free database on Chinese herbs and proprietary medicine covered by medical insurances in China. Useful for programmers in Chinese medicine systems.
dyhp.com.cn/fcl/fjx/fjx.htm	Free lecture notes on Chinese herbs and formulas.

Table 13.2 *(Continued)*

Website	Contents
dyhp.com.cn/yssz/yssc.htm	Free. A hospital website in China with strong emphasis on Chinese medicine.
chinaeh.com	Free. Provide information on wholesale prices of Chinese medicine
Chinesemedicines.net	Free sites offered by Chinese medicine traders. Information on grades and prices of Chinese herbs.
nicpbp.org.cn	Official website of the Chinese National Institute for the Control of Pharmaceutical and Biological Products.
yy2000.com/xinyaodongtai/ xinshengban.htm	Learn how China approves and regulates a Chinese medicinal product.
gb.ibucm.com	Distant learning opportunities for Chinese medicine in Beijing.
herbasin.com/herbs.htm	Free English database on Chinese herbs.
usetm.com	Free. Clinical Chinese medicine and herbs in traditional and simplified Chinese.
Cnm21.com	Free. Information on proprietary Chinese medicine.
c11.unihan.com.cn/Index.htm	Provide links to related websites, though some require id and password.
bandh.com.hk/index.htm	Free. Basic theories and clinical Chinese medicine. Good for students.

13.9 Net-teaching and E-learning in Traditional Chinese Medicine

As discussed recently (Broudo and Walsh, 2002), net-teaching differs from simple display of website contents in several ways. In addition to a content-display platform, net-teaching must have additional components to track student progress, assess student proficiency, and facilitate student-to-instructor interaction. Same coin with different sides, e-learning is defined as "a learning environment for delivering interactive multimedia education using the World Wide Web as a communication medium"

(CUHK, 1999). The two terms "net-teaching" and "e-learning" are usually interchangeable.

13.10 The Net-teaching and E-learning Environment in Hong Kong

The rapid technology changes in the last decade, especially the fast proliferation on the use of the Internet and the World Wide Web has indeed transformed the way we live, work, communicate and learn. The Internet population in the Greater China Region (Taiwan, Mainland China and Hong Kong) has reached 15,200,000, currently in the third place behind only the United States and Japan (Chen, 2001: pp. 56–58). The number of domestic web stations dedicated to net-teaching and e-learning has also increased. Like in all other countries, the trend of this new kind of teaching and learning mode has been established in Hong Kong and continues to prosper.

With the advancement in technology and improvement on the macro environment in bandwidth, equipment and teaching system platform, we believe that net-teaching and e-learning will become a dynamic alternative to the traditional teaching and learning mode in the near future.

13.11 The E-learning Course Series of Chinese Medicine

Net-teaching and e-learning on various biomedical disciplines have been described, and they can be functionally categorised as curriculum-oriented or education-oriented (Veldenz and Dennis, 1998; Dwyer *et al.*, 1997; Wallis *et al.*, 1995; Gurwitz *et al.*, 2003). For Chinese medicine, there have already been many similar courses offered by mainland universities or local organisations. In 2000, the first e-learning course on Chinese medicine offered by local tertiary institutions, titled "The Online Course Series of Chinese Medicine" (中醫藥學網上教學系列), was launched by the School of Continuing Studies of the Chinese University of Hong Kong (SCS, CUHK). There are also similar net-teaching/e-learning facilities available for enrollment. Table 13.3 shows a list of net-teaching resources on the Internet, all of which charge a fee for enrollment.

Table 13.3. A list of net-teaching/e-learning facilities available on the Internet.

Website	Programme
www.scs.cuhk.edu.hk/tcm/	Chinese University of Hong Kong.
www.hkcyberu.com/study/ welcome.htm	Polytechnic University Hong Kong in collaboration with China Academy of Traditional Chinese Medicine, Beijing. Curriculum-based.
big5.ibucm.com/wywq/ wywq_8_1.html	Beijing-based net-teaching facility; curriculum-based.
www.gd-edu.com/class/zk/28.htm	Examination-based net teaching programme in Guangdong.
www.njutcm.edu.cn /yuanchengjiaoxue/zyx/zyml.htm	A Chinese pharmacology net-teaching programme in Nanjing.
tmc.topcool.net/ycjx/	TCM distant-learning programmes in Nanjing.
cte.medchina.net/	Offers distant learning programmes in Chinese medicine.
www.bhmai.edu.cn/english/	English online learning and examination programmes in Chinese Medicine. For foreign students.

13.12 Interactive Knowledge Bases — Making Syndrome Diagnosis Based on Symptoms and Signs

The interactive knowledge base discussed in this section has been demonstrated in several recent international conferences (Xu *et al.*, 2002; Hui, 2003a and b).

For centuries, description of Chinese medicine syndromes has been highly structured and concise. In the description of a syndrome, symptoms, signs, tongue findings, and lastly, pulse findings follow the name of the syndrome. This highly structured format makes TCM syndromes particularly suitable for building databases. At Kwong Wah Hospital, we built an interactive Chinese medicine database that enables users to differentiate a Chinese medicine syndrome by entering symptoms and signs.

On designing an interactive database on Chinese medicine syndrome, the following points were considered:

(1) *No additional software:* The backend database is a flat file text database. Users can build or modify the database using text editors.
(2) *Source of knowledge:* Users can choose own source of information. For education, practice and quality control, it is suggested that the source of information be limited to current professional guidelines at users' sites of practice. When used for research or implementation of corporate policy, users can build their own knowledge base. There is a category of distinguished and senior TCM physicians in China, whose personal experiences in TCM syndrome diagnosis can also be used. For this project, we built a syndrome database comprising of 806 syndromes based on several bilingual (Chinese-English) university-level textbooks, professional guidelines and national examination questions.
(3) *Language barriers:* Conversion of a Chinese knowledge base to other languages is easier than translating lengthy documents. A two-column Chinese-to-English glossary was made, which enabled conversion of the Chinese knowledge base to English using the widely available software *sed*. This program is a non-interactive stream editor that can convert text files from one language to another using a pre-defined glossary.
(4) *Synonymous descriptions:* To ensure effective search, synonymous descriptions and translations were encompassed rather than unified. For example, the diagnostic symptom of Yin deficiency "feverish sensation of palms soles and chest" is synonymous to "five center heat", and therefore the two descriptions were encompassed under Yin deficiency.
(5) *Illustrative descriptions:* Illustrative descriptions are fairly common in TCM writings, some of which are of diagnostic specificity, e.g. the sign of Yin deficiency "flushed cheeks" and "flushed cheeks like wearing cosmetics" are synonymous and therefore both are encompassed under Yin deficiency.
(6) *Operating system independence:* We use JAVA2.
(7) *Fonts:* This is not an issue for non-Chinese alphanumeric display. For Chinese characters, it is necessary to save the backend

database in UTF-8 encoded text files, which enables simplified Chinese characters (used in China) and traditional Chinese characters (used in Hong Kong and Taiwan) to be visualised on any Chinese operating systems.

(8) *Search strings:* As many signs and symptoms are indigenous to TCM, a list of search strings is made for users to select. Examples of TCM-specific signs include the tongue and pulse signs.

13.13 System Description and Screen Shots

For demonstration, a traditional Chinese version is shown below.

In flat file text database, each syndrome is represented by a row of text. The name of the syndrome is at the beginning of a row, which is separated from the rest of the row by a comma. The description of the syndrome follows the comma, and individual symptoms are separated by a pipe "|". Each row of text is ended with a line break.

The software system, which is developed in Java, supports three languages: English, traditional Chinese and simplified Chinese. It provides a graphical user interface for users to search syndromes by symptoms and vice versa. The screen showing the syndromes returned given a number of symptoms and that showing the symptoms returned given a syndrome are given in Figs. 13.3 and 13.4, respectively.

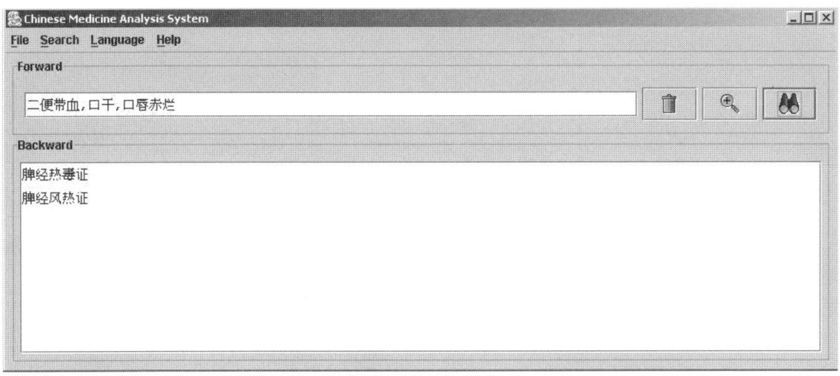

Figure 13.3. The screen showing the syndromes returned given a number of symptoms.

Figure 13.4. The screen showing the symptoms returned given a syndrome.

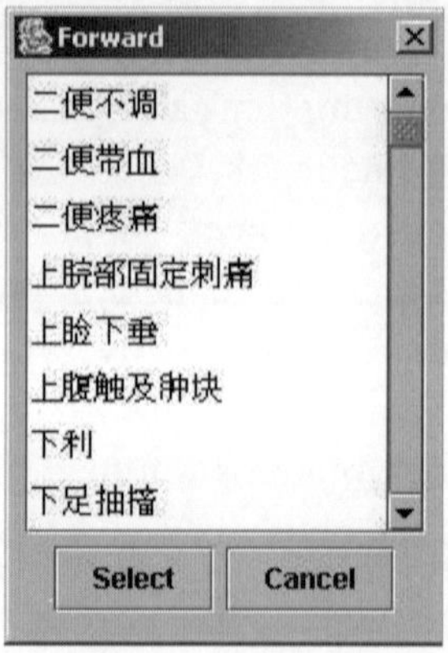

Figure 13.5. The screen showing a list of symptoms for users to select.

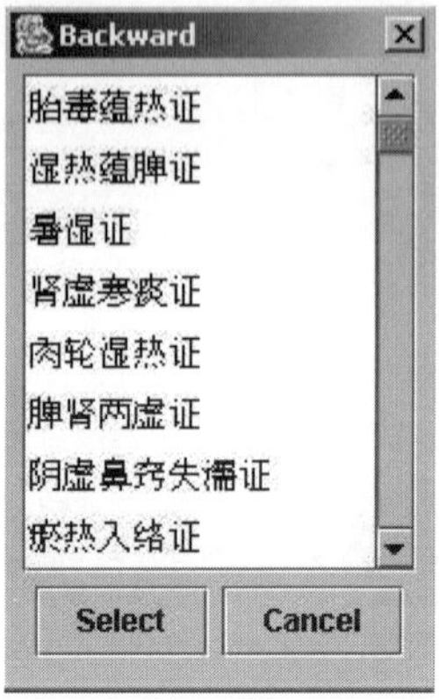

Figure 13.6. The screen showing a list of syndromes for users to select.

The software also allows users to select from on existing list of syndromes and symptoms for searching. Figures 13.5 and 13.6 show the screens displaying a list of symptoms and syndromes for users to select, respectively.

Furthermore, the system allows users to provide his/her own flat file text database for searching and printing search results.

13.13.1 *Availability*

The software is compatible with Windows 9x/NT/2K/XP/Linux/Unix. There are versions for simplified Chinese, traditional Chinese and English. To request for test versions, please contact Dr. P.K. Hui at pkhui@ha.org.hk.

13.14 Conclusion

Medical informatics has become one of the central components of hospital management (Frisse, 1999). As Chinese medicine researches and services are gradually emerging in conventional medical settings (MacLennan and Wilson, 2002), the application of medical informatics in Chinese medicine will inevitably be increasing. This article outlines the designs of various information systems actually running in a Chinese medicine clinic in Hong Kong. Listings of Internet resources and net-teaching/e-learning opportunities are provided for those who want to pursue self-learning of Chinese medicine. Readers who are interested in tele-diagnostic systems of Chinese medicine and chemistry databases of Chinese herbs can consult relevant references (al-Taei *et al.*, 2000; He *et al.*, 2001). They are not included in this article because they are similar to their counterparts in Western medicine.

References

Access Asia Company Profile (2001) *Sanjiu Medical and Pharmaceutical: A Company Profile.* Access Asia Limited, London (also available at http://www.chinaonline.com/estore/publishers/AA.htm; http://estore.chinaonline.com/acascomprof.html)

al-Taei, M.K., Pan, Y. and Lu, D.M. (2000) An Internet-based telediagnosis system for Chinese medicine. *J. Telemed. Telecare.* **6**(Suppl. 1), S63–65.

Anonymous (1983) Lectures on essentials of traditional Chinese medicine. VII. Differentiation of syndromes. *J. Tradit. Chin. Med.* **3**(2), 163–168.

Broudo, M. and Walsh, C. (2002) MEDICOL: Online learning in medicine and dentistry. *Acad. Med.* **77**(9), 926–927.

Chen, C.F. (2001) *Learning Trend Web Site — New Realm of Online Learning.* C Trend Seasonal, 3.

Chen, Q.Q. and Hou, C. (1988) Clinical disagreement of traditional Chinese medicine physicians in treating patients according to syndrome differentiation for chronic persistent hepatitis. *Chung Hsi I Chieh Ho Tsa Chih* **8**(3), 132, 144–146.

Cross, P. (1990) A classification of health computer systems and how it could help in deciding investment requirements. *Health Serv. Manage.* **86**(6), 284–286

CUHK (1999) *Report of the IT Strategy Committee.* The Chinese University of Hong Kong.

Dwyer, T.M., Fleming, J., Randall, J.E. and Coleman, T.G. (1997) Teaching physiology and the World Wide Web: Electrochemistry and electrophysiology on the Internet. *Am. J. Physiol.* **273**(6 Pt. 3), S2–13.

Frisse, M. (1999) Medical informatics' promised land: Are we there yet? *Acad. Med.* **74**(12), 1301–1306.

Gurwitz, D., Weizman, A. and Rehavi, M. (2003) Education: Teaching pharmacogenomics to prepare future physicians and researchers for personalized medicine. *Trends Pharmacol. Sci.* **24**(3), 122–125.

He, M., Yan, X., Zhou, J. and Xie, G. (2001) Traditional Chinese medicine database and application on the Web. *J. Chem. Inf. Comput. Sci.* **41**(2), 273–277.

Hong Kong Hospital Authority Annual Plan 2002–2003, pp. 25 (http://www.ha.org.hk).

Hui, P.K. and Chan, M.H. (2003) *Cancer Patients Using Chinese Medicine* (Abstract). Academic paper collection, Cancer Conference: Chinese Medicine and Modern Medicine Approach, Hong Kong, p. 182.

Hui, P.K. (2003a) *Information Systems in Chinese Medicine.* Proceedings of the Hong Kong International Medical Informatics Conference, 23–25 January, pp. 47.

Hui, P.K. (2003b) *Information Systems in Chinese Medicine: Opportunities and Challenges.* The BioIT World Conference, 25–27 February, Hong Kong.

Kaptchuk, T. (1982) The holistic logic of Chinese medicine. *Sci. Dig.* **90**, 32, 34.

Lee, M.P. (1995) Automation and the future practice of pharmacy — Changing the focus of pharmacy. *Pharm. Pract. Manag. Q.* **15**(3), 23–35.

Li, Y., Qian, R., Huang, X. and Zhu, G. (1995) Treatment of idiopathic thrombocytopenic purpura based on TCM syndrome differentiation. *J. Tradit. Chin. Med.* **15**(2), 83–86.

Lin, Y. (1994) Study on application of the principle of eliminating stasis and refreshing spirit for acute stage of hemorrhagic apoplexy. *J. Tradit. Chin. Med.* **14**(2), 92–97.

MacLennan, A.H., Wilson, D.H. and Taylor, A.W. (2002) The escalating cost and prevalence of alternative medicine. *Prev. Med.* **35**(2), 166–173.

Marietti, C. (1997) Robots hooked on drugs. Robotic automation expands pharmacy services. *Health Inform.* **14**(11), 37–38, 40, 42.

McGinnis, P.J. (2002) The scope and direction of health informatics. *Aviat. Space Environ. Med.* **73**, 503–507.

Muller, M.L., Ganslandt, T., Eich, H.P., Lang, K., Ohmann, C. and Prokosch, H.U. (2000) Integrating knowledge based functionality in commercial hospital information systems. *Stud. Health Technol. Inform.* **77**, 817–821.

Schwid, H.A., Olson, C., Wright, P. and Freund, P.R. (1990) Microcomputer-based data acquisition system for clinical research. *J. Clin. Monit.* **6**(2), 141–146.

Tung Wah Group of of Hospitals Annual Report 2002–2003, pp. 67–71 (http://www/tungwah.org.hk).

Veldenz, H.C. and Dennis, J.W. (1998) The Internet and education in surgery. *Am. Surg.* **64**(9), 877–880.

Wallis, J.W., Miller, M.M., Miller, T.R. and Vreeland, T.H. (1995) An Internet-based nuclear medicine teaching file. *J. Nucl. Med.* **36**(8), 1520–1527.

Wang, Q., Li, H. and Zhang, Z. (2001) Causes and countermeasures about adverse reaction of traditional Chinese medicine. *Zhong Yao Cai* **24**(6), 430–433.

Wong, E.T. and Abendroth, T.W. (1996) Reaping the benefits of medical information systems. *Acad. Med.* **71**(4), 353–357.

Xu, B.J., (Hui, P.K.) and Lai, S.L. (2002) *Application of an Interactive Database on Chinese Medicine Syndromes* (Abstract). Second World Integrated Medicine Conference, Beijing.

Yu, E.C. (1998) The basic clinical diagnostic framework synergized. *Chin. Med. J. (Engl.)* **111**(5), 460–465.

Yu, G., Chen, J., Wang, J. and Hou, J. (1990) New progress in the four diagnostic methods of cancer. *J. Tradit. Chin. Med.* **10**(2), 152–155.

Zhao, Y.K., Tsutsui, T., Endo, A., Minato, K. and Takahashi, T. (1994) Design and development of an expert system to assist diagnosis and treatment of chronic hepatitis using traditional Chinese medicine. *Med. Inf. (Lond.)* **19**(1), 37–45.

Zhong, J. and Shi, D. (2000) Treatment of unstable angina pectoris based on disease- and syndrome-differentiation. *J. Tradit. Chin. Med.* **20**(2), 141–146.

Zhou, H. and Li, Y. (1999) Relation between modernization of traditional Chinese medicine and syndrome differentiation of integrated traditional Chinese and Western medicine (Chinese). *Zhongguo Zhong Xi Yi Jie He Za Zhi* **19**(2), 117–118.

Zhou, C., Yu, Z., Li, R. and Tian, Z. (2001) The principle and technique of using Chinese drugs in the treatment of hypertension. *J. Tradit. Chin. Med.* **21**(1), 7–11.

Zhu, G.D. (1982) Treatment of vitiligo based on the principle of pacifying liver by resolving stasis and activating blood circulation, plus exorcising "wind". An observation on therapeutic effects in 100 cases. *J. Tradit. Chin. Med.* **2**(1), 71–75.

Chapter 14

The Future

Ping-Chung Leung & Charlie Changli Xue

14.1 Introduction

With the global adaptation of the concept of evidence-based medicine, the future of Chinese medicine cannot be considered outside the future of medicine at large, since all streams of medicine are catered towards the maintenance of human health and they all complement and supplement one another.

Unlike Chinese medicine, the trend of development of modern medicine is in a state where it is increasingly more and more dependent on science and technology. Diagnosis will become more and more accurate, hence diagnostic tools become indispensable and specialisation earns more popularity. Medical services including diagnosis and treatment cost will also become more expensive. The experience of the healer becomes less and less important (Richardson, 2001; Hannallah *et al.*, 2002).

There is, therefore, a likely situation that technical advancement and technical dependence further jeopardise human touch, and personal care for diseased organs may soon be equivalent to the repair of machine units and change of spare parts. With the further decline of the art of healing, some patients become even more disillusioned. In contrast, the strength of Chinese medicine such as emphasis of individualised treatment and practitioner-patient interaction may attract greater proportions of patient population to consider Chinese medicine as a viable alternative (Bensky and Gamble, 1993).

In the current regimens of modern medicine, when the outcome of accurate diagnosis is simple, management is easy and thus patients are satisfied. On the other hand, when diagnosis is not clear even after the most sophisticated investigation and the utilisation of the most updated technology, it may result in frustrated and disheartened patients. Chinese medicine will then be considered as another option of health care (Leung, 2001).

It seems that modern medicine is effective only in cases when the mysterious nature of some pathologies are easily unveiled and when subsequent solutions are straightforward. Thus, despite tremendous advances, modern medicine remains defective.

One area of unpredictability lies in the development of genome studies and the stem cell research. If diseases can be tackled at the molecular level by manipulating the responsible genes, how will this new specialty affect the overall practice is still subject to speculation. It may mean the shrinkage of specialties like pediatrics or some branches of medicine. The dramatic success of locating the "death gene" will rewrite the whole text on cancer treatment and degenerative diseases (Chinese Medicine Post, 2002).

If stem cell cultivation can lead to the creation of human organs and tissues, then once again surgery becomes mainly a service for the changing of spare parts!

However, assuming that science, no matter how promising, will stay being short of almighty, unsolved problems still require alternative treatment, and in the Chinese communities, Chinese medicine will remain the most popular alternative.

Thus, the demand for alternative supplement will remain. In fact, with more advanced specialisation and higher costs, the need for alternative medicine is expected to increase worldwide — this has already been demonstrated by studies conducted in Western countries such as the United States and Australia (Eisenberg *et al.*, 1993; MacLennan *et al.*, 1996).

14.2 Healing Services

When hospitals in China, not only those labeled "Chinese Medicine Hospital" but all hospitals, provide alternative treatment upon request, one takes it as something natural for China. In fact, Chinese medicine delivers approximately 40% of total health care in China mainly via the public hospital system. When Massachusetts General Hospital provides special acupuncture services upon request, its implication is a lot more significant, since it means that the American Health Administration has developed trust in acupuncture and endorsed that patients can make use of it as a means to control pain. Similar situations have occurred in other Western countries including Australia and Germany (Goldbeck-Wood *et al.*, 1996; Fisher and Ward, 1994).

Everywhere in the United States, medical schools are already providing students' choices for courses of alternative medicine. One expects, therefore, that service hospitals will likewise provide alternative services. As long as modern medicine remains as the mainline, integration between the two will be unnecessary.

Different branches of alternative medicine, notably Chinese medicine, will rapidly grow. Professional groups and associations will be formed to take care of their colleagues and lead the way into the hospitals and clinics.

However, in the West, the public acceptance of Chinese medicine as an effective health care option will rely heavily on the scientific evidence concerning its efficacy and safety. The public in the Chinese communities may not demand the same level of proof at this stage, as it appears to be part of the Chinese culture and the belief that the long clinical use of Chinese medicine as a healing art in China has already proven its efficacy. This situation will soon change as Chinese medicine practitioners are now facing more educated and better informed public who would like to be more involved in the process of their health care.

As a result, research into the efficacy and safety of Chinese medicine should be set as a priority for the overall development of Chinese medicine. In addition, research outcomes should be incorporated into educational programmes in Chinese medicine training to ensure that graduates and future practitioners are well equipped not only for Chinese medicine practice, but also for the ability to pursue scientific scrutiny.

Therefore, the quality of the practitioners in Chinese medicine or integrated medicine remains a critical issue to be addressed. The public will expect that their practitioners be conversant in modern medical diagnosis and be knowledgeable in clinical therapeutics in both modern and Chinese medicine so that their practice at large can be on a more evidence-based basis.

Practitioners will therefore be expected to carry out continuing education, and update their knowledge in new research findings related to scientific evidences on efficacy and safety of the interventions recommended to their patients.

14.3 Education

In Australia, Chinese medicine education has been introduced into the public-funded university system since the early 1990s. Currently, there are four public universities in Australia offering degree programmes in Chinese medicine, including acupuncture and Chinese herbal medicine. In addition, acupuncture components have also been incorporated into the curricula in modern medical programmes in some universities in Australia. This is consistent with the development in other parts of the world such as the U.S.A. Over 90% of medical schools in the U.S.A. are already providing elective curricula of alternative medicine. The trend will most likely continue to strive (Studlert *et al.*, 1998).

Some medical schools will probably run special integrated courses through which students will get the best of the two systems. The higher cost will most probably prevent integrated courses to be run and delivered on a regular basis but rather, ambitious students will be encouraged to go into such pursuits.

Now that alternative medicine becomes generally accepted, both by the clients and health providers, general knowledge and short enlightening courses for the health workers will become more and more popular. Electronic learning and provisions of net courses, either on general enlightenment, or on specific topics like acupuncture and massage, will thrive.

The qualification standards for alternative medicine practitioners are already well defined in China, Hong Kong as well as Australia. Likewise, the educational pathway and qualification requirements are well documented and being practiced. Cities and places outside China will find good value in the Oriental examples. Such global movements would generate good supportive forces in support of the traditional art of healing which has been suffering a real decline under the pressure of the successes of science and technology.

14.4 Research

Evidence-based clinical trials on apparently promising herbs and herbal formulae offer the only future to a genuine development of Chinese medicine. The established methodologies will be applied. Good clinical practice will be followed, using assumably uniform herbal preparations. Compromises are inevitable because quality control of the herbs is not possible, and the exact chemical equation of the active ingredient is not known. Most frequently, even the active ingredient itself is not known.

Future Chinese medicine research still depends on compromising efforts. It would be naïve if one expects that the active ingredients can be identified and made into pharmaceuticals. However, more and more herbs will be grown strictly according to one standard; thus conforming to good agricultural practice (GAP) and simple efficient tests will emerge for the quick testing of the true identities of different herbs; thus making good manufacture practice (GMP) more feasible.

Concerning acupuncture, with its existing popularity in the West as an alternative means for pain management, the public acceptance will remain. Further studies on its effectiveness on conditions other than pain will benefit the clinical application of acupuncture for a wider range of conditions. For example, recent studies have demonstrated the clinical value of acupuncture for hay fever, nausea, morning sickness and tension type headache (NIH, 1997).

As far as clinical assessments are concerned, the two different streams of practitioners will reach a consensus on the common objective data and common subjective data like the different aspects of quality of life. With a conceptual harmony, the modern scientific stream can be less insistent on science-led planning while the traditional worker will be more capable of making compromising suggestions.

14.5 Drugs

The problems with herbal drugs are that producers care more about their marketing needs rather than the efficacies. The producers are obviously taking advantage of the cultural attitude which tempts the individual with personal testimonies or trials, instead of agreeing on an objective scrutiny.

The convenience and ease of sale, has hindered the proper clinical tests required to arrive at a more general call for practical utilisation.

Now that many clinical trials basing on evidence-based needs are underway, their results are expected to affect the attitude of the drug manufacturers. Hopefully, successful results will provide more confidence and enthusiasm towards more solid, evidence-based development of drugs.

Successful results may also activate the market for "drugs of botanical origin". Apparently, since the recognition of this category of drug as an entity in the U.S. market, to date, more than two years after, no new creation has been granted official license when this chapter is being prepared. When more evidence-based clinical trials offer phase II efficacy and reliable safety profiles, more licenses will be expected. In Australia, guidelines on therapeutic claims concerning complementary medicine including Chinese herbal medicine have been sent for registration or listing of new therapeutic products.

14.6 Recognition

The recognition of alternative therapies including Chinese medicine will rely on the level of evidence that can be produced for efficacy and safety. In addition, the training of practitioners will also play a critical role in attaining the public's confidence in Chinese medicine. It has been the perception of the Western medical profession that the recognition of alternative medicine as a supplementary means of healing has run a tortuous course. Since the old ancient days when "quacks" moved around deceiving sick people, practitioners with recognised qualifications had been running their exclusive infra- and supra-structures. Patients and the general public encouraged the qualified practitioners to be exclusive, since it helped the patient to feel more secure, and thus be protected from the "quacks" (Harrington, 2001).

In the past decade, the same group of patients and the general public realised that qualified practitioners may not fulfill their expectations and they felt uneasy to be tightly bound within the practitioner's practising circle. People who felt that way have joined together and demanded for alternative treatment (NIH, 2001).

When the demand for alternative treatment gathered momentum, the practitioners and the administrators felt the need and responded to it, by either actively participating (a few) or quietly accepting the trend (the majority).

In spite of the change, embarrassment still exists between the two different streams: who belongs to the mainline and who belongs to the alternative? Does the mainline deserve all the recognition while the alternative stays the subordinate?

If this awkward relationship is not settled, not only will the suffering patient be affected by it, the proper development of both streams and their future cooperation will also be ruined.

A practical way to solve this dilemma is to recognise alternative medicine like Chinese Medicine as a separate specialty capable of providing a special medical service. The specialty should have its own right to set its own professional requirements and qualifications, and establish its own professional code of practice. Once recognised as a separate specialty, the mainline against alternative issue becomes unimportant. Like any other medical specialty, Chinese medicine specialty will enjoy its existence and contribution, will accept referrals from other streams and refer their own patients to other specialties. Collaborations in day-to-day service, education and research thus becomes natural.

Once Chinese medicine becomes a recognised specialty, market forces will lead to a higher demand, a genuine "integrated" entity will emerge. The service providers may mean a new breed who go through separate trainings in modern and Chinese medicine, or may simply include a close cooperation between qualified modern and Chinese medicine practitioners. Such integrated entity can take the form of clinics or hospitals. A practical system of genuine sharing will be developed. Unlike such entities one finds currently in China, the system of genuine sharing offers an unexemptable integrated treatment programme, rather than leaving the choice to patients.

The many "pure" practitioners of Chinese medicine will still be practicing since the demand for their service, although expected to decline, will still persist. At some stage, either patients themselves or regulating bodies may insist on a referral from the modern medicine practitioner so as to make sure that there will be no controversies on the diagnosis and recognition of special pathology.

References

Bensky, D. and Gamble, A. (1993) *Chinese Herbal Medicine, Materia Medica.* Eastland Press, Seattle.

Chinese Medicine Post (2002) *Chin. Med. Post*, 18 November 2002.

Eisenberg, D.M., Kessler, R.C. and Foster, C. (1993) Unconventional medicine in the USA — Prevalence, costs and patterns of use. *New Engl. J. Med.* **328**(4), 246–252.

Fisher, P. and Ward, A. (1994) Medicine in Europe: Complementary medicine in Europe. *BMJ* **309**(6947), 107–111.

Goldbeck-Wood, S., Dorozynski, A. and Lie, L.G. (1996) Complementary medicine is booming worldwide. *BMJ* **313**(7050), 131–133.

Hannallah, D., Peterson, B. and Lieberman, J.R. (2002) Gene therapy in orthopaedic surgery. *JBJS* **84**, 1046–1061.

Harrington, A. (ed.) (2001) *The Placebo Effect.* Harvard Medical Press.

Leung, P.C. (2001) Editorial seminar series on evidence-based alternative medicine. *Hong Kong Med. J.* **7**(4), 352–353.

MacLennan, A.H., Wilson, D.H. and Jaylor, A.W. (1996) Prevalence and cost of alternative medicine in Australia. *The Lancet* **347**(9001), 569–573.

National Institutes of Health (1997) Consensus conference statement on Acupuncture. *NIH publication* **15**(5), 1–34.

National Institutes of Health (2001) *National Centre for Complementary and Alternative Medicine. Five-year Strategic Plan 2001–2005.*

Richardson, W. (2001) *Crossing the Quality Chasm: A New Health System for the 21st Century.* The National Academic News.

Studlert, D.M., Eisenberg, D.M. and Miller, F.H. (1998) Medical malpractice implications of alternative medicine. *JAMA* **280**(18), 1610–1615.

Index

Y

Z